Chewing the Fat

... IN MY WORDS... AND THEIRS

MARCO LEWIS

THAT'S A FACT PUBLISHING

Copyright

Copyright © 2024 by Marco Lewis / Marcus Brown

All rights reserved. No part of this publication may be reproduced, distributed or transmitted in any form or by any means, including photocopying, recording, or other electronic or mechanical methods, without the prior written permission of the publisher, except in the case of brief quotations embodied in critical reviews and certain other non-commercial uses permitted by copyright law. For permission requests, write to the publisher, addressed "Attention: Permissions Coordinator," at the address below.

THAT'S A FACT PUBLISHING
CHEWING THE FAT... IN MY WORDS... AND THEIRS

Publisher's Note: This work is non-fiction and covers a period of time in the author's life. All experiences are his own. Interviews conducted with other individuals have been cleared for inclusion.

CTFIMWAT / Marco Lewis – 1st Ed.

ISBN: 9798345948552

Dedication

To Jonathan... I can breathe easy knowing you're always beside me.

What is BMI and what does it measure?

(Source. www.nhs.uk/conditions/obesity/)

The body mass index (BMI) is a measure that uses your height and weight to work out if your weight is healthy.

The BMI calculation divides an adult's weight in kilograms by their height in metres squared. For example, A BMI of 25 means 25kg/m2.

BMI Ranges

For most adults, an ideal BMI is in the 18.5 to 24.9 range.

For children and young people aged 2 to 18, the BMI calculation considers age and gender as well as height and weight.

If your BMI is:
- below 18.5 – you're in the underweight range.
- between 18.5 and 24.9 – you're in the healthy weight range.
- between 25 and 29.9 – you're in the overweight range.
- 30 or over – you're in the obese range.

Accuracy of BMI

BMI considers natural variations in body shape, giving a healthy weight range for a particular height.

As well as measuring your BMI, healthcare professionals may take other factors into account when assessing if you're a healthy weight.

Muscle is much denser than fat, so very muscular people, such as heavyweight boxers, weight trainers, and athletes, may be a healthy weight even though their BMI is classed as obese.

Your ethnic group can also affect your risk of some health conditions. For example, adults of South Asian origin may have a higher risk of some health problems, such as diabetes, with a BMI of 23, which is usually considered healthy.

You should not use BMI as a measure if you're pregnant. Seek advice from your midwife or GP if you're concerned about your weight.

Check your BMI: https://www.nhs.uk/health-assessment-tools/calculate-your-body-mass-index/calculate-bmi-for-adults

WORDS, BUT WHAT ARE THEIR MEANINGS?

FOOD: something that people eat to keep them alive.

DRINK: a drink or beverage is a liquid intended for human consumption.

COMPUSLION: a very strong feeling of wanting to do something repeatedly that is difficult to control: a strong feeling of wanting something.

GLUTTONY: a situation in which people eat and drink more than they need to.

SATISFIED: pleased because you have got what you wanted, or because something has happened in the way that you wanted.

NUTRITION: the substances that you take into your body as food and the way they influence your health.

OVEREAT: to eat more food than your body needs, especially so that you feel uncomfortably full.

GUILT: a feeling of worry or unhappiness that you have because you have done something wrong, such as causing harm to another person.

TEMPTATION: the wish to do or have something that you know you should not do or have.

DIET: an eating plan in which someone eats less food, or only particular types of food because they want to become thinner or for medical reasons.

HUNGER: The feeling you have when you need to eat.

CHEWING THE FAT

REMORSE: a feeling of sadness and being sorry for something you have done.

FAT: a word used to describe a person that is overweight.

SELF-CONTROL: the ability to control oneself, in particular one's emotions and desires or the expression of them in one's behaviour, especially in difficult situations.

ABSTINANCE: the fact or practice of restraining oneself from indulging in something.

SYNS: For members of slimming world, it means SYNERGY, and shows how foods like healthy extras, Syns, and free foods work together to help with weight loss in people.

HEXA: Healthy Extra A - Foods that provide calcium. Milk & cheese (including dairy and non-dairy options).

HEXB: Healthy Extra B – Foods that provide fibre, minerals and other important nutrients. They include high-fibre cereals, wholemeal bread, fibre-rich crispbread and cereal bars. dried, canned and cooked fruit, and nuts and seeds

AND THE BADDEST BITCH OF THEM ALL...

ADDICTION: an inability to stop doing or using something, especially something harmful.

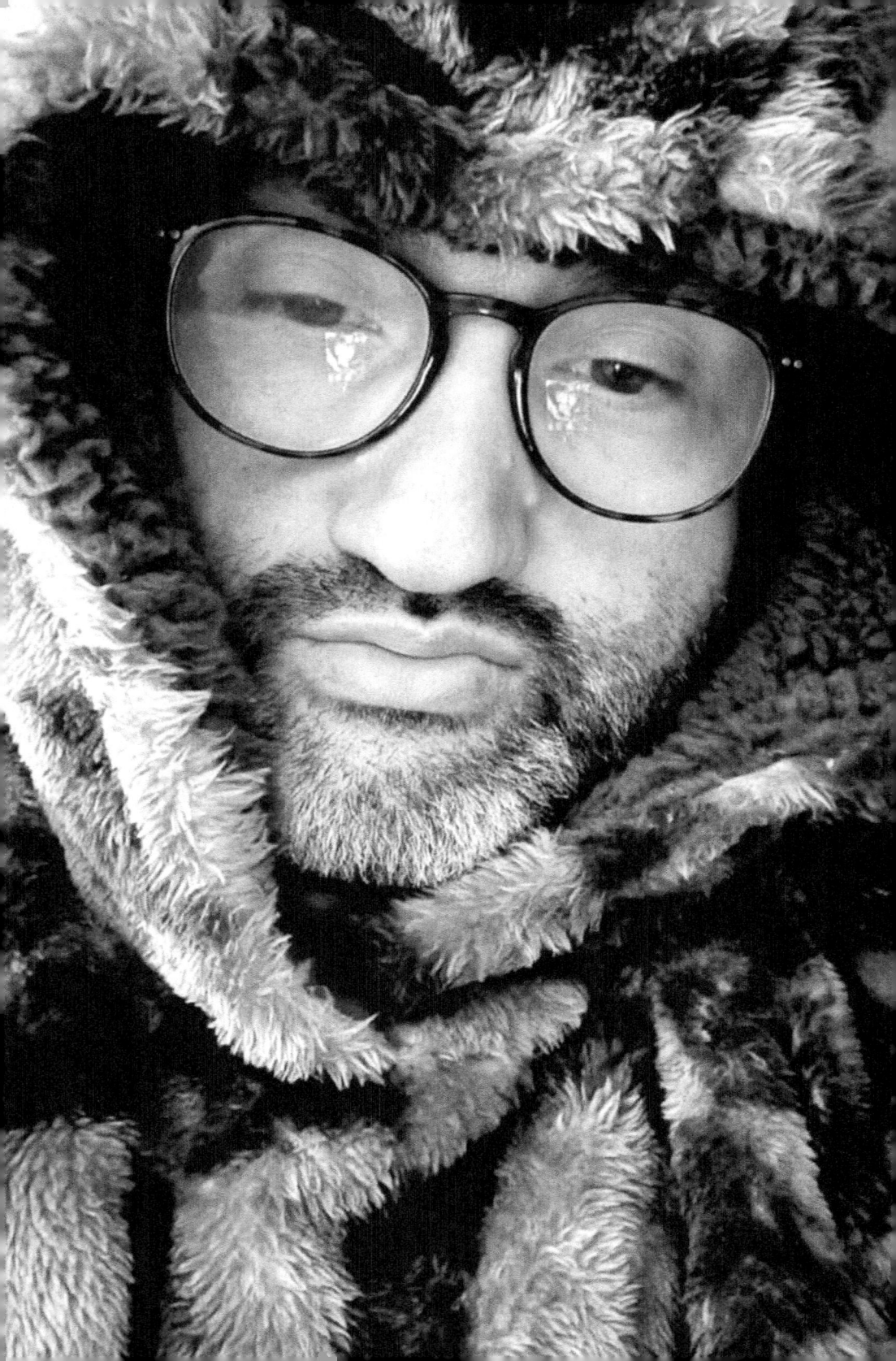

FOREWORD

The aforementioned words and their descriptions have been a part of my life for as long as I can remember. I'm certain most, if not all, of them will have infiltrated your world too.

Why?

Because I have an addiction to food.

And so do you, or you probably wouldn't be reading this book.

But my story is only one of many millions who understand the daily struggle. For those, like me, who spend their days over-eating, then experiencing the tsunami of guilt that follows the over-all-too-quickly high brings an endless cycle of misery with no end in sight.

I know what compels me to eat. There are many triggers, but the one thing sitting amidst my misery, whispering temptations at me, are a myriad of conflicting emotions. I am an emotional eater, though not just limited to times when I am fed up, bored or unhappy. I consume just as much when I am happy or mundanely watching the TV.

Nothing beats that feeling of slipping under the duvet, binge watching my favourite *Netflix* programmes and tucking into chocolate, crisps, and my favourite, cakes, to name a tantalising tasty few.

I like what I like. It's part of what makes me, me.

Granted, there are many things that I would change, particularly my sweet tooth. But I'm not the only one.

Do you, dear readers, find that once you're at the top of that slippery slope, with the bag of goodies calling out from the finish line, you've chomped your way through the lot?

Do you then want more?

Often, when I give in to that little voice telling me that the shop is only two minutes away, that is exactly what I do.

Go on, you'll be back and tucked up in bed before you know it.

Giving in to temptation might seem like a good idea, but it always ends the same way for me—the immediate high hits me, just like heroin, galloping through my veins. As a result of this drug of choice, I might spend an hour squirming on the toilet the following morning. It's a small price to pay for those few minutes of absolute bliss.

I tell myself enough is enough, but it never is.

It's part of a vicious never-ending circle of dieting—remaining in control, feeling good about oneself, then falling off the wagon, stuffing my face, then berating myself for not knowing any better as a nearly fifty-year-old man.

Some people tell me that I should learn to accept myself for who I am. While I appreciate the sentiment, and their encouragement, it's an easy statement to make when those offering their pearls of wisdom are sliding into a 30" waist pair of jeans while I'm having to launch myself off the top of the wardrobe to jam myself into a 44" pair. It doesn't get much better once I'm fastened in as my circulation is almost cut off—the biggest pair don't fit me comfortably, but I refuse to buy a larger size.

So, I suffer in clothes that look awful, and physically hurt me.

I know that I'm not the only person that breathes a sigh of relief when getting undressed.

As well as bruises caused from wearing certain garments, there is the constant compulsion to breathe in, hoping passers-by in the street won't somehow notice I'm fat.

And yes, I know the word fat isn't considered to be politically correct in these crazy times of wokeness, but I will offer a first and last word of warning because this book will not be politically correct and will deliver my truth, and your truths, warts, and all.

I endeavour to say it as it is, and for those who have volunteered their own story, I hope you will too.

The fact is, I am fat, and the woke can dress it up however they like; fat is fat is fat and while I know it is factually incorrect to say that *I* am fat, what surrounds my flesh and bones *is* fat. I've done the research and what sits under my skin is not pretty.

I hate my reflection because mirrors, unless they are of the Fun House variety, never lie.

Mirror, Mirror
On the Wall
Who's the fattest of them all?
You fat bastard, you fast bastard... you are, you are.

I loathe having my picture taken from any angle. I hate my smile. When forced before a camera, even for something as humdrum as renewing my passport, I cringe. All my mind finds in the photo is a cross between Captain

Pugwash and a convicted felon staring back at me. I have never been photogenic, and pictures rarely present me as I truly am.

Photoshopping, ugh, what's the point?

I once knew a guy that would only have his photograph taken from one side. He was a well-known TV personality, and apparently, many celebrities take the same stance.

Maybe I should try it.

Do I even have a good side?

If I do, I've never seen it.

I detest clothes shopping because it's impossible to find clothes to fit me in the stores I want to shop in. Instead, I drag myself to the nearest Big 'n' Bouncy (not the true brand name but for the purposes of this book and not openly endorsing or promoting clothes shops that think the larger amongst us have no fashion sense, let's call it that!) and hope nobody I know spies me buying items of clothing I detest. The embarrassment of being forced to purchase clothing not available in mainstream shops is one more knife in my heart because I cannot control my compulsion to over-eat foods that are bad for me and will cause weight gain.

Websites exist in today's world that cater to the larger person. Click on most of them and find the link that screams the word, PLUS or in my case PLUS AND TALL; yippee, wonderful, yes, the clothes look halfway decent and admittedly fashion for fatties has come on leaps and bounds over the years. The problem remains that no matter how good they look in those airbrushed pictures, when I put them on and stand in front of the mirror, it's akin to rolling dog poo in glitter—*what's the point?* I still feel fat and hate the way the clothes hang on my frame.

As the old saying goes, "You can't polish a turd, *or* throw glitter at it."

I know people reading this will think I am too hard on myself, and that may be true, but it's how *I* perceive myself. If you were being totally honest, you have those moments too. Oftentimes, the negatives outweigh any positives, and that's an easy rabbit hole to find yourself falling down.

Maybe it's strange reading a warts-and-all account from a man... we're not supposed to vent our feelings or care that much about our appearance, size, or self-esteem, are we?

Well, in these times of metro-sexuality and gender fluidness, looks absolutely do matter, not just for ladies, but men, and all those who sit in between, and outside of, genders too.

Men, in general, tend to brush things off, but inside, all we want to do is to present our very best selves.

Take a quick look at the guys passing you on the street; sporting trendy hairstyles, wearing expensive, fashionable clothes, outfits that co-ordinate from ear piercings to footwear, and realise it's the world we now live in.

FASHION RULES THE WORLD…

And with that knowledge comes the requirement that we all must be a certain size and shape.

IMPOSSIBLE… that's if you aren't viewing the world through rose-tinted spectacles.

Ask yourself; when was the last time you saw a woman wearing a size 24 dress, or a man in 46" waist jeans strutting the catwalks at London, Paris, Milan, or New York Fashion Week?

NEVER… and it's for one simple reason; the major fashion houses of the world refuse to present people that look like me, or you, or use people they see as aesthetically inferior, advertising their considered superior, high-end brands.

It sends out the wrong message, but the truth is, beauty sells; fat doesn't.

Don't get me wrong, I do have days when I think I look presentable, and I do scrutinise myself, almost believing my face looks smaller, that my belly is a little flatter, or my legs look less chunky…

But is it wishful thinking?

As I inspect my current choice of attire, I tell myself I look okay but whatever weight I have managed to lose, when I cast a glance at myself, I still believe that clothes rarely look right on bigger people.

"You're just big boned," people fondly remark.

Erm, no, a Tyrannosaurus Rex had big bones…

"You've just got broad shoulders."

Bollocks!

It's very nice when people try to use decades-old adages to bolster confidence and to spare negative thoughts and feelings, but let's call a spade a spade, excuses is what they are.

Admittedly, we do all come in different shapes and sizes, and excess fat does not form due to big bones or a big frame; it's caused by consuming more calories than the body requires or consuming vastly more calories than you are burning off.

For me, that is about to change, especially after today's experience.

Earlier this afternoon, I was having my hair cut and beard trimmed in the local barbers. This isn't anything new, and something I do every two weeks, but today, I caught a glimpse of myself as the stylist tilted my chair back. To say I was shocked is an understatement... *Turkey neck*, I thought to myself, before immediately wondering what lotion or potion I could buy to get rid of it. *Save your money, Marco.*

Cosmetic surgery aside, nothing I do will combat the problem because the skin covering every part of my body has been stretched over the years due to weight fluctuations. Plus, I am approaching the big 5-0, and the days of skin that pings back to perfection are long gone.

My skin simply won't have the elasticity it had when I was a teenager, but that doesn't mean I have to walk around looking as though I don't care about what is presented to the outside world.

So, my journey begins...

MY WEIGHT-LOSS JOURNEY

I thought long and hard about sharing these statistics, and when wrestling with the need to share it, ultimately, I feel it is important you do see my journey in full.

You can see my progress, both positive and negative, but also the large gaps in between some weigh in sessions, which will be openly and honestly explained at relevant parts of the book.

Please see below conversion.

1 Stone = 14 pounds

1 Stone = 6.35 kilograms

1 Stone = 224 ounces

In the UK, we tend to use stones and pounds. Kilograms, and ounces are used elsewhere.

Date	Weight	Loss	Gain
22.02.2022	22, 6		
11.03.2022	22, 3	3	
18.02.2022	21, 13	4	
25.02.2022	21, 12	1	
04.03.2022	21, 8	4	
11.03.2022	21, 3½	4½	
18.03.2022	21½	3	
25.03.2022	21	½	
01.04.2022	20, 10	4	
08.04.2022	20, 9½	½	
14.04.2022	20, 12		1½

CHEWING THE FAT

Date	Weight	Loss	Gain
22.04.2022	20, 4	8	
29.04.2022	20, 5½		4½
13.05.2022	19, 13	6	
20.05.2022	20½		1½
10.06.2022	19, 12½	2	
01.07.2022	19, 7	5½	
08.07.2022	19, 6	1	
15.07.2022	19, 7½		1½
22.07.2022	19, 7	1½	
19.08.2022	19, 6½	½	
23.09.2022	19, 7		½
30.09.2022	20, 2		9
07.10.2022	19, 10½	5½	
14.10.2022	19, 8½	2½	
04.11.2022	19, 4½	4	
24.11.2022	19, 8½		4
09.12.2022	19, 5	3½	
29.12.2022	19, 11		5½
19.01.2022	19, 12½		1½
27.01.2022	19, 9	3½	

Date	Weight	Loss	Gain
03.02.2023	19, 10		1
17.02.2023	19, 11		1
10.03.2023	19, 11		
24.03.2023	19, 9	2	
31.03.2023	19, 6	3	
21.04.2023	19, 2½	3½	
12.05.2023	19, 7½		5
26.05.2023	19½	7	
16.06.2023	18, 10½		4½
07.07.2023	19, 1½		4
28.07.2023	19, 1	½	
17.08.2023	19, 11½		10½
25.08.2023	19, 4	6½	
15.09.2023	19, 3	1	
05.10.2023	19, 11½		8½
28.10.2023	19, 8½	3	

| 17.11.2023 | 19, 12 | | 3½ |
| 07.12.2023 | 20, 3 | | 5 |

Date	Weight	Loss	Gain
04.01.2024	BLIND		
12.01.2024	BLIND		
19.01.2024	BLIND		
26.01.2024	BLIND		
02.02.2024	BLIND		
09.02.2024	BLIND		
16.02.2024		½	
23.02.2024			1½
01.03.2024	20, 0		
15.03.2024	19, 7	7	
22.03.2024	19, 4	3	
28.03.2024	19, 4½		½
05.04.2024	18, 11	7½	
12.04.2024	19½		3½
26.04.2024	18, 7½	7	
03.05.2024	18, 7	½	
10.05.2024	18½	6½	
24.05.2024	17, 12	2½	

January 1, 2023

I've been thinking about writing this book since I restarted my weight loss journey in February 2022.

Despite my best intentions, I have stopped and started work on the project for various reasons. Now it's time to get it finished.

Start weight date: 22nd February 2022.

Start weight: 22.6 stones (310 pounds)

How did I get here?
To cut a decades long story short, *Weight Watchers* worked for a time, but eventually their plan failed, or as I should say, *I* failed, again and again and again. I wasn't ready. My leader, Alison, was an angel, heaven-sent, and a

tower of support and strength. I felt I could call her anytime I needed guidance or a few kind words, and she would be there for me. But as wonderful as she was, and still is, only I can make the decision to lose weight and keep it off.

After so many disastrous attempts, I was too ashamed to return to *Weight Watchers*, so the only other alternative was *Slimming World*—a diet plan I had tried ten years previously.

I remember the hot, summer's day like it was yesterday.

My partner, Jon, and I plucked up the courage to defect from *Weight Watchers* and picked a class that was held in the cricket club of my local park. We reasoned that we could take a nice leisurely stroll and begin our journey together and throw in a hint of exercise too.

Lovely!

Nope, it was anything but. In fact, after that awful first experience it took another decade for me to try SW again.

Why?

The group leader was pleasant enough, as they always are on the surface, but spent the entirety of the class comparing SW to *WW* and criticizing the latter. In her unique and skewed opinion, target and the perfect waistline could only be found at the end of the yellow brick road, where the *Slimming World* Wizard would be there to pat us on the back. However, dare diverge off plan and the Wicked *Weight Watchers* Witch of the Northwest would be waiting to turn us all back into fatties.

Nothing about her attitude to losing weight or the contents of her class sat well with me, or Jon. We hated every minute of being her captive audience. The first week of SW, we both gained, so neither of us returned. We knew for certain that if the group leader had spent less time slagging off the competition, and instead buoyed the nervous new members who seemed confused by the plan, as it was back then, we both would have had better results.

Anyway, let's jump ahead to that weird time when the first COVID lockdown ended, and SW classes finally re-opened. I decided to bite the bullet, even though I had no intention of staying for class or sitting around with strangers, largely due to the fact Jon and I had avoided contracting coronavirus when the pandemic struck and were eager to maintain the status quo.

Aside from the obvious health risks of a class with so many others sitting nearby, Jon and I have very different personalities. Whereas he comes to life with an audience, I am shy and do not thrive in group settings and am forced to put on an act to hide my discomfort. This awkwardness is nothing new and has been embedded in my personality since I was a little boy. Aside from meeting new people, which I still struggle with, situations I can't control unnerve me. Those reasons aside, I loathe public speaking and being the focus of attention. So, without prejudice, rushing in to get weighed, then scooting off into the shadows with a loss, gain, or stay-the-same suited me fine.

After rethinking everything and glancing again at myself, I re-joined. Encouraged by a lovely chat with Donna, my consultant at her temporary group home, and thoroughly confused with the plan despite her best intentions to explain it to me, I skipped off with all the bumph and paraphernalia to get me started. This time with an ironclad determination to succeed.

And I did try my hardest, for a while at least.

Then, life got in the way, and I had my second COVID vaccination, which is when disaster struck.

Three days later, I felt unusually unwell, convinced I had a bout of indigestion or heartburn, which was a rarity for me. But no matter how many Rennie's I chewed, or glasses of milk I guzzled, the burning sensation sitting like a dead weight in my chest didn't seem to want to go away.

Quite quickly, my symptoms worsened. I became seriously ill with Pericarditis, which then led to symptoms of Fibromyalgia, which have since been fully diagnosed by a Rheumatologist.

To my shame, I was one of the many who believed that Fibromyalgia was 'all in the head' and that it was something the lazy amongst society dreamed up to avoid having to work for a living.

I am quite happy to hold my hands up and admit that I WAS WRONG!

Though I tried to mask how awful I truly felt to my nearest and dearest, I felt like I'd been hit by a steam train. Almost every horrible symptom I'd read about this largely unknown and incurable disease walloped me.

For those in the know, it can be debilitating, and for a while, it ruled me entirely. It still does, but I fight back against it with everything I have.

Below are the symptoms which impact my daily life:

Widespread pain.

Extreme Sensitivity to bright lights, smells, and sounds.

Stiffness in my neck, back, legs and arms.

Chronic Fatigue.

Poor Sleep Quality (Non-Restorative Sleep).

Cognitive Problems (Fibro Fog).

Irritable Bowel Syndrome.

Clumsiness.

Dizziness.

Problems with attention and concentration.

Restless Leg Syndrome.

Inability to regulate body temperature.

Tingling, numbness, prickling sensations in my hands and feet.

Burning sensation of the skin on my feet, ankles, and legs.

Arthritis / Arthrosis.

    The diagnosis left me in an extremely unhappy place physically, but not mentally, because I refused to surrender that part of me to this wretched illness. At that time, I was unfit, dangerously, and morbidly obese, and to make matters worse, pain racked every part of my body.
    Sod this, I thought, defiantly, unwilling to allow it to drag me to the pits of despair or let it get the better of me. Yet, despite my ruthless determination, to this day there are more symptoms than not that I have no control over.
    Bright lights hurt my eyes forcing me to exist in the dark. Even though I am partially deaf in one ear, I found I became hypersensitive to noise. Whether those sounds come from the traffic outside my house, or just having the television on in the background, I can't handle the enhanced stimulation. Every smell seemed to make me nauseous. As a lifelong non-smoker, walking past somebody in the street who blew smoke my way made me gag more than I had before. Every smell seemed to be heightened, from food, to cleaning products, and as disgusting as it is, I continue to make my partner's life miserable whenever he uses the toilet. I have developed such sensitivity to most smells that I stocked up on air fresheners, and developed a nervousness every time I heard him close the bathroom door—that hasn't

changed. In fact, I told my brother off last week for using my toilet which seems totally irrational, but my brain seems to have been re-wired, and things that never used to bother me, cause me to feel extreme anxiety.

"SPRAY," I bellowed, pulling my T-shirt over my nose, just in case the smell hit me.

"You'd think your shit smelled like roses," my brother yelled back, furious with me.

I had no comeback, but anyway, with Fibromyalgia comes irrationality...

Lying in bed at night, my legs throb, my feet and toes sting, and my skin itches and burns to the point I feel like I'm losing my mind. So bad is the latter, I bleed profusely from scratching myself unknowingly in the night.

"You need to slow down, Marco," my GP warned at my last consultation.

"I know." I *was* listening but I didn't have the luxury of slowing down, especially with a partner that had been extremely poorly and was still unwell.

Eventually, and at odds with my GP, I found my own routine. In time I discovered the more I do, and the more active I am, the less pain I feel, most of the time anyway. It works for a while then I relapse and want to sleep for a month before the cycle begins all over again.

My GP advised me to spread my household chores across weeks, rather than days.

It seemed a sensible, yet impossible request because as I said above, Jon has been very poorly, with several ailments for a couple of years, and wasn't physically capable of doing even the simplest things. So, everything fell to me.

The absolute truth: Jon was very ill, suffering from a disease that could have killed him had it not been picked up accidentally. While my illness is non-life threatening, it is chronic and will only get worse, not better, especially if I don't take care of myself. But if the carpets needed hoovering and the floors mopped, or we needed food shopping, I did it.

Every night, the dogs demanded to be walked, so I did that too.

Often, these non-stop activities took a terrible toll on me. I struggled, but I won. I was exhausted.

What other choice did I have?

To be frank, *none*.

So I got on with it and nothing has changed.

Yes, I still have bad days, but less weight puts less stress on a body already screaming for mercy.

But something had to give. The axe fell on SW again, and my second attempt became yet another failure in a long list of failures.

I hated that I had been beaten. The plan on paper is so easy to follow, but back then, one more thing on top of everything else weighing me down seemed too much to bear.

But I made it back, eventually, as do many others.

And now, I am writing this book.

Why?

Because I am still fat, hefty, overweight, big boned, call it whatever you want, and need to overhaul my lifestyle, this time permanently.

Looking back, I can't say for sure when I first realised that I had gained a massive amount of weight. It seemed to creep up on me like an enemy assassin.

What I do recall very strongly is being a teenager, standing in the kitchen in my childhood home, and listening as members of my extended family chatted away. I soon became the topic of conversation.

"You need to put a bit of beef on…" my aunty said.

Followed by…

"You're going to waste away…"

Yes, I was *that* kid, and my weight was deemed a problem in my teenager years, but from the opposite end of the spectrum.

Too fat, lose weight.

Too thin, put weight on.

Who can win?

I never imagined I would be looking at weight issues from both sides—I've been fat, thin, and everything in between.

But it's easier to remember the fatter times, or to be truthful, the unhappiest times, of which there have been many.

Families are supposed to be supportive, and a few members of mine have been. Some not so much, but those aren't worth naming.

I can distinctly remember my parents driving to Lancashire to pick up my Aunty Vera. She had not long lost her husband, my Uncle Don, and as it was Christmastime, I suggested inviting her down, not wanting her to be alone, or to spend the holidays with her own children who seemed to care less at that time.

So, on the day in question, I went to my parents' house and prepared a casserole.

It was freezing outside, and as my nan had once declared with disgust, "Vera can eat one more potato than a pig," I made sure I used the biggest pan I could find.

A few hours later, Aunty Vera strolled into the kitchen.

"Hello, Aunty Vera." I'd always been fond of her, despite others being less so, and was genuinely pleased to see her.

Instead of giving me a hug or returning my greeting, she hit me right between the eyes with her opening shot. "My God, you're obese."

I was shocked, and still am when I think back to how rude she was. There was no hello, no hug, or any kindness shown to me. The person she once declared her favourite nephew now a punching bag.

The malice and disgust in her tone, plus her condemnation hurt my feelings. I wouldn't give her the satisfaction of seeing that, so I turned to my mum.

"The casserole is cooked. I'm off." My blood boiled because I'd busied myself with peeling, chopping, and cooking to make sure Vera had a decent meal to sit down to, and all she offered me came in the form of a criticism of my size.

Did being 'obese' change the person I was?

Had my weight gain stopped me from being concerned that she would spend her first Christmas alone without my Uncle Don?

In response to the above, the answer is no… I was still the same person inside, although unforgiving where she was concerned.

Rude old bag.

She was right though! I was obese, although it didn't need to be pointed out in such a degrading and offhand manner.

My dad, never my biggest fan back then, did put her in her place later that day when she said. "I think I might have offended Marco."

Rightfully and something I have always appreciated, he told her that she had been extremely rude, which was decent of him. I never showed my face for the duration of her mercifully short visit, and the next time I saw her she had flown in on her broomstick for my mum's funeral. Fortunately for me, I was going through a slimmer period.

Not once did she say, "My God, you look good," or "My God, you've lost weight." But that wasn't a surprise because people are often keen to criticize but can't find the simple words to offer praise. Putting others down seems to make certain people feel superior—says more about them I feel, and their own insecurities wreaking so much havoc within themselves that they have to deflect it to others.

Due to the heartbreaking circumstances and other things being more important than my hurt feelings, I skated over my hatred of her, kissed her powdered cheek and offered my begrudged greeting. Underneath it all, what I really wanted to do was shove the old battleaxe into the nearest grave and pay somebody to quickly shovel the dirt on top of her.

She's still with us, and sadly, suffering from dementia. That makes me sad, but I never could bring myself to forgive her or make the effort to visit her again.

Anyway, at which point in my life was I happiest?

Right now, I'm not exactly doing cartwheels, but I am happier than I was in February 2022. Although, this weight loss journey seems to have me trapped in a vicious cycle and twists me in knots.

You see, as the tall, skinny kid, it's not ingrained in a person to worry about being underweight, but God help any person that suddenly tips the scales. You're viewed differently, stared at, judged by every echelon of society, and while those casting judgement might not be brave enough to comment, condemnation seeps from every pore.

In September 2022, my sister and I went to Kim Wilde's 40th Anniversary Greatest Hits show in Liverpool. It had been postponed many times due to the pandemic, but the wait really didn't bother me. I always had something to look forward to and from my perspective, the delays served me well, especially since I'd lost weight and valuable inches. I didn't seem to take up as much space as I used to.

But my sister is what many would call a big girl but still beautiful inside and out, and while others don't see that, I do. So, as we were shown to our seats, only two other seats in that row were occupied.

Sods law that the two faces gawping at us in horror were to be our concert neighbours.

So, I ushered my sister in first, knowing there was an empty seat next to her, and I took the seat next to Mr and Mrs Judgemental.

Hushed whispers told me they weren't happy sitting next to the 'fatties', but I didn't care. I sat there quietly seething, biting my lip, wanting to tell them if they had something to say, then to say it out loud.

But my sister hates it when I cause a scene in public, so although it went against my nature, I kept schtum, for her.

After more whispers and side-eyed glances, followed by an accidentally-on-purpose-elbow-in-his-side from yours truly, Mr and Mrs Judgemental moved two rows down when it was apparent Kim wasn't going to be playing to a full house.

So, with the Devil on my shoulder egging me on, I hauled my sister to her feet and followed them onto the empty row they had decamped to. The look of abject terror on their faces was priceless, then sheer relief as we passed them by.

"Wankers!" I hissed as I sashayed past them, head held high while my sister stared down at the floor.

That is one example of how society treats overweight people, not caring one bit how we are made to feel.

To the many 'big boned' of us who have suffered long haul flights, I'm convinced other passengers would be less offended if we had a dump in the aisle then stuffed ourselves into the seat next to them.

As I was once a prolific traveller, I bought my own seat belt extender to avoid the shame of having to ask for one in front of other passengers. Some might think that a step too far, but most cabin crew members that I've encountered wouldn't know discretion if it bit them on the arse—they make a big fuss and hullabaloo and wave it about the cabin, ensuring most of cattle class can see the fatty needs an extender. Anyway, I would pack it in my hand luggage for every flight and never had a problem, until I flew to Goa via Bahrain and my bag was searched as I left the plane on my layover.

How unnerving it was to be pulled to one side by a lady covered from head to toe, where only suspicious and hateful eyes could be seen, and questioned. As mentioned earlier, I am partially deaf and still tend to lip read, so was buggered from the start when her many questions began.

The dog sniffing at my crotch was particularly unnerving. I wanted to tell its mistress, "There's nothing down there that doesn't belong to me, love," but I held my tongue.

Throw in her broken English and obvious dislike of anybody not from the beautiful state of Bahrain, she was convinced I'd stolen the extender from the flight.

Of course, I protested my innocence; my mind conjuring images of Bahrain's version of the Bangkok Hilton. But she didn't seem to care, and her mind was made up... I was a thief.

Would I be arrested and forced to sleep on a cockroach and rat-infested concrete floor and survive on pig swill?

What if they somehow discovered I was gay? Would I be beaten, or worse, hung?

It would have taken one heck of a strong rope to lynch me, but every terrible scenario filtered through the cracks in my mind.

Thankfully, somebody with a shred of common sense informed the harridan that Monarch Airways branded their equipment and what I had been accused of stealing was property that I had legally procured.

No apology came my way. She simply wafted me away with contempt like an annoying mosquito.

Embarrassed, but relieved, I found the nearest *McDonalds* (I was surprised to find a branch inside an airport which screamed opulence and wealth—most have cars to give away, usually Skoda's or a Vauxhall Astra... not here—the first prize was a gold Lamborghini) and ordered large fries, a hamburger, and a large full fat coke.

When my statement arrived the following month, my jaw nearly hit the floor when I saw the charge...

EIGHTEEN POUNDS for three paltry items.

Highway robbery!

I wondered if the cow that produced my burger had been plucked from the King of Bahrain's prized herd.

Who knows?

Maybe I should relocate permanently to Bahrain. At those prices, I'd soon have the figure of a catwalk model.

Is Being Fat a Crime?

In today's world, where the vacuous and beautiful seem to reign supreme, I would say the scales are tipped in their favour.

But who says I'm not beautiful, or handsome, or that I don't make others weak at the knees? My partner of nearly twelve years, Jon, thinks I'm hot… and yes, I question if his eyesight is failing, but he loves me, chunky and all.

It's a comforting thought, knowing he is fond of my wobbly bits, but I'm sure he'd love it even more if I had a body like one of his favourite WWF wrestlers, or Henry Cavill.

What I do know for a fact is that he wouldn't be attracted to me if I was skinny because he prefers a bit of timber on a man.

He struggles with his weight too, more so than I do right now.

The simple truth is he understands me, and I understand him, and as much as he drives me bonkers (definitely vice versa), I am lucky to have him. He is luckier to have me though—Ha!

Most people don't see overeating or the compulsion to eat as an addiction, but he does, and let me address that confusion and make it abundantly clear… it IS an ADDICTION for me, him, AND millions of others.

In my opinion, to those of us fighting the battle, an addiction to food is just as debilitating as heroin addiction, if not more so. I do not say that lightly, lack sympathy, or wish to take away from others' struggles, but for me, my addiction is made more difficult because I see my downfall everywhere I look; in every shop, supermarket, leisure centre, and service station to name but a few.

I can't be in the minority here; when trying to lose weight, a supermarket is the worst place in the world to have to visit. Everything that can derail our attempts to lose weight is under that one roof, which is why so many of us have learned which aisles to avoid.

TRUTH: We MUST eat food to survive.

TRUTH: We DON'T have to use recreational drugs and can survive without them.

TRUTH: We DON'T have to smoke and can survive without cigarettes.

TRUTH: We DON'T have to drink alcohol and can survive without it.

TRUTH: We CAN survive without gambling.

TRUTH: Sex is wonderful, but we CAN survive without that too.

I have never smoked.

I drink in moderation.

I know nothing about casino's, slot machines, or horse racing to name a few.

And yes, admittedly, in my younger days I used recreational drugs most weekends, but not once did I ever consider myself addicted. It was a tool to thrust me into party mode, and so off my face, I didn't care who stared at me as I wobbled on a podium in syncopated rhythm with a gaggle of other gays to *Tragedy* by Steps.

Am I addicted to sugar, sweets, cakes, chocolate, crisps?
Does a bear poop in the woods?
Yes, I am, which is another reason to write this book. I hope that those who read it, on the same journey, or who might just be curious to see what I am waffling on about, will believe the struggle is real for millions of us, and it will be until the day we die.

As is the case for most addictions, there is no cure. We can only manage it.
So, where am I on life's highway now?
I feel as though I'm stuck on a rollercoaster ride going round and round the same track.

I am desperate to get off this ride.

This is a lifelong fight, and I'm already decades in. But I am wiser now, and as the years have passed, I have finally cottoned on to something simple; perfection does not exist.
I might yo-yo diet and gorge on the wrong foods for the rest of my days, but I will get to as healthy a point as I possibly can.

DONNA'S STORY

When meeting Donna, a fifty-seven-year-old, married, mother of one from Manchester, you would be forgiven for assuming she is as she presents herself. Displaying bravado that packs an almighty wallop, it soon becomes apparent that the loud personality which greets you is only a shade of who she really is.

Warm, effervescent, vivacious, and enthusiastic, she welcomes you into her world with open arms, a beaming smile, and a flutter of her long, dark eyelashes. You might take a step back and say to yourself, *wow, she's a lot*!

And you would be right to think that, but there is a valid reason why... past, present, and her hopes for the future have shaped the woman Donna is and will become.

Working tirelessly for *Slimming World* as a consultant since 2005, she joined the race and ran for her life. Eighteen years later, she's still at breakneck speed in the fast lane, learning as she navigates her way through what will essentially be a lifelong journey, gaining valuable and insightful knowledge and experience, delivering truths to those who walk through her doors, desperate to turn their lives around.

Donna has earned the right to stand in front of her many groups and share her life's lessons simply because she has been there, done it, bought the T-shirt, lost weight, stuffed herself sick with chocolate, drowned her sorrows in Vodka, re-gained weight, ate the pies, and stayed the same. She is a fighter, and survivor of food addiction.

Currently weighing in at a svelte ten stone, thirteen pounds, happy in a size twelve dress, yet overweight according to what she believes is an outdated BMI chart, she is quick to tell me; "I'd be happy at ten stone, seven pounds." While those who have never experienced issues with their weight might say, *but it's only six pounds...* to Donna, and to many like her, that figure makes the difference between self-acceptance and endless scrutiny of oneself.

This is Donna, as she is today, but how did she get here?

At seventeen, when most of us are still deciding what path to take in life, Donna joined the army, wishing to escape the council estate she had been raised on. Most might call it a brave choice, because serving one's country is certainly no walk in the park. Still, in that disciplined environment, she thrived. Attaining peak physical fitness, she found she could eat whatever she wanted and at no point did she worry about her weight. Thanks to the daily exercise regime the army demanded, cognitive equilibrium ruled, and a healthy weight was maintained.

Upon deciding to leave the army four years later, Donna's hearty appetite remained but she was no longer exercising enough to burn off the calories. And like many people, combining that potent mixture of overeating with lack of physical exercise, excess weight crept on.

Matter of fact, she tells me, "At my heaviest, I was twelve stone thirteen and a half pounds."

Unhappy, she took forty laxatives per day while surviving on one Rich Tea biscuit. Thankfully, she had the foresight to realise this destructive pattern of behaviour couldn't continue. So, she visited her GP, desperate for support and understanding, walking out of the consultation feeling truly devastated to be told that she was morbidly obese.

After being prescribed Ponderax, now banned in the United Kingdom because it caused heart valve, and other issues for some patients, Donna continued to eat and drink alcohol to excess, while simultaneously remaining on the drug for a few months.

Some might see this as a low point, but happier times loomed on the horizon.

Meeting, Ade, the man who would later become her husband, she remembers their first date. "I refused to eat fatty foods in front of him, so I ate a salad, when I really wanted pie and chips."

At twenty-five, madly in love, happily married, and pregnant, she told herself what countless women have over the years, that she is eating for two. She gave birth to Chloe, yet, she still struggled with her weight, at her heaviest during this time.

So, she found a local clinic in the Northwest of England who prescribed her slimming tablets, or 'speed' to call them by their true name. At a weekly cost of £25 per week, including a weigh-in, she found herself awake all night, either cleaning ferociously, hoovering, dusting... or playing Casper on her brand-new *PlayStation* console.

Suddenly losing her mum, Donna weighed in at nine stone, slipping into a size eight suit from *French Connection* for the funeral. During this sad time, she undressed in front of her sister who noticed Donna's protruding ribs.

"You've gone too far," her sister warned.

Sensibly, she stopped taking the prescribed slimming tablets and regained the weight she had lost, and more. But fate was to step in when Donna met a girl in her local pub who had lost a lot of weight.

"You look great," Donna complimented. "How did you do it?"

"*Slimming World*," the girl replied.

"I've never heard of it." In truth, Donna had never heard of any slimming organisation or the many groups out there.

Curious, she researched *Slimming World* and found mutual friends who had joined and successfully followed the plan. Wanting to try but worried about taking the plunge, she arranged to go with a friend. After three weeks of excuses from this same friend, Donna knew she had to act and decided to go alone. It could very well be one of the best decisions she had ever made.

Accountability

the fact or condition of being accountable; responsibility:

Accountability is the backbone of *Slimming World* and as Donna readily agrees, nobody can be forced to diet, or to adopt a healthier lifestyle... that never works. But if a person does embark on that journey, with the ups and downs presented by the plan and one's humanity, accountability is key. If a person loses weight, fantastic, but if they gain, accountability is also vital, as is honesty and transparency to oneself. We can all follow the plan, it's quite simple, but we have all fallen off more times than we care to remember, as has Donna.

So, with determination, and the fact she had not weighed herself for a long time—she knew she weighed more than her husband, which mortified her—Donna joined her local group and spoke candidly with her consultant, Di.

"I want to lose a stone first, then tell me what I weigh."

Di agreed, and Donna's journey began.

For a while, and still on plan, she would stand on the scales backwards to avoid seeing how much she weighed.

Finally, celebrating the loss of her first stone, Di delivered the news Donna had been waiting for. "Well done, you weigh eleven stone, thirteen and a half pounds."

Shocked and confused, Donna replied. "No, I've lost a stone." In *her* mind... and remember that she had not been weighed in a long time... she had told herself she was only twelve stone.

Di repeated her weight. "You weigh eleven stone, thirteen and a half pounds."

Horrified by the realisation that she had begun her journey at twelve stone, thirteen and a half pounds, and even though she had done amazingly well, Donna went home and cried her eyes out, relying on old faithful to cheer her up—goodies. She sobbed while scoffing a packet of biscuits, until her husband returned home.

"Why are you crying?" Ade asked.

For the first time, ever, Donna revealed her true weight to him. "Because I've lost a stone and I'm still eleven stone, thirteen and a half pounds."

"Right, you've got two choices. You put the stone you've just lost back on or realise you're halfway there."

Her husband's wise words gave her the kick up the backside she needed, and she continued her journey. But his words highlighted the fact that he, like a lot of others, did not understand the concept of over-eating, or the thought process behind polishing off a whole packet of biscuits or a multi-pack of crisps. He would often leave food on his plate, something a person addicted to food can never understand.

She smiles when she remembers reaching target. "The emotions were indescribable. That feeling that *I'd* achieved it." And then a look of pride settles, and I see in her eyes how much it meant and continues to mean to her. "It took me a year to lose two and half stone, but I'm still here nineteen years later. The proof is in the pudding. This plan works."

Discussing her victory in more detail, she explains; "There is no right or wrong way of doing *Slimming World*. It's your way that matters."

Wise words indeed and some might think she did it with ease. Nothing could be further from the truth. Addiction is ALWAYS there, whispering temptation, *go on, eat it... go on, you can worry about it tomorrow.*

Not only do you fight with yourself, but reactions from friends, family and strangers affect your mindset, often nudging people off their chosen path.

"I learned people are very quick to judge... they don't understand..." With that, her voice tapers off, and I wonder how much damage has been done by the negativity of others. Quickly, she changes the subject, "I eat the same things all the time... I'm happy, and I like what I like."

For those people who do struggle with their weight, the judgement Donna glossed over so expertly is glaringly obvious and is a bitter pill to swallow. Many of us have been there. Donna obviously has but forges on, determined not to be beaten.

"I've been a target member for eighteen years and like a lot of people, lockdown screwed me up. I ate *Slimming World* chips for every meal during lockdown with the only variation being the type of sauce I poured over the chips... I know the plan inside out, and work on *me*, which is an everyday job. I learned what my weaknesses and triggers are, I had to. I haven't had crusty bread, and butter for nineteen years now..." As Donna is aware, we all make sacrifices because sacrifice is required to maintain some semblance of balance. Still, she knows the plan works. Admiring her slim frame, more often than not shrouded in baggy clothes, regardless of the continuing fight, it's obvious she is a winner. I just hope she sees it herself. "You can go to any supermarket and eat in any restaurant and the plan works if you want it to. *Slimming World* helps with accountability."

Her words resonate with truth, and I tell her so. "I totally agree, and my weight hasn't been as stable as this for years."

"Social Media slates *Slimming World* as toxic. It is not. Essentially, it is a calorie-controlled diet, that's how you lose weight. We're saying you can still eat all this food and feel full. Because of this, people think something is wrong. But what we are doing is maximizing those low-calorie filling foods to keep you full for longer."

"It makes perfect sense to me." Following the plan, and putting my journey on paper, I too know that it works.

"Think of it this way. Food is fuel for your body, and it's taken me twenty years to realise this. It's *not* a reward. Food can be the best or worst medicine.

Say you have a car... This is where SYNergy comes in.

Step One, which is your free food and the bulk of your plan, that's the petrol for your car.

Step Two is your Healthy Extra, the water.

And then the more minimized is the oil, which is your SYNS, spelt with a *y*. It stands for SYNergy."

While it might sound too scientific for some, the plan is easy to follow, and like a lot of people, I assumed SYN was spelt SIN. It is a common misconception, and one Donna is keen to explain. I wonder how she retains this vast knowledge, then remember she is nearly two decades into this lifestyle and its ever-evolving plan. And while she is a 'pro', she is under no illusion that she is cured of her addiction to food.

"We're never cured, we just learn to manage it." She is brutally honest. "My downfall is still Vodka and crisps, chocolate, and everything else. Yes, you can have it, just not lots of it. I can't have open chocolate in the house and tell my husband... 'any open chocolate, eat it, or put it in the car'. We both know I would eat the whole bar."

Food addiction wasn't Donna's only vice. "I used to smoke and stopped six years ago, but I could never do drugs because I have an addictive and obsessive personality. I've just been diagnosed with ADHD which answered a lot of questions about why I do things that I do."

Out of respect, I won't delve into the specifics of her ADHD diagnosis because there are parts of Donna's world that should remain private. She already gives so much of herself during her many weekly group meetings. Still, she offers insights into her personality.

"I wore the same clothes on every night out. Black pants, black shirt, the only things I felt comfortable in. Yes, I would've loved to have worn different clothes, but..." She is distracted and dragged down memory lane. "... I once tried this dress on in *Top Shop*, and while trying to pull it over my head, my back seemed to swell, and I couldn't get it off. I had to rip the dress to get it off." She isn't the first, or the last person that will happen to, but at the time, shame was all encompassing. She exited the changing room, hid the damaged dress, and rushed home, dissolving into tears.

That was then, and now she can reflect on hitting *her* perfect weight. "When you get to target, it's you who has done it which is why I decided to become a *Slimming World* consultant. All because of that feeling. I cried when I got to target because it meant so much. Finally, I was able to look in the mirror and smile at my reflection, rather than despise this girl, which I had done for so long. That feeling... I wanted somebody else to feel it."

It's an emotional moment listening to Donna bare her heart and soul, because I have been there many times. She isn't alone in experiencing that feeling and digs deeper into her psyche at the time.

"I despised myself because of low confidence and self-esteem. I was always loud and would get the fat jokes in first before anyone else. If I was in the pub and somebody called me fat I'd go home and get into bed, stuff my face with two Hollands Meat and Potato Pies, and cry."

"We've all done that," I remind her.

"I still binge. When I'm angry, or upset, food is it... stuff it, I'll have it, and I get to the point where I can't shovel anything else in and want to be sick. The only way I can describe it, that self-harm, when people cut themselves, that release, I get that when I eat."

Once more, it's something I have experienced myself. That quick rush, almost like a surge of adrenaline, although it's over as quickly as it begins. "I get it." I can empathise, most people addicted to food know that feeling all too well.

"I am not binge free. I am binge better." What a corker of a statement, and one that should be used to convey realism on *Slimming World*'s various promotional materials. "But I realised, the more I chastised myself, the more I binged, and it took me a long time to stop doing that. I've still got the same insecurities, at target. I still look in the mirror and see a cheater. My last binge was four days ago."

"Wow, really?" I had never imagined Donna would still suffer the curse of binge eating but her honesty is refreshing, which is why she is a long-term, successful leader. You can't kid a kidder, as the old saying goes. She has heard every excuse in the book.

"Every relationship you can have with a human I've had with food. It's been my best friend, my worst enemy, lover, hated it, loved it... sometimes I look at myself and tell myself I look alright. I'm still a work in progress and always will be. I'm still that fat person inside and if you were to put a load of cakes on that table and told me they were ten SYNS per cake, I would find the one with most chocolate in, or the biggest. That never changes."

She is a woman after my own heart. "So would I."

"I've hit another stage in my life where I want to wear modern clothes, but I can't 'cos of my body shape. I don't think I will ever be satisfied. In my head I am twenty, but my body says *no, not a chance.* I've given up running due to problems with my knees—they would pop if I ran anywhere."

"Is there anything else you do to maintain your weight, *Zumba*, Yoga...?"

"Oh, God, no. I couldn't sit down and meditate—I've got ADHD, my brain can't do it. Running was my sanity, and I was addicted. Because I know what type of person I am, I have got to keep working at it all the time. I can't exercise, but I dance—Northern Soul. Dancing makes me happy, and feeling happy in my own skin makes me happy. I'm not perfect by any means. I know what food is to me, but I've learned. I'm happy with who I am."

I must admit, I am envious that she has found a shred of self-acceptance because I am still adapting, re-wiring thought patterns long since embedded in my brain. "I understand." And I do, even though I am not there, yet.

"Luckily, I've had no health issues due to being overweight because I nipped it in the bud before it came to that. Still, in twelve months, I know I will still be doing this because I will never be cured."

"Do you think you will always be a consultant?"

"Yes, I would like to think so because it's a tough world where people are judged. If you're fat, you're lazy. No, we're not." Her tone shifts lightning fast from light to dark, and quickly back to light again. "I want people to be happy. I did it, I still do... I got more confident. I can't change if somebody calls me ugly, as long as they don't call me fat, 'cos I'm not. Confidence is the most attractive quality to me, but I still have my down days. Anger compels me to eat, or sadness. If I'm happy... it's emotion, but mainly anger and sadness."

"I'm exactly the same as you, but I stuff my face when I'm happy too."

She is quick to reply. "Like I said, I'm not perfect... chocolate and crisps are my downfall. And at Christmas, I have a pie butty. Two pies. One must be hot, and the other has to have brown sauce and salt on it. Both on bread..."

When asked what advice she often gives to her members, she answers without pause or thought, "We're all human, and I would rather be consistently decent than inconsistently perfect. Just work on being consistently decent."

"I've never, ever heard that said before, but it makes sense."

She briefly touched upon common decency, and kindness, to those casting negative judgement. "People should keep their mouths shut and opinions to themselves."

"Exactly!"

And like Mother Hen, she tells me what I wasn't aware of before our chat. "I'm very protective over my members."

Rightly so, and when I ask her what her ultimate goal is, she answers with a twinkle in her eye... I wonder what is coming and so unprepared am I to hear so profound a response, I am covered in goosebumps, leaving me speechless, and our chat over.

"My ultimate goal is to stay happy. It costs nothing and yet it's the hardest thing to achieve."

The Journey so far...

August 5, 2022
London, England.

The weather is glorious, and the sun shines high in the cloudless, blue sky. People mill about laughing, smiling, singing, and dancing.

And I'm one of them.

Tomorrow, I will be forty-eight (how did that happen?) and with three stone already shed, I haven't felt this good in years.

But it's not my birthday that is on my mind because tonight is *the* night... I've waited six years to see the ABBA Voyage concert in Stratford, and I am beyond excited.

I've loved them since I was a small child and born the same year as they won the Eurovision Song Contest with *Waterloo*, I don't remember a time that their music didn't fill my life.

So, as a treat for my birthday, Jon and I travelled down on the train.

It's not even lunchtime but Jon is starving and moody having been deprived of a scoff at Liverpool Lime Street (I had no idea that *Burger King* had been replaced by a *Krispy Kreme,* so I'm already in the doghouse). As I don't have the hormone that tells me I am hungry, I can take or leave eating, but to move forward, Jon *must* eat. Or else.

Me being me, I have limited patience, and in a rush to get to the hotel, which is conveniently next door to the ABBA Arena, I buy a traditional Cornish pastie for me and a chicken one for him at Euston Station (SIX POUNDS, FIFTY PENCE EACH... Howdy, Bahrain prices... stand and deliver, your money or go hungry...) and we eat them on the hop.

This might not seem unusual, aside from the exorbitant price, but I have always, up to that point, refused to eat in public, aside from an actual restaurant, thinking others would look at me and think *he's fat enough, look at him shovelling that pastie in.*

But that wasn't the worst part.

Anybody who has navigated the London underground will know it's a maze of lines with people rushing to get to their destination, and with Jon, who suffers from extreme anxiety, it wasn't an easy feat, dragging a suitcase behind me with various outfit choices inside, while clinging onto a red-hot pastie with the other.

It was stressful enough to make the Pope swear.

As I'd lived in Brixton around 1997/1998, I was used to the underground but for Jon, a novice, it was a lengthy, sweaty experience that meant train hopping in the blistering summer heat. Neither one of us was prepared to dump the pastie in case you were wondering, not at six-and-a-half-quid-a-pop thanks very much.

But despite the outrageous price, I enjoyed the pastie, even though I typically dumped most of the filling. Delicious! The only thing missing was salt and lashings of brown sauce slathered all over it.

PastieGate over and done with, we arrived at our destination and stepped onto the platform at Pudding Mill Lane station, thankful that the last stage of our journey had been above ground.

Opposite the station to our right was the ABBA Arena, and to the left was our hotel, or what I thought was our hotel.

I'd chosen the Snoozebox because of its proximity to the arena.

So far, so good, or so I thought.

Checking in, the bar area impressed me most. Beautiful people milled about the spacious area. The buzz instantly ignited the mood to party within me, and my mind targeted on one thing, ABBA.

Walking along the landing toward our room, a more subtle notion took hold, and the ambiance changed. Reminded of those metal crates, you know the kind hoisted onto the back of trucks, stacked on top of the other, that transport goods up and down the country... but the biggest surprise awaited us when I pulled open the door to our room.

The impression the bar held morphed into something different. "They should have called this place the Rabbit Hutch."

Talk about small... bloody hell, I couldn't believe I'd paid £103 to spend the night here.

Our living quarters for the night was eight by ten foot at most, and I swore that HMP Belmarsh inmates would have more room in their cells.

I wondered how Jon and I were going to comfortably fit inside this tiny space.

A double bed mocked us in the corner of the room—Jon is six foot one while I stand at six feet on a good day, not to mention our combined width when lying side by side.

But I didn't want it to dampen my mood; it was only for one night, right.

Strangely, about two feet above our bed, a single bunk bed dangled from the ceiling. Three people in this tin can—no way! Neither of us would risk sleeping on that, and it only added to my growing claustrophobia.

The bathroom (think Harry Potter's cupboard under the stairs but smaller) consisted of a shower to the left, with the toilet on the far right, with a small sink placed weirdly too close to the toilet. I soon discovered that, for the hefty amongst us, hanging my right leg over the sink was the only way to carry out one's ablutions.

If I had any intention of having a number two (I wasn't), it would have taken a miracle squeezing my backside into the space designated for it, but then what do I do with my thighs? It's Sods law, but as soon as I spotted the toilet it was turtle head time, so I needed to go, which meant closing the door in the tiny, windowless space. It was a terrible experience, and by the time I'd finished, I couldn't see a thing because the closed door trapped in the sweltering heat, and as I was sweating like a glass blowers' arse, my specs had fogged up. I could barely see a thing.

As awful as it sounds, I made the best of it, opened the bathroom door then flung open the hutch door, gagging for fresh air.

Poor Jon lay naked on the bed, trying to cool down after the jaunt across London while I unpacked and decided what outfit and shoes I was wearing. You might laugh, but this was a moment for me. I'd waited years, and despite my closet-like surroundings, excitement bubbled inside.

There was also the bonus of meeting up with my good friend Jill after the show, who I hadn't seen for about seventeen years.

I just wish there had been a camera inside the room filming us while we tried getting ready.

We showered but had to keep the bathroom door, and the hutch door open, to keep the air circulating. Then once dressed, we stepped out onto the landing looking the absolute business, ready for a drink or ten.

Music pumped from the bar area... I arrived slimmer, tanned, my hair freshly cut and stubbled shaped.

For the first time in years, I felt a surge in confidence.

Brand new blue ripped jeans, which I bought and couldn't fit into a year before, new suede loafers and tie-dye T-shirt; I felt good, while Jon looked handsome and smart in his chosen outfit. Don't ask him about the suede loafers I bought for him... stylish, but by the end of the night he walked like he'd been hobbled.

With the sun beaming down upon us, Jon and I sat having preshow drinks in the bar area. But Jon quickly ushered me into a shaded area. Pfft! I love feeling the sun on my skin while he loathes it.

What do they say about opposites attract?

That aside, the Prosecco cocktails (Awful! I swear dishwater with a Clit Bang chaser would have tasted better) and the Gin and lemonade (yummy) flowed despite the £24.00 price tag for two doubles. I'd forgotten about London prices, but hey, the anticipation of ABBA charged about me... I could live with it.

We had a fantastic time and hadn't even stepped foot inside the arena by this point.

Our moods transformed from buoyant, upbeat, to celebratory. And it wasn't just us. It seemed the people of London joined with us in coming out to have the time of their lives.

We entered the arena, amazed by the design. Futuristic neon lights sat nicely against the wooden structure surrounding us. I could only describe it as old meets new, industrial meets nature, but I was amazed, and eager for the show to start.

Jon treated me to a tank top with ABBA emblazoned across the front, which we could pick up after the show. When he saw the £70 price tag, he nearly fainted, but I had to have it although I knew it wouldn't fit me. But it would do by the time I intended to go again in the summer of 2023.

After buying a couple of drinks inside the arena we stood on the dance floor in front of the stage.

"Halfway back and just off from the middle is the best place to stand," the lady I bought the ABBA scarf from advised.

And right there I stood waiting, on tenterhooks.

The atmosphere felt like an electric charge, and I glanced around at happy, smiling faces.

A journalist, in his review of the Voyage show said something along the lines of, "It's the greatest ABBA performance the world has never seen. Until now." And they were right, but it was so much more.

The lights faded and the live band struck up the first notes and despite the technology involved, I really didn't know what to expect or how I would feel.

Excitement was at fever pitch and seemed to permeate from person to person, then from the blinding white light four figures could be seen rising out of the stage.

It was ABBA presented as they were in their 1979 heyday, well not really them, but as good as.

The crowd roared their approval as the spotlight settled on Frida.

She took the lead on the first song of the night, *The Visitors*, and my brain instantly kicked into gear.

Oh, my God, it's Frida.

Although it really wasn't.

But yes, it is.

I argued with myself, then the three other band members stepped into the spotlight to thunderous roars.

Tears fell, and I don't know why because I am not overly emotional by nature, certainly not at concerts.

It's usually Jon who bawls at gigs, but rather than crying with emotion, it was the brand-new suede loafers crushing his chubby trotters that almost brought him to tears.

But nostalgia kicked me good and hard because my mum should have been there watching it with us. Sadly, she died of breast cancer in 2012 but would have loved every moment of it. I hoped that somehow, she danced and sang right next to me.

Agnetha twirled around the stage in front of me whilst singing her heart out to *Mamma Mia*, then Benny and Bjorn spoke to the crowd, and there was nothing that could have convinced me that they weren't there.

It was astonishingly realistic, and the songs sprung to life by a ten-piece band and three backing singers who really should have a show of their own someday.

At various times during the ninety-minute show, I was reduced to tears. The music transported me back to my childhood and the memories those songs triggered, both good and bad, played like a timeline film in my mind.

Watching transfixed as ABBA performed *Chiquitita* in front of an eclipsing moon, or singing *Fernando* underneath the Northern Lights, or giving their all to *Dancing Queen* while surrounded by the most dazzling and spectacular light show I've ever seen at any concert, must be seen to be believed. Those are only three moments that spring to mind, but the show brought many more.

I sang from start to finish (out of tune, and in keys yet to be invented), danced (adequately, *my* feet were fine), clapped (like a demented sea lion), cheered (until my throat screamed at me raw and irritated), and cried (unashamedly) along with the rest of the audience (apart from Jon) who found ABBA's performance as majestic as I did.

So, when the opening lines, "I don't wanna talk, about things we've gone through," boomed out of the speakers, emotion swelled and tears fell again. *The Winner Takes It All* was always a favourite and to see it performed 'live' was a rare privilege.

And then it was over.

When the four band members, as they are now, in their mid to late seventies, walked on at the end for their curtain call, it was like the second coming for many of us in attendance. A touching end to one of the best nights of my life.

Still on a high, it was a treat to catch up with my friend, Jill, who looked wonderful but after a few hours, Jon and I were both ready for bed so reluctantly said our goodbyes.

Back in the hutch, it was a squeeze, but we finally fell asleep.

But too soon my eyes fluttered open and I lay wide awake. When I lifted my leg and bashed my shin on the curiously placed bunk bed it reminded me never to stay there again.

To put our stay at the Snoozebox into context, Jon and I were checked out and at London Euston by 7 am and back home, approximately 181 miles, by 10:30 am. To our dismay, the pastie shop was closed.

I'd go back and see ABBA time and time again but would find another hotel.

To sum up this trip, for me at least, it highlighted my newfound confidence, only gained by losing weight. How funny is that—to gain the courage to do something that came to mean so much, I had to lose what I truly hate.

That weight loss is the only reason I felt able to make the trip and enjoy it. Refreshingly, I felt people looked at me for other reasons than my size. I appeared presentable in my chosen outfit, rather than busting out of my jeans or tugging at my top, trying to hide my moobs (man boobs).

Used to my jeans bruising my waist, I found I could slip in and out of them without undoing the button. Now, that might cause a shrug and a mocking giggle from the beautiful people, but for an overweight person who has lost significant inches, it is a minor miracle.

Saying the above, and as comfortable as *I* felt, I'm certain Jon didn't feel the same way, and offered the choice, would not have come with me. But I can't really speak for him. His tale is his own to tell.

August 6, 2022

Today marks my birthday, and though Jon spoiled me again, I have no desire to celebrate. The night before with ABBA at the helm was everything, and after all, I am forty-eight. That is nothing to bang on about.

At Jon's urging, upon arriving at Liverpool Lime Street, I treated myself to a box of twelve *Krispy Kreme* doughnuts. I'd never had them before and thought, *what the hell, you can claw the Syns back...* but to my dismay, they were far too sweet, even for me, so I shared them with my lovely neighbours Kath and Phil.

I fell back into the wrong cycle and missed weigh-in that following week, and over the next few weeks, found myself locked in failure.

August flew by, as did September.

September 30, 2022
WEIGH-IN DAY

A major setback this week, but not entirely unexpected because I had missed weigh-in for three weeks.

Have I avoided it?

Yes, and no.

After the high of the concert, losing weight seemed less important to me. I had basked in the moment, but ultimately, I ignored the main reason for wanting to lose weight. Yes, that concert sat as an aim, but was now in the past. I lost motivation, temporarily forgetting the endgame. The horror erupted deep down inside in me when the scale noted a whopping nine-pound gain post-concert setback. Mortification filled me, and I could have kicked myself, but the scales hadn't lied. My self-sabotage had done its dirty work.

So, I went back to it with renewed vigour and the aim of losing three stone (42 pounds) by Christmas.

Would I do it?

Right now, I clutched at hope, but I refused to be too hard on myself if I don't quite get there.

What I did strive for was to be healthier, slimmer, but most important, regain that confidence I had at the ABBA concert.

But for the remainder of the year, my mojo deserted me entirely. I desperately wanted to lose 4, 5, 6, 7 stone. I just couldn't get there.

I did hit the three stone mark by the way.

DANNY'S STORY

Danny read about this book on social media and contacted me to discuss the possibility of contributing, and while I was only too happy to hear his story, just as he was to tell it, he insisted on one caveat—that his identity, and those he mentions, are given pseudonyms.

I've never met Danny, but his accent tells me he is from the north of England. He is approaching "dirty thirty", as he calls it, and is in a long-term relationship with his girlfriend, Emily.

I readily agreed to his terms, so while this may read differently to the other interviews, it is no less remarkable a read.

This is *his* story, so it is only fair that he gets to tell it *his* way.

"I never, ever, ever saw myself being fat, it just wasn't who I was, and to my shame, if I saw a fat person walking down the street, I'd stare at them, wondering how they had let themselves get so big. Now, I see things from the other side because I am stared at now, and worse, judged and mostly by total strangers who don't even know my name not to mention my story.

How could they?

I don't shout about myself from the rooftops, and they don't stop to ask why. They just snarl, or snigger. I can almost hear it... *fat fuck*... but maybe that's in my imagination and a manifestation of the misery I feel being overweight?"

There is nothing Danny says that many of us haven't experienced, but what was the trigger to his weight gain? I tell him that some members of my family struggled with, and still struggle with, their weight. "Is that the case with you?"

He is quick to answer. "None of my family are overweight, in fact, my dad, mum and brother, they're all gym freaks. My girlfriend, she's always been slim too but doesn't like, or go to, the gym." Thoughts of his girlfriend seem to stop him in his tracks. I wonder what he's thinking. "She's stunning, I'm punching, I know that... but weight just crept up on me..." Hesitation seems to be his bedfellow. He's lost in his own world. "You know, I was the typical sporty kid at school. In fact, if I wasn't man of the match, I got mad, thinking that I'd failed somehow."

"Why was failure your first thought?"

"My dad taught me and my brother from an early age to win at all costs, that second best meant failure, so it was always there, instilled deep down. Winning was good, losing was out of the question. Don't even go there... I wanted to do better, be better, to overachieve—get the best grades, bring home the medals, get the hot girlfriend, get a well-paid job and a huge house... and to be honest, I thrived on it all—it made me who I was, so when I left school with nine A-Stars, then went onto college and passed everything with flying colours, my dad was so proud that he bought me a brand-new car."

"That was very generous of him."

"It was, but that night, I lost control of the car and smashed into a lamp post."

"Okay..."

"Are you surprised by that...?"

"Well, yes, but you won't be the first or last," I reply. "Were you drunk?"

"Worse."

"How so?"

"I was smashed off my face on drugs."

"Can I ask what drugs you had taken that night?"

"It wasn't so much what I had taken that night, but what I'd always used."

"Okay." I wait for him to open up.

"Weed. I'd been smoking it since I was twelve, but the funny thing was, I'd never even tried a cigarette. Hated the smell, and still do."

"So, you'd been smoking marijuana while driving, or before?"

"Before I got into the car, I smoked a couple of spliffs at the bottom of the garden. Dad was out but he'd always been anti-drugs, so I made sure he didn't know I was doing it. He'd have knocked me from one end of the house to the other if he realised. Anyway, not thinking I was unfit to drive, I spent hours racing around town, you know the score—typical dick head, boy-racer-type. Spotting a couple of girls, I pulled up, showing off with my mates, then had another couple of spliffs with them, and tried a line of coke. I didn't realise how affected I was because I'd been doing weed for years. But this was the first time I'd ever used coke and been in charge of a car on my own."

"So, you crashed?"

"My mate, Jeremy, was in the passenger seat and the two girls were in the back. Jeremy went through the windscreen, and I found out later that he died instantly. Thankfully, the girls had buckled up, but they were hurt, whiplash, things like that."

"Were you injured?"

"Not badly. But it wasn't me I was worried about—it was Jeremy. He was my best mate, and I'd killed him."

It's hard to hear his confession, but with his words, I feel that he is waiting for my judgement. "I'm sorry. It must be hard to live with that guilt."

"It is, I think about him every day and prayed I would go to prison."

"You actually wanted to go to prison?"

"How else could I pay for what I'd done?"

"Were you given a custodial sentence?"

"Even though my dad begged me not to, I pled guilty—what else was I gonna do? How could I stand in a courtroom in front of Jeremy's parents, and family, and lie about what I'd done? I knew I couldn't shit on his memory like that."

"Many would have done," I replied. "... to escape a prison sentence."

"Not me. I can still see his face clear as day. I climbed out of the car, and he was lying on the road like one of those dolls whose strings had been cut, his limbs splayed at a weird angle. I knew he was dead before I reached him 'cos no way would he be lying there in that position."

"I don't know what to say..."

"What can you, or anyone, say? It's his eyes I can't forget—that look, fear I think, that he knew he was gonna die... he knew I'd lost control of the car before I did. His eyes captured how scared he was, just like a photograph... I did that to him."

I'm at a loss for words right now, and don't want to push him to reveal anything that isn't comfortable for him. I can tell by the quiver in his voice that he is crying yet trying his hardest not to let me hear. So, I give him a minute to compose himself then continue. "How long were you in prison for?"

"I was sentenced to thirteen years, with three knocked off because I pleaded guilty and showed remorse in court. Remorse, what a joke! Of course I was sorry, but it wasn't gonna bring Jeremy back, was it? I was also banned from driving, which meant nothing because I wouldn't be driving anywhere while locked up in prison, would I?"

Anger laces his words, but I understand why. "So, how long were you in prison for?"

"Just over six years because I had time knocked off for good behaviour. But even walking out of the gates, my sentence hadn't ended."

"Why do you say that?"

"Because *I* lived, and Jeremy died. His parents came to see me you know, in prison, quite a few times."

"That was very gracious of them."

"They forgave me, even though I couldn't forgive myself."

"Surely, their forgiveness meant something to you?"

"Yeah, it did, and it still does. They are better people than I could ever hope to be. Didn't help though, not in the long run."

"It was an accident." I'm trying to play Devil's Advocate because I have no right to judge or to make him feel any worse than he already does. As far as society is concerned, he has paid his debt, but no sentence will erase the guilt gnawing away at him. "You didn't actually mean to kill anybody."

"I was off my face, stoned, coked-up, of course it was my fucking fault, whether I meant it or not."

"Some would see it that way, but even if they did, you served your sentence in the eyes of the law, and Jeremy's parents forgave you."

"It didn't matter anyway—I came out of prison a different man that went in?"

"Is that when your weight problems started?"

"No, while I was in there."

"Prison you mean?"

"Yeah."

"Why?"

"I could get whatever I wanted, food, drugs, anything as long as I played their game."

"*Their* game… would you please elaborate?"

"A load of men locked up, gagging for sex. They can't have it off with their wife or girlfriend, so where else are they gonna stick it? Get me… I was the new boy, pretty boy, knew jack shit about how the system worked, never saw the signs, and assumed them being friendly was just that. The screws weren't interested. But then I used it to my advantage."

My blood runs cold, because abuse within the prison system is endemic, but usually glossed over in favour of pristine reports to the governing bodies. "I'm so sorry."

"It happened, doesn't bother me. I'm well over it. But it made my mental health worse, and I was already going downhill after killing Jeremy."

"Did you discuss what happened with anybody?"

"Nobody knows, well, only my doctor, and I see a shrink sometimes. Doesn't do well to be a grass in prison, and I wanted a quiet life, to serve my sentence and get on with it."

"You see a psychiatrist—is that because of what happened to you in prison, or a mixture of things?"

"A mixture of things, helps me try and compartmentalise my thoughts, but being in prison, aside from being used and passed around, drugs are everywhere—what I wanted, I got, and I stupidly thought that being off my face would make the time go faster."

"So, you had access to illegal drugs in prison?"

"And then some, yep."

"How often."

"As often as I paid for them."

"Did you have cash in there, or was payment made some other way?"

At this point he laughs, and it is the first time that I notice he is not monotone. "My dad always used to tell me to 'use what God gave you', so I did."

"I see."

"Like I said, I was the new boy, pretty, athletic with a good body... I was popular and knew how to work it to my advantage."

"So, you used sex as a way to pay for drugs, right?"

"Yep, and food, but without the drugs, I'd have lost my mind sooner than I did."

"Were you using drugs throughout your sentence."

"Inmates came and went, but I had no problem making friends to get what I wanted."

"Did your parents visit you?"

"At first yes, then no."

"Why did the visits stop?"

"Cos my mum cried every time which made me feel worse, and my dad was angry with me for giving in and shoved it in my face as often as he could. So, I stopped their visits and refused to see them."

"That must have upset them."

"Only three things consumed my mind—Jeremy, food, and drugs."

"I understand."

"I put myself inside, but I did what I did to survive in there, do you get what I'm saying?"

"I think so, yes."

"You ever been inside, Marco?"

"No, never."

"Well, whatever you've seen on the telly, its way worse, trust me. If there is a hell, I can't see it being worse than nick (prison)."

"You did survive though." At this point, I am still clueless about Danny's weight gain, and how it happened, as well as its impact on his life now. So, I ask him as bluntly as I can, and only because he requested that I not pussyfoot around him, "Why are you overweight now?"

"Simples... my mind is a mess, gone, kaput, I'm used to it."

I have no idea what he looks like, but I picture him tapping the side of his head. But his words don't ring true because despite the obvious pain, his mind isn't as 'gone' as he thinks it is. "How so?"

"Schizophrenia, bipolar, manic depressive, OCD, I had it all thrown at me—the antipsychotics screwed me up big time. I didn't wanna do anything, so I sat on my backside day after day and did nothing. When I got out, nobody wanted to employ me, so all the A-Stars in the world meant nowt. My mum fussed over me like I was a baby, trying to convince me that my prison sentence was a miscarriage of justice." He laughs again, but I hear a touch of anxiety and know that reliving his sentence is harder than he imagined it would be. "Nah, I deserved it, and more. I killed my best mate—she knows it, I know it, everyone knows it. But she buries her head to make it easier. I love her to bits, but I couldn't live with them hovering around me and treating me like some fragile wreck, so I moved into my own place."

"How was life after moving out?"

"My parent's paid for the flat and the bills, so I spent my days smoking weed, and shovelling whatever food I could in. Add all the meds into it and I didn't stand a chance. Before I realised, I was the size of a house and before long, I couldn't even fit in trackies that were once too big for me. I can't get jeans to fit me now, well I can, but I'm not spending money on something I still look a mess in."

"Taking the medication, how are you now?"

"Stable. More stable than I've been in a long time. I've had a few wobbles, but not for a while. For the first time, I can see a light at the end of the tunnel, but I've been here before and crashed and burned. Took me a long time to recognise the signs for what they were. This time, I'm fighting back. I've got to, or that's it."

"Why this time in particular?"

"I'm gonna be a dad." I hear happiness and am genuinely pleased for him.

"Congratulations. When is the baby due?"

"Thanks. December."

"Boy or girl?"

"I don't know yet. We want it to be a surprise."

"Your girlfriend knows of your mental health problems, I assume?"

"She does, but she's never judged me, not for my past, my mental health, not anything. She's been amazing."

"How did you meet her?"

"Online. We chatted for ages, and to be honest, I wasn't planning on ever meeting her looking like this, but I told my brother about her, and he forced me to take the chance."

"Do you have a good relationship with your brother?"

"Yeah. He drives me to the gym every night after he finishes work?"

"You must be close."

"We are, but it's not like it was before I was sent down."

I don't want to delve any more than I have to. If Danny chooses to reveal the intricacies of his relationship with his brother, that's his choice. "So, you have plenty to look forward to."

"Yeah, but I worry that social services will think I'm nuts and take the baby away."

I'm not qualified on how social services operate, nor am I about to offer advice on it. "Keep taking your medication and seeing your psychiatrist... be honest with how you're feeling because there are people out there who want to help you and will do given the opportunity."

"I hope so, but I'm determined not to crack again."

"You can only do your best, but I have high hopes for you and wish you the best."

"Thanks, this is easier than I thought it was going to be."

"As I explained in our first chat, we all have our reasons for gaining weight. Not one person is perfect, and we all fall at times. We've led different lives, but neither experience negates the other."

"I worried you would be some stuck-up writer and judge me."

"I'm far from perfect and definitely not stuck up, or in a position to judge anyone."

"A lot of people do judge me unfairly... yeah, I messed up, but I don't wanna pay for it for the rest of my life, not when I've got a kid to take care of." For the first time, I hear his fragility so step back to explain as clear as I can.

"We're all here for different reasons. I'm fat because I prefer sweets and chocolate over salad. My sister is big because she overeats the wrong types of food and doesn't exercise, there are others featured in this book who are still overweight, and some who are at their target weight—not one of us is the same, so don't ever worry I am going to judge."

"I appreciate that."

"I'm just a writer trying to share a part of his world, and highlight that food addiction is real, no matter how I and others got there. I'm here to listen, never to condemn or patronise…"

"Yeah, I get it. Food never used to bother me one way or the other… what was it my nan used to tell me, eat to live, well, I live to eat now, but I am slowly changing my mindset and going back the other way."

"That's good to hear, but please remember that whatever is in your past, I am no better than you, and you are no better than me, okay."

"Okay." He seems more settled and sounds less agitated and anxious.

"Can I ask what you weigh now?"

"I'm just under nineteen stone."

"And how tall are you."

"Five foot ten."

"What was your weight when you went into prison?"

"Eleven stone-ish—I was lean but muscular, no fat on me."

"So, the medication you're taking, is that known for causing weight gain?"

"Yeah, it can happen, but 'cos I sat around eating and not exercising, it was worse. Self-control is my problem but sometimes I can't control what I need to control. My brain doesn't let me. It's like it's going a hundred miles per hour, and I can't catch up with it. And the voices, it's like being stood in a room surrounded by televisions on at full volume. Sometimes, I just want silence, and the only way I can drown it out is to put my headphones on and blast my ears with music, you know. One voice is better than a hundred. Exercise helps drown out some of the noise too."

"What is your exercise regime now?"

"I've just got back into the gym but feel embarrassed walking in, especially when I see somebody I used to know. Maybe when I lose some more weight, I might try other things. I loved football and jogging but I'm too fat and out of shape now. I'd probably have a heart attack."

"I know how you feel, and although I wasn't the sporty kid, I feel as though people stare at me in the gym even though others say I'm imagining it."

"They probably do stare, and anybody that says otherwise is a liar." His honesty is refreshing.

"What's your ultimate goal?"

"To shift the lard, get fit, get my mind more balanced but most of all, to be the best dad I can be. That's the most important thing to me, and I won't be raising my kid like my dad raised me either. It's not about winning at all. It's about doing the right thing even though the odds are stacked against you. It's about manning up and owning the mistakes. That's one thing I can teach my kid if nothing else. Face up to stuff. One thing about me, I never lied about what I did and how Jeremy died. I tried to make something good out of something horrible. I owed it to Jeremy and his family. Still do."

"Are you still in contact with Jeremy's family?"

"Nah, it's too hard for me, and for them. Seeing them, and I did once when I got released, pushed me right back to that night, you know, all his pictures on every wall smiling back at me. It was like he was taunting me, but I was halfway gone when I got out and sliding down that slide into a black hole. Seeing his smile reminded me that I was the idiot that took his smile away. I felt like I was jumping on his grave even walking through his front door. What right did I have? I'd known them since I was five, they knew me, knew how much I loved them all. They forgave me, and to this day, I don't know how they could bring themselves to do it, or even say we forgive you. It broke me all over again because I didn't deserve to be absolved, I think that's the word. I was honest and told them I couldn't come back, and they said they understood. Secretly, they were probably glad to see the back of me. Religious, yeah, I forgot about that part, and Jeremy was too... they were all about forgiveness but what's the point in them forgiving me when I will never forgive myself?"

"Do you think you ever will forgive yourself?"

"I can't see it happening."

"Surely, you deserve to put the past behind you and live a happy life with your partner and child?"

"I want that, so much."

"Then take what you want. In the eyes of the law, you've served your sentence, and Jeremy's parents forgave you—anybody else's opinion, who cares? There is a saying I try to live by... other people's opinions of you are none of your business."

"I don't feel I have the right to it, not fully."

"What would Jeremy say?"

Danny laughs again and takes a moment to answer. "He'd tell me to get off my fat arse and stop wallowing."

"Really?"

"I think so, yeah. He was like that, get up and go, shut up and do it. He never sat still for a minute."

"He was your best friend, right?"

"Still is, and I'll go to my grave hoping I will see him again on the other side, and that he doesn't hate me."

"And you trusted him, I assume?"

"100%."

"Knew him better than most I imagine..."

"He was closer to me than my own brother."

"So, you know how his mind worked…"

"He'd say, it is what it is, Danny lad. He always said it, kind of his catchphrase, it is what it is… drove me nuts… not as nutty as I am now though."

"May I make an observation?"

"Go on…"

"You're remarkably self-aware."

"Am I?"

"Don't you see that in yourself?"

"I just say it as it is and how I see things. Sometimes, my thinking is skewed, the meds, guilt, there's a lot I keep hidden… I'm not who I was, the kid who had it all. Just the other week, I was walking down the road, and some kid yelled fatty at me … forget I went to prison, they only see what's on the outside and assume what's in my head—usually a jumbled mess, but I do have feelings. I was judged for killing my best mate, and I deserve that, but why judge me just because I'm fat?"

"I wholeheartedly agree with you, but you have already been judged by the court and served the sentence that they imposed. Always remember human nature—that people are ignorant and judgemental. Humanity is still not enlightened enough to know better. But you did the right thing back then… you're trying, you're struggling, you hate what stares back at you in the mirror because it is another part of you that you no longer recognise. Aside from that, you made a terrible mistake, and your best friend lost his life…"

"Yeah."

"But you held your hands up, admitted what you did, knowing you would go to prison… not many people would have had the courage to do that."

"I know, but…"

"No buts, Danny. You served your time and dealt with some terrible things while inside."

"I knew what I was doing."

"My point is, you did all that, suffered a serious breakdown, was diagnosed with schizophrenia amongst many other things… you met a girl I assume you love…"

"Loads, yes."

"And now you're going to be a dad, but you're going into the future with your eyes open. You know your life will never be the same again, that you could potentially relapse, but there is positivity there I think you are too easily overlooking."

"I didn't think of it like that."

"You're struggling with a myriad of issues from fluctuating mental health to being overweight and add to that the responsibility of impending parenthood... you're scared, and understandably so. You told me you want to be the best dad, and I have no reason to doubt you will be everything you want to be."

"I don't want my kid to be bullied because people see me as the crazy, fat shut-in who killed his mate."

"Kids are bullied for many things... sometimes, you can't protect them from it. As long as your child knows you're there for him or her, you can only do your best. Parents aren't perfect, I know that, and you know that from your own experiences."

"It's still my kid though, I've got to get my head on straight."

"Are you a shut-in?"

"Not anymore, no."

"And are you working as hard as you can to lose the excess weight?"

"Yeah, I really am trying but I'm fatter than my girlfriend and she's pregnant. Even now, knowing that I need to get fit for myself and my kid, I'm starving and want to pig out."

"So what? We all go through that, but you're still trying, and when the baby is here, although the incentive is already there, holding your baby in your arms might be the catalyst that pushes you to your goal weight."

"Are you sure you're really an author and not a shrink?"

I can't help laughing at the absurdity of it. "If I was, I wouldn't have made so many mistakes in my own life."

"You seem to have your head screwed on."

"I'm nearly fifty—I've learned a few things along the way but not nearly enough. I'm still learning, and you won't be any different."

"You've given me a lot to think about."

"Let me ask you a question..."

"Okay."

"Does being overweight make you a bad person?"

"No."

"Does the fact you eat too many burgers or kebabs, or whatever your pleasure is, mean you are less deserved of happiness and contentment than anyone else?"

"Sometimes, I can't help it, and I eat until I'm sick."

"Join the club—been there, done it, and thrown my guts up many, many times."

"Kebabs, pizza, chips, I'm not overly keen on sweets and prefer savoury stuff. It's become a habit."

"For me too, habit, but I prefer sweets and chocolate. I am not a fan of what you would call normal food like kebabs, burgers, or takeaways, but I'm still in the same boat as you are—watching TV, I need that bag of goodies."

"Me too, and since I quit weed, I struggle more which is weird because people associate the munchies with people who smoke weed."

"I've never smoked weed, or tried it any other way, so I'm out of my depth there. I just know that I prefer cake to pizza."

"I wish I could go back, that's my only wish, to that day, and talk some sense into myself, not get into the car—my mind is chocka trying to file away the mess—Jeremy, trying not to think how good I felt smoking weed, what my life was then, trying not think about walking to the shop to buy ten bags of crisps... sometimes I feel like my head is going to explode and it's too much for me to take."

"You can't change the past. Why bother tormenting yourself over it? You have a future, a baby on the way, and better days with your mental health."

"I hope so."

"Staying off weed and taking control of your eating habits... you have so much to look forward to, but if you keep one foot in the past, you're denying yourself that future."

"Are you sure you're not a shrink?" He laughs. "Come on, you can tell me, I won't freak out."

"I swear I'm not. But for the record, it's always easier looking in from the outside, and if you knew half of the things I have done and been through, you would offer advice that I never thought of. I'm also a lot older than you and with age comes clarity—and no, life is not suddenly crystal clear, but age allows us to pass on pearls of wisdom, sometimes."

"It's so easy talking to you."

"I'm glad you think so because not one person who has contributed has found this a walk in the park. You, and they, are giving away a part of yourself, and not one of us knows who is going to pick up this book, or what their opinions are going to be. If just one person says, *ah, yes, I get it*, then my job is done."

"Can I read it when it's published?"

"Of course, I truly hope that you do, and I will make sure you get a copy to read, as will all the contributors."

"Thanks..."

"When you read it, you will see my story, and my deepest insecurities, and biggest victories... then hopefully you will believe I am what I say I am—I read it back sometimes and cringe but there is no point doing it if I'm going to lie my way through it. I have made some almighty cockups over the course of my life. I've learned the hard way and there are things, like you, that I wish I could take back. But history is called history for a reason and not there to be changed. Live and learn, I did, and it's not that bad really. Forget Z, it's just getting from A to B that should be the focus."

"I wonder who will play me in the movie?"

"Take your pick, but I've already bookmarked Rik Waller to play me."

"Who's that?"

"Gosh, I am really old."

We both laugh, and chat bubbles for a few minutes. Then, he tells he has an appointment that he is already late for and should go.

Although I probably won't ever speak to him in depth again, unless he instigates it, I hope that our chat helped him to realise that working towards tomorrow is always better than trying to find a way back to yesterday.

MY JOURNEY - JANUARY 2023

January 16

Re-reading Danny's interview, and the others featured, a common thread weaving through every story is judgement. I have been judged negatively for my weight too many times to count, but only on rare occasions have I been judged positively for it. I can't say I was thrilled by this particular encounter, and that it doesn't embarrass me upon reflection, but I will share it with you regardless.

Before meeting the love of my life, I'd signed up to *GAYDAR*, a well-known 'dating' website.

With trepidation, I'd put up the best picture of myself I could find—no nudes, or naked shots, not ever. But a few decent face pics taken at good angles, and always close-ups. I truly believe that I resembled Sloth from *The Goonies* in most photos, so finding anything remotely decent was not easy.

I wasn't sure I'd even agree to meet up with anyone if it came to it, but whatever I chose to do, or not to do, it didn't take long before my first message arrived in my inbox.

YOU HAVE 1 NEW MESSAGE.

I clicked it open, read it, and sat pleasantly surprised.

Hey! Wanna meet?

I looked at his profile in disbelief—a stunning specimen of the male species; blonde, blue-eyed, tanned, muscled, and packing in all the right places, which is obviously why he had no problem sending NSFW (Not Safe for Work) pictures.

It begged the question, why would somebody who looked like him want to meet somebody that looked like me?

But I played along anyway. *Yeah*, I replied, certain it wasn't going to happen, and that his profile was one of many fakes.

Cool. What are you into?

Anything was my standard response, though I later realised that it opened me up to guys asking if they could wrap me in clingfilm, tin foil, spank my bare bottom with a spatula (yes, that offer came in, too) or partake in other such weird and wonderful kinks I'd never given a moment's thought to.

But I'm not here to kink shame. Each to their own and no judgements, but not for me, plus at that time, it would have meant a trip to *Costco* for a catering pack of whatever was needed to successfully prepare me for plucking.

I'd already selected *LARGE* when asked to specify my body type, so he should have seen it when viewing my profile. I felt it better to be transparent and mention it anyway, just so there was no misunderstanding *if* we did meet. *But I just want to let you know, I'm not skinny*. A gargantuan understatement that would read so much better than me writing, *you won't fancy me because I'm a lard arse*.

I waited for him to block me as most did, because in gay world massacring a whole town is preferable to humping a fatty.

But to my surprise a reply came right back. Years later, I can still recall it word for word because he had the audacity to write it.

*That's okay. I'd rather f*ck a fat guy anyway–they're always more grateful.*

With my self-esteem at its lowest ebb, I could take that backhanded compliment on the chins. *Okay*, I replied.

It got progressively worse with his following messages.

I prefer fat guys because it means I'm always the better looking one, and besides, shagging fatties is less hassle.

"Dickhead," I grunted, but not to him.

What did he mean by less hassle? I never did ask. Perhaps his over-inflated ego could only cope with people he deemed less attractive than him. I really don't know. But as I considered him a bona fide hottie, I was still prepared to go through with whatever he had planned.

Then he sent another message. *I could bring my mate with me.* He swiftly sent me a picture of this friend who was just as fine as him. *As you can see, he's fit, and he likes fatties too. We're both feeders.*

Ugh, you almost had me!

But then The Death Knell Ringeth.

The idea of a threesome with two muscle studs was the stuff of fantasy, but I was instantly turned off because for the first time in my life I'd been fetishized. Nothing about it felt right, or decent, and if possible, I felt even more worthless than I had before starting the conversation with him.

He only wanted me because I was fat, and he considered me easy pickings, not because he found me attractive, and aside from that, he wanted to feed me cream cakes (Victoria sponge, thank you very much) and get his jollies at the same time.

While I'd gladly tuck into the cakes, he could keep his meat and two veg to himself.

Despite thinking little of myself, I hadn't sunk so low, nor did I fancy being rogered by one hottie while the other licked fresh cream from, as he so eloquently described it, *my moobs.*

So, I blocked him and went straight to the shop for a bag of goodies.

My faithful old friend *Cadbury's Dairy Milk* cheered me up in no time at all.

But suffering with low self-esteem, I went on dates with people I never would dream of entertaining now; I am certain that if I found even the smallest plus in whoever I was talking to, regardless of alarm bells ringing warnings, that would be all that was needed for me to give them a chance.

Grindr struck again, this time sending me on a date that didn't end too well.

I'd agreed to meet this guy, and while he wasn't specifically my type, we seemed to get on, and anything was better than nothing, or sitting at home wishing and wondering when I would meet the man of my dreams. So, with arrangements made, we'd planned on going out for a bite to eat, then a few drinks afterwards. Nervous that he would run when he saw the fatty waiting, I met him at the top terrace in Liverpool One.

As silly as it sounds, I hadn't taken much notice of his hair, or lack thereof when he sent me his pictures initially. What I did know; he was an Italian jockey living in the UK, very slight of build, which put me in mind of David and Goliath, and that he was prettier and more feminine looking than I usually liked. I do recall his head seemed very shiny, but I put that down to moisturiser. But like I said, we seemed to get on, so I thought what the hell. It wasn't as though I was cursed with Brad Pitt or Harry Styles good looks, nor could I afford to be uber-fussy.

CHEWING THE FAT

To my relief there was no awkwardness between us.

We found a place to eat and waited to be shown to our seats. Everything was going swimmingly, until halfway through the meal. Talk was animated and flowing, and we were really getting on, and I found I was enjoying myself despite initially wondering why I agreed to go. Then the most bizarre thing happened. I saw it, almost in slow motion, but didn't really know what it was that I'd seen.

It was apparent that he had seen it too, although he tried to play it cool.

Perhaps I should have let it be, but it's not in my nature. "Something just dropped into your food," I said.

"Did it?" He was playing dumb—I know he saw what I had.

"Yeah." I had my eyes fixed on the contents of his bowl, then gasped, because it looked like a caterpillar sitting on top of his food. "Oh, God, is that a—" The thought of insects and creepy crawlies in general horrify me, but in a restaurant, my absolute nightmare! My mind went to one place; if they were in his food, they had to be in mine too, right?

Wrong!

"It's my eyebrow," he sheepishly replied, dropping his voice to barely a whisper.

"I beg your pardon?" I leaned in, a bit deaf, remember, thinking I'd misheard him.

"My eyebrow has fallen off."

Thoroughly confused, it took a moment for his words to sink in, and then I cast a glance at him. At the start of the meal there were definitely two eyebrows present, and I knew that for certain because it's a thing for me— nice shoes, teeth, and eyebrows, it's a pre-requisite—but one of his eyebrows was missing, or more to the point, sitting on top of his main course.

Quickly, he scooped it out of his bowl and rushed away from the table, and into the toilet.

I put my fork down, wanting to be polite and wait for him. But all the while, I was wondering how his eyebrow had fallen off. I rarely made eye contact with anybody, but they'd looked perfect to me when I cast a glance his way.

When he returned to the table, he appeared flushed and embarrassed, and the conversation had stalled, so I tried to skim over it, despite his eyebrow now being back in its proper place.

Itching to ask the specifics, I didn't want to upset him, so I went with a tried and tested question that might open him up to talking about it, "Are you okay?"

"I have alopecia."

"Okay." It's only then that I noticed he didn't have a single strand of hair, or stubble, on his head, or indeed anywhere—face, arms, or chest. *So that's why your head is so shiny.* I had initially thought that he chose to shave it all off as some are inclined to do, or perhaps less hair made the horse go faster. I have no idea, but his condition was something he had no control over, nor did it bother me in the slightest. Had he told me, I probably would have still met him because he appeared to be a nice guy; I wasn't beating men off with a stick. "I didn't know."

"I've had it since I was a kid—I'm really embarrassed about it, sorry."

"There's no need to be embarrassed, or sorry. It is what it is." I empathised with him, knowing something made him feel so bad about himself, but it didn't stop my brain from working overtime. For those who know me well, I have the strangest sense of humour and while I am sure the John Bishop's and the Ricky Gervais' of this world tickle some funny bones, they don't tickle mine at all. Instead, I am amused by slapstick, and the ridiculous, so an eyebrow dropping off mid-meal would usually be enough to induce convulsions of howling laughter. Instead, and battling against my true nature, I fought hard and kept myself together. But he carried on talking about it which made it worse. For those who think me wicked, I can't help it—it's a nervous thing, which is why I usually avoid funerals because I find myself laughing inappropriately.

"I don't have any eyebrows, or eye lashes. In fact, there isn't a single hair on my body."

"Ah, right." I hadn't noticed the missing eye lashes, but then again, why would I expect them not to be there? He hadn't told me about the alopecia during our initial conversations and some might say I am unobservant, but something amiss usually must smack me in the face for me to notice.

"So, I buy these particular eyebrows from Milan because they look realistic, and the glue comes from a shop in London."

"They do look good, very realistic," I added, honestly, trying to soothe his embarrassment. "I had no idea they were stick-ons." For once, and as difficult as it was to do so, I looked into his eyes, wishing to convey my sincerity.

"But it's so hot in here, the glue has melted."

His words lit my bizarre humour like touch paper. Laughter bubbled inside. I instantly lost any eye contact I'd forced with him and lowered my gaze. Then, I snorted loudly into my food and knew I was losing it. So, I excused myself from the table and sat locked in the cubicle for five minutes desperately trying to compose myself.

When I returned to the table, I was surprised, and a tad disappointed that he was still there, and only because I was terrified that I'd burst out laughing and make a fool of myself, and worse still, make him more self-conscious than he already was. Anyway, we enjoyed the rest of the meal and thankfully his wandering eyebrow remained in place for the duration.

He drove me to my mum's and came in to meet her. But you might not be surprised to learn that we didn't see one another again. They had a good chat about his profession, and though my mum knew as much about horse racing as I did, she enjoyed his company.

"Whatever happened to the jockey?" she asked me weeks later. "He seemed like a nice lad."

"He was, but his eyebrow fell off halfway through the meal."

"You what?" Busy completing a crossword puzzle at the time, she peered over her glasses at me, probably thinking she had misheard me.

With her mouth turned up, I told her the whole story, and by the end, the pair of us were in peals of laughter. Her sense of humour was as warped as mine.

"I bet you laughed," she accused, still tittering.

"Not in front of him I didn't, but I went to the toilet and laughed in there."

"Wicked sod." All the while her shoulders bobbed up and down.

"I couldn't help it."

"I bet." And then, she was off again, and she abandoned her crossword puzzle. "I wish I'd been there. Your face would have been a picture."

She knew me too well.

Date night with the jockey wasn't my only embarrassing moment, in fact, most of my dates have been Bridget Jones-style disasters, and it's a wonder I plucked up the courage to meet Jon.

In my younger days, I could be found shaking my bottom and anything else that wobbled on podiums in and around Liverpool's gay scene. The Escape, which was on Paradise Street back then, was a particular favourite, so every Thursday and Friday, and sometimes Saturday, I could be found shimmying away to Kylie, Steps, S Club 7 or The Vengaboys, you name it, I wobbled to it.

The Escape always crackled with a carnival-esque atmosphere and somewhere I looked forward to going. Ten quid all in and drink however much I wanted (I will never drink Strawberry Vodka Milkshakes ever again), and I usually did.

This one night, I seemed to have caught the eye of a hot young guy whose name escapes me, and after flirting across the dancefloor, we got to chatting. *Chubby Chaser*, I thought. *He likes a bit of timber.* One too many Strawberry Vodka Milkshakes later and his unexpected invitation to accompany him back to his place was greeted with an enthusiastic yes, let me get my coat.

No judgements please. I was young and full of hormones. Yes, I admit that I was a big, fat trollop when the mood called for it... so what.

Anyway, back at his place, a dodgy high rise in Bootle with a lift that juddered too much for my liking, especially after a belly full of booze, he showed me into his bedroom.

Grateful of the opportunity to sit down before my knees buckled, those of us who carry excess weight will understand, I took a seat on the edge of the bed, then he flicked the light off.

He's shy, I thought to myself. But works for me because the less flesh of mine he sees, the better.

I had no idea why because he was utterly gorgeous. But his place, his rules. It didn't stop me from stripping off. When sloshed, I seemed to adopt a porn star personality—no fear at all. Now sprawled naked on his bed like a starfish, I could hear him shuffling about, but the room was pitch black, so all I could see was his shadow dancing about.

"What are you doing?" I slurred.

"Just putting my leg on the chest of drawers."

"Oh, okay." The room spun, and I was sloshed, probably not interested in what he was saying because I was ready to get cracking.

"Won't be a minute."

I lay back on the bed, ready for action when I felt him on the bed.

He slinked across me like a panther, and with me raring to go, things got weird.

As he crawled up my person, I felt something brush my plums, and assumed he had a massive willy.

I remember briefly asking myself, *what was that?* But too drunk to focus or give it much more thought than that, we got down to the nitty gritty. The next morning, I woke before him, eyelids stuck together because I'd forgotten to take my contact lenses out and with my mouth drier than an Arab's sand shoe, I just wanted to go home, shower, take two Paracetamol, drink a litre of water, and sleep it off in my own bed.

So, I slipped out of his bed as quietly as I could, and it was then that I noticed it with a gasp... *No, it can't be...* But I wasn't seeing things. His artificial leg sat on top of the chest of drawers and the *Nike* trainer and sock was still attached to the prosthetic limb.

He suddenly moved and groaned.

I turned to look then froze, praying he wouldn't wake up. As the duvet moved, I could clearly see that his leg had been amputated from the kneecap down.

While he had been packing more than adequately where it mattered it wasn't his appendage that had brushed my crotch, but his stump.

Now, I have nothing against amputees, or those with different abilities, far from it, but the shock of it almost floored me. Some warning before agreeing to escort him home, just as the case with my hairless Italian jockey with the wandering eyebrow, would have been appreciated so I could get my mind around it. I didn't fare well in unknown and surprise situations because I was inclined to laugh out of nervousness. Thankfully, on this occasion, sozzled, I didn't.

Then again, he did tell me he was putting his leg on the chest of drawers but in my drunken, horny, carefree, wannabe porn star state, I'd assumed he was being sarcastic.

His words came back to haunt me. *Just putting my leg on the chest of drawers.*

How was I to know he was being serious?

But hindsight is a wonderful thing.

Anyway, I rushed out of there as fast as my chubby legs could carry me, then when I got home, I called my friend and told her what had happened. As expected, she screamed with laughter at my lack of understanding.

I can see the funny side now, but at the time, I felt like the world's worst for hot footing it out of there. But in my defence, leg, or no leg, I'd have snuck out anyway.

I did see him around the club scene many times through the years. I apologised, and there was no frostiness, in fact, we always had time for a hello and a hug. Just as I had consistently experienced negativity for being me, he had experienced it too but for other reasons. His attitude was; if people don't like me, I'm not going to lose sleep over it, and I admired that about him. He was a lovely, decent guy; handsome with a great body and not in the least bit interested in body shaming me or anyone. I soon got the idea that he was more the one-night stand type, so the absence of round two wouldn't have been unusual in his world.

I am reading this back and thinking to myself, *God, you've lived*, and I have, whatever weight I've been.

I'm cringing at the memories for many reasons, so let's get back to the present.

Three weeks ago, I fell off the wagon and have been dragged kicking and screaming behind it, trying to climb back on one leg lift at a time.

I told myself that I would return to group on the 20th of January 2023, but it's been so long since I was weighed, fear stalls me. My time off the wagon led me to being thrown out of the *Facebook* group. Initially miffed, I understood due to confidentiality concerns, and no matter how many times I told my leader I wasn't leaving, she did what was right. In all fairness, my pleas lined with the same records she's played from other clients thousands of times over the years.

But I decided that I would show my face on Friday and face the scales.

I knew I gained, but whose fault was it anyway? Mine!

In preparation for getting back on track, I drew up my shopping list for the week's meals on Sunday night and set my alarm for the ungodly hour of 9 am. When it rang the following morning, I groaned. I had things to accomplish and buried underneath my warm, comfy, teddy bear bedding, I would achieve nothing.

So, I faced the biting cold and trotted round ASDA, avoiding the best (sweets) aisles. Ten minutes later, my trolley slugged along, overflowing with the following items:

Potatoes. Onions, carrots, red cabbage, white cabbage, courgettes, stewing steak, baking potatoes and stock pots...

And many other items which were basically Syn Free, and not because I was on a mission to claw back, but more to do with the fact I prefer vegetables, fruits, and tiny amounts of lean meat, to other food items, if I have to eat.

When I write about *having* to eat, I know it is not possible to survive without food, but I take no enjoyment from it, only nourishment. For some, sitting down to a full roast dinner, an Indian or Chinese, or something as simple as steak and chips is satisfying, and the nutritional value doesn't come into it—gratification does. I don't even have pleasure to fall back on. Food does absolutely nothing for me, so when it comes to mealtimes, it is more of a tick box exercise, in fact, it has become a nightmare having to partake in something several times a day that I don't want to do. When I do eat 'normal' food, I will always choose fruit and vegetables over all else, even going so far as to pick the meat off the plate and give it to the dogs and cat. I choose this because I prefer it, and I know the benefits of eating it.

And here lies the conundrum: I have no appetite for and get no satisfaction from nutritious food but can and will eat cakes, sweets, and crisps without limit. Another anomaly to my odd personality; when I don't eat junk food, I know I don't need it and can survive without it, but because I can't have it, or shouldn't have it, I want it.

Will I ever get to the bottom of my own muddled mind and relationship with food? I don't think so, and it doesn't help that my aversion to nutritious food is a byproduct of the addiction to over-indulging in the junk items.

Fighting with that inner voice, trying to cajole me into journeying down the sweet aisle, and approaching the Rotisserie Chicken counter, I bumped into Donna, my group leader.

Well, thank God it wasn't Friday because the above items would have been replaced with doughnuts, French fancies, Roast Beef Hula Hoops, Creme Eggs and Haribo... basically all the good stuff.

Donna smiled and gave me a hug, then cast a suspicious glance into my trolley, akin to eyes of the Supreme Leader of *Slimming World* upon me.

"That's a damned good shop." She smiled, approving of my choices.

"I told you I wasn't leaving." I should have those words tattooed across my forehead.

She took a photograph of the contents of my trolley, after I'd sidestepped, reminding her that my chins wouldn't fit into shot.

I don't know what she did with the picture. Perhaps she put it into the *Facebook* group, but as she kicked me out, I couldn't say for sure.

We had a quick chat about Jon and his health issues (this past week he had a severe case of gout, and the medication he is on for other ailments have given him an upset tummy, and that is putting it mildly, so he hasn't strayed too far from the loo, nor left the house), then the remaining aisles beckoned.

"See you *both* Friday." It wasn't an order, not really, but the steel in her tone couldn't be mistaken.

"Yes, you will."

And see us both, she would, and for you, dear readers, I shall honestly report how much damage I have managed to inflict upon myself in three short weeks.

I am adamant. 2023 is here, so I want to shift the remaining weight and keep it off. That summer body is mine, and Jon's if he's lucky.

January 19
WEIGH-IN DAY

As Jon and I were already out and about for his diabetes check, we decided to weigh-in a day earlier than planned. Brave I know, but it was easier to do it there and then as the doctor's surgery is opposite the meeting hall.

I worried because I wasn't wearing my usual weigh-in clothes, so I made sure my pockets were empty then I hopped on the scales.

"One and a half on," Donna whispered.

"I know it's a gain but it's not as bad as I thought it would be."

"It's a new week now."

"I wonder how much this belt weighs."

"Don't worry about last week, focus on now."

"If I hadn't got back on plan three days ago, it would have been much worse."

As an added incentive, I paid for a six-week subscription and stocked up on SW bars.

Following weigh-in, we dined in a local café, where I partook in my usual of bacon medallions, fried eggs, mushrooms, tinned tomatoes... all cooked in fry light, therefore all Syn Free.

I also ate two pieces of dry white toast. As I don't like butter or margarine anyway, I don't feel like I've been punished. I counted 8 Syns for the toast.

Add in a large pot of tea, with full fat milk (I am not keen and usually have 1% milk at home, but it was all that was on offer, and I used my healthy extras (HEXA – for dairy / cheese), and sweetener tablets, so Syn Free again.

It's time to buckle down and get into the next stone bracket.

January 27

I probably haven't mentioned it, but if I have, forgive me. Late last year I was diagnosed with Ankylosing Spondylitis. It's more than a mouthful to say, a bugger to spell, and a nightmare to navigate. Basically, it means I have a condition that affects my spine which renders my neck too stiff to move as it is designed to. I've been aware of this lack of movement for years but put it down to what I call Fat Neck Syndrome... some will laugh when they read this but the larger amongst us don't always move in the same way as our slimmer counterparts. I wrongly assumed my neck muscles were buried so deep in fat that movement had been restricted. But I should have sensed something more sinister afoot because there was little change as I lost weight.

So, I was seeing a physiotherapist, a lovely young lady named Phoebe, at Arrowe Park Hospital, and after the second visit, I noticed some improvement.

Then, Jon and I were floored by the dreaded Covid at a Sugababes gig in Liverpool which meant I couldn't attend my appointments for a few weeks. Christmas happened, and then I was transferred to Clatterbridge Hospital for further sessions as Phoebe was taking up another position in another part of the trust.

Yesterday, I met my new physiotherapist and to say I was unimpressed with him would be an understatement.

After arriving for my appointment, a whole hour too early (my fault), then sitting there for a further eighty minutes, I was led into a cubicle. He drew the curtain, affording me an element of privacy.

He was suitably professional and introduced himself. Immediately I felt like Nellie the Elephant compared to his dainty, slim frame. (I've never seen such small hands and wondered how he was going to treat me—my neck was bigger than both of his hands together).

Anyway, my issues aside, he looked over my notes, and x-rays, and asked me many questions, repeatedly, which bothered me because it appeared he was trying to catch me out, although I couldn't fathom why.

"Do you have swollen fingers?" he quizzed.

Immediately, my thoughts shot off on a tangent and I thought of ET and his glowing finger. I was itching to laugh, but this wasn't the time, or the place for my peculiarities.

"No."

"What about your toes… are they swollen?"

"No," I replied.

"So, you don't have swollen fingers or toes?"

"No." I held my fingers up to show him they were quite un-sausage-like. I hate showing my feet and toes so kept my footwear firmly in place.

"Does anyone in your family have swollen fingers and toes?"

"No." I was teetering on annoyed by this point. Did he think my family had some sort of genetic predisposition, or mutation, to fat fingers and toes?

"What about your knees, are they swollen?"

"No, not swollen either." My tone switched to sullen at this point.

"Are they painful?"

"No! Why would they be?"

"Any diabetes in your family?"

"No."

"What about arthritis?"

"Nobody in my family has it."

"Well, *you* have severe arthritis in your neck." He delivered this surprising news exactly as I have written it.

"Do I?"

"Yes."

"Will it get worse?"

"It might not get any worse, but you won't ever have movement in your neck like you did when you were eighteen."

I wasn't expecting to be as limber as I was in my teenage years. "So why am I having physiotherapy?"

"To be honest, I don't think it will work for you anyway, so I'll need you to see a Rheumatologist."

"I've already seen one."

"When?"

"September 2021 when I was diagnosed with Fibromyalgia."

"Did you self-diagnose, or did the Rheumatologist diagnose that?"

"*He* did." My surly side came on stronger with each passing minute. "I don't diagnose anything because I'm not a doctor."

"And what did he say about your neck?"

"Nothing, because I didn't mention my neck."

"Why not?"

"Because I thought it was just fat neck syndrome, and as I was bigger than I am now, I thought nothing of it. It's only since losing a lot of weight that I noticed how bad it was."

He laughed, which was the first time he expressed any shred of personality. "And did you tell him about the pain in your neck then?"

"No."

"Why not?"

"Because there was no pain in my neck."

"None at all?"

"No, and I told my GP and Phoebe the same thing when they asked me, but in the last two weeks it has been hurting a lot."

Cue more questions about swelling and pain.

"Can you take your top off please."

Oh, no, I felt sick. *I really don't want to show my body.*

"And your shoes too." Probably to check I didn't have mutant feet. I really wanted to say it but restrained myself. Still, mortified at having to flaunt my flabby bits, I reluctantly did as he asked.

"Stand up and face the curtain, then bend over as far as you can."

I complied.

He stood behind me as I bent over, and I worried how undignified it must look. Then, I don't know why the movie *Carry on Camping* popped into my mind, (Bend, Barbara...) but it did. I crossed my arms to stop my moobs from hanging but he told me to try and touch my toes.

Yeah, right!

He observed how low I could go before jabbing his finger into the small of my back. "Can you feel that?"

"What, the finger in my back?"

"Any pain?"

"No."

"Fine. Now, sit on the bed and put your hands like this."

"Okay." I followed his lead.

"And do this, and this."

I copied him, and typically, my mind travelled to the strangest of places. Some of these moves were reminiscent of The Macarena. Instantly, I felt a right tit. But he was only doing his job. But my inner voice had more to say. *What's next, The Time Warp?*

"You can relax now."

I sat with my arms crossed over my moobs, assured he would realise how displeased I was, but thankful I had a tan at least.

"You can put your top and trainers back on now."

"Okay."

"So, as I said earlier, I need to refer you back to see the Rheumatologist. It could be swelling on your spine which means we can put you on anti-inflammatories which could help improve your movement. We also need blood tests... swelling would be much better than the alternative. If it's degenerative, there's little we can do."

"I've already had blood tests."

"But the one thing I need to look for wasn't tested and going back over your notes for the last three years, I can't see anything."

"Right. One question if you don't mind..."

"Of course not, go on."

"You're telling me that physio won't work, so why did Phoebe bother to treat me with it?"

"Well, I'm more of a spinal specialist physiotherapist." He avoided answering my question, which only dug him deeper into the hole he plonked himself in.

"So, she shouldn't have been treating me at all."

"I didn't say that."

"Fine, but she *was* treating me and you're telling me it won't work when I've already told you numerous times whatever she was doing had improved my condition and given me more movement and flexibility."

"You can't have massages on your neck for the rest of your life."

With the line crossed, my temper was severely stretched. "I didn't say I wanted massages with a physiotherapist for the rest of my life but to be honest I am very disappointed."

"Do you mind if I ask why?"

"Because I walked in here his afternoon with hope, and now, I'm leaving with none."

"Okay."

"I thought you could help me regain some movement and you're basically telling me what has been done was a waste of time, even though I know it was helping."

"I'm not saying we won't continue with physio once we get these results back, and I've spoken with the Rheumatologist."

"Oh." He could have told me that earlier, but it all felt a little hopeless.

"So, what I want you to do is book in with me at reception for my next available slot and when I see you again, I should have more answers for you. I'll arrange blood tests and call you with the time and place."

"Does that mean I'm going to be waiting a year to see the Rheumatologist again?"

"No, I don't think it'll be that long."

Seething and feeling like I had been fobbed off, completely ignored, and the fact he had not even touched my neck, or tried the exercises Phoebe had, I left it at that and booked into see him again, on the 22nd of February. I am not looking forward to it.

I came home in a thunderous mood because it seemed my world had come to an end. I was terrified I'd have to walk around hunched and with restricted movement forever.

I'm not moody or a sulker by nature, but I woke up at 2:30 am the following morning, still annoyed and angry. *Stuff this.* I Googled sports masseurs and finding Ian Perry minutes from where my SW class was held, I booked in for later that day.

At 3:45 pm, nervous, I walked in, took a seat, and felt that Ian listened to me and was interested in what had been happening to me.

After the massage, Ian warned me I would be sore the next day. But I immediately noticed the difference and walked home, which took me ten minutes. I had more movement in my neck. Thrilled, I booked four more weekly sessions which would drop down to fortnightly then monthly.

Ian promised he would be able to help me, and I had no reason to doubt him.

But a raging fire burned inside me, that I had come so far in my journey, and nothing was going to derail my plans. If I had to pay privately to hopefully overcome my condition, I would. The so-called physiotherapist can frig right off. Yes, I knew my weight would rise and fall, and that the struggle was not, and never would be, over, but this neck issue was proving to be a never-ending nightmare. Sorry for swearing above, but there are occasions when nothing else can adequately describe the ebb and flow of emotions especially when things are not going one's way.

No surprise, but anger sat like a dead weight because I was doing everything within my power to move forward and take back my life with two hands and obstacles seemed to appear from thin air, desperate to thwart my efforts.

Nothing speaks the truth like that old saying... no pain, no gain... well, if I had to suffer a little pain, so be it.

January 27
WEIGH-IN DAY

Crikey—as far as a good night's sleep goes, that was anything but.

As predicted, soreness and stiffness settled right in just as Ian said it would. Relief came with a few stretches, and the locked in tightness subsided. Yes, my body felt tender, but my neck definitely had more movement.

"Are we walking?" Jon asked.

"I'm calling a taxi." Although I usually would, I couldn't face the ten-minute walk.

Jon faced the scales first while I had a laugh with Dawn, the lady who booked me in and took payment for my HiFi bars.

He lost three and a half pounds, and I was thrilled for him.

Now, it was my turn.

The fleece hoodie was once again cast aside and horrible feet or not, off came my trainers.

As per usual, I had not put underwear on and had virtually wrung myself out, squeezing the last drop of pee out.

I was thirsty and my mouth was like an Arab's sand shoe, but I thought a cup of water would be counterproductive.

"... three and a half ..." I only heard the number and assumed the worst.

"On?" I was instantly disappointed.

"No, you've lost three and a half."

"Oh, brilliant."

So, that's where I am. I'd gained seven pounds, so I've got four and a half to shed to be back to where I was. Then it is upwards and onwards.

MY JOURNEY - FEBRUARY 2023

February 1

This week hasn't been a good one for a multitude of reasons.

My neck has given me so much trouble; the stiffness and locked in feeling returned with a vengeance. But I plodded on regardless. I sat at my desk working on a new crime fiction book with my writing partner for release in May, all the while buffing this title up into something worthy of releasing.

It's easier said than done right now as sitting in this position for hours was not ideal. Every turn of my head left or right, even up and down, hurts, so I might have to invest in a riser for my keyboard and screen so I can stand and type. I should also use my new laptop more, but I'm not used to the keys or the mouse pad yet.

That's not all.

The clock shows 12:58 pm and I'm not in the least bit hungry. Not one morsel of food has passed my lips since I troughed through a whole box of shortbread last night.

Do I feel guilty?

Yes!

Did I enjoy them?

Of course.

A sense of relief washed over me that they are gone and no longer tempting me. I'm trying to forget about the Terry's Chocolate Orange I've hidden in the dining room, but we shall see. Anyway, forgetting the not-so-hidden goodies, I am learning to move on and accept responsibility because nobody forced the biscuits into my mouth.

Weight gain on Friday was now inevitable, and only a minor miracle could save me.

I'm not perfect and the journey to target will be a rollercoaster.

I've got a few things to do today: haircut, beard trim, sunbed, then I need to get this house into some sort of order before my cleaner comes on Friday. Yes, I am that person who cleans before the cleaner comes.

Something good, and unexpected, did happen today... I ordered a new pair of trousers from ASOS, in readiness for my next stop at the ABBA Arena in London. This time I'll leave Jon at home and party with my friend instead.

I'd decided on the black leather look skinny trousers in a 36" waist... Well, they arrived early this afternoon and aside from the realisation they might be a little too trendy for me to carry off at nearly fifty, I like them, a lot. So, fighting the urge to send them back and purchase a nice pair of brown corduroy slacks (Not in a million years!), I decided to try them on, and to my surprise, they *almost* fastened.

Damn you, gunt!

I wasn't disheartened because I saw it as a small victory.

Why?

I hadn't anticipated getting them past my knees for a start, let alone anywhere near my waist. I showed Jon, who cocked his eyebrow.

"They'll look nice."

"Is that it?"

"What do you want me to say?

I wasn't expecting him to do cartwheels, but a little encouragement wouldn't hurt.

Miserable fecker!

Anyhow, I am determined that by the time I visit the ABBA Arena again, they will fit comfortably. Perhaps I should have ordered a size smaller? I'll take some pictures on the day, and you can judge for yourself.

Haircut. Tick.

Beard Trimmed. Tick.

Eyebrows (What on Earth is happening with them? Whereas they used to be nice and neat, they seem to want to sprout of in every direction.) Trimmed. Tick

Food Shopping. Tick. (I walked past shelves filled with easter eggs, Cadbury's Mini Eggs, Frangipanes, you name it, I wanted it, but I resisted. Damn you, Cadbury's Crème Eggs... you nearly got me, but I stayed strong.)

Exercise. 45-minute walk. Tick.

Sunbed. I decided it was too cold to get undressed, so I abandoned plans, deciding I'd go on Friday after weigh-in.

Dinner was a success as far as I was concerned. I enjoyed what I ate and have only used five Syns today: Roast potatoes with *Fry Light*, carrot and turnip, sweetcorn, onion and mushroom gravy, and Aunt Bessie's Yorkshire Puddings.

After dinner, Jon and I took the dogs for a walk, but the wind howled around us. My previous workout had me sore so we didn't go as far as we usually would. As the dog's dislike adverse weather and wanted to turn back after doing their business, I didn't feel too guilty.

The kitchen was clean, and the dishwasher had been stacked, so I sat back down to do a little more on this book and the other work in progress.

Will anybody be interested in anything I have to say?

Will they even care?

I really don't know, but my aim from the beginning was to share my journey until I hit target... brace yourself, readers, because this could well end up longer than the *Lord of the Rings* trilogy.

February 2

It's just gone 10 am, and I'm up and about.

I'm tempted to go back to bed and continue watching *Teen Wolf*.

But I don't.

Instead, I've hung my washing on the line for the first time since winter kicked in. Knowing Spring is around the corner is a comforting thought. The kitchen is spotless, and I've faffed about for too long. I need to knuckle down and get some writing done.

Being self-employed is a Godsend because I choose my own hours, but it means that if I don't work, I don't get paid. Still, it beats being a slave to the wage and working for somebody else. My writing partner feels the same way, and typically our working week looks like this:

Monday to Thursday: 12:30 pm – 3 pm (10 hours)

It doesn't seem a lot, but that ten hours is the time we are live on Skype (Audio only because I look a total dog on camera!) working in sync even though I live thirty-eight miles away from her. It works for us but times those hours by ten and it still doesn't come close to the hours we actually put in to writing our novels. We often make plans to meet up in Chester and huddle up with our laptops in a bar or café, but it hasn't happened yet. But, as well as being my writing/business partner, she is also my friend and mother-in-law (Not the dragon type). So, we do see one another, although it is socially, and work is rarely mentioned unless pre-planned.

My little fur babies (the dogs) are due to be groomed today, and both, although sixteen and fifteen respectively, and therefore should be used to it, HATE it with a passion. Ellie, the lady who grooms them is adorable and the dogs do like her, as far as other people that aren't Jon and I are concerned. As Shih-Tzu's, grooming is unavoidable and must be done regularly, but I am not prepared to groom them myself as doing their nails and the other fiddly bits would be impossible. And anal glands—forget it!

Although Jon and I both work from home, they have never been left alone for long periods of time. Their separation anxiety remains off the charts, mainly from Sally. I admit I am stressed when I am away from them too. But for those forty-five minutes, neither are far from me as Ellie parks her doggie van outside my house then hooks up her cables to my mains and does an exemplary job.

Then I have an appointment for my second sports massage with Ian. I'm hoping he has some sort of technique for loosening and shifting fat, plus helping expel the calories from that whole box of shortbread I shovelled in a few days ago. As it stands, the clock ticks down from twenty hours until I weigh in. I need all the help I can get, and I don't care if it involves witchcraft, voodoo or hocus pocus. I might even bribe the lady on the scales.

What's her price, I wonder?

SEX

Okay, while I dread my next weigh-in, please bear with me while I speak some truths.

SEX: *sexual activity, including specifically sexual intercourse.*

Most of us do it. We like it, love it even... want it often... perhaps morning, noon, and night.

Right now, I don't.

But my partner would like it more often than he gets it and recently informed me how long it had been since we last played hide the sausage—November 2022—far too long.

Was it really November?

Apparently so.

Wow! Time flies when you're not having fun.

Have I gone off sex?

No, not really.

But as I have pointed out to my other half, it's not nearly as enjoyable as it used to be.

Why?

Because fat gets in the way, and the bigger and more out of shape a person is, the more it compromises mobility and affects one's libido. Not only that, but things can get a little more difficult for men, especially where the dreaded gunt is concerned.

GUNT: the flabby area below the stomach, and just above a man's penis.

Not only does it look unsightly, but this particular spot is a bugger to circumvent.

Worse still, it also robs a man of vital inches because the penis buries itself in that little hair-covered mound of fat, and no matter the amount of weight loss, exercise, or prayer, the only way to flatten it to pre-weight gain status is surgery.

Surgery, hmm, I'm all for it and have had the odd procedure, but I am yet to decide if gunt surgery is worth it. Ask me once I've hit target and I might have a solid answer.

Who knows?

I might do a full Dolly Parton, start with a facelift then have everything that's sagging and dragging stitched back to where it once was.

Jon is adamant that he doesn't want me to do anything surgical, but it's my body. He doesn't need to worry because I don't want to look radically different or remove the bandages and premiere a stretched face with lips that look like a cross between a puffer fish and a swollen arsehole, no thank you very much. I would just like to look and feel refreshed. Less saggy would be a nice bonus.

Anyway, back to sex.

Yes, it is still moderately enjoyable, and admittedly Jon and I aren't shy about nakedness, especially around one another, but it's the logistics, of what goes where, or if we can get into the position to put it where it should go.

How times have changed.

Years ago, Jon could wrap his legs round the back of his head like an oven ready turkey, as could I, well that was before his legs, and mine didn't weigh the equivalent of two tree trunks.

Factor in the excess weight, our flabby gunts, my Fibromyalgia, his gout, my wonky neck, swollen spine, his varicocele, and everything else going wrong between us, and we're hardly going to be competing in the next Olympics, never mind throwing one another around the bedroom with vim and vigour.

The truth is, Jon would need a crash helmet to give me a gobble or risk concussion from slapping his forehead off my gunt.

It does make me sad because I miss those days of heady, sweaty, breath-robbing, athletic sex, where we could bonk like *Duracell* bunnies, have a little nap to refuel the tanks, then go back for more.

Those were our glory days, and I know Jon misses that side of things too, especially as he is only in his mid-thirties and still raring to go.

Love is still there in abundance and while the mind is willing, the bodies are not able, right now.

I hope that will change and when I (we) hit target, expect to hear the bang, and crash of fireworks, and the headboard crashing against the wall.

Once more, Jon's story is his own to tell and while I know he has the same aspirations as I do, his many health issues derail his plans, and that vicious cycle is the game he is locked in.

To break that cycle, something has to give with said health problems and right now, he is far from being back to his best. For him, one of his conditions means he struggles to walk, so when he is immobile and overeating, he is gaining weight while also losing whatever fitness levels that remain.

Until doctors can fix the mobility issue, he can't exercise so it becomes all-consuming, and he does lose hope, most people would. And while it seems like he is walking along an endless road right now, I have no doubt Jon will get to where he needs to be.

I try my best for him, and always to support him, but sometimes a journey has to be started alone before another, even a life partner, can fall into step.

February 3
WEIGH-IN DAY

I'm so nervous, about weigh-in because I know I've not followed plan. But I will man up and face the music.

Wish me luck.

"One pound on," Shelly relayed.

"Could have been worse." Although I guessed that there would be a gain, the disappointment gnaws at me.

Total loss: 2 stone, 9½ pounds. I had managed to lose three stone, one pound so I need to do everything I can to get back there and beyond.

After weighing in, I quickly fell into the same old trap again. We went to the local café and later that night, and the following two days I gorged on candy sticks, crisps, chocolate, homemade fudge… I forgot what else, but there was definitely lots more.

Did I enjoy it?

Absolutely, but if truth be told, I enjoy my bowl of fruit, natural yoghurt, and tropical granola just as much.
So why do I do it?
Simple.
I'm human, and we make mistakes. And that's not some hippy-dippy excuse, but something my SW consultant pointed out to me when I had a small gain. And she was right—unless I start to see myself for what I am—human—I would spend more time berating myself for failure than praising myself for success.

February 9

Wow, what a busy week! Starting last Saturday when I journeyed across the water to Liverpool One, with my friend Sandie, the first time we'd met up socially in ten years.

It was lovely seeing her again, and it felt like no time had passed at all. We picked our friendship up right where we left it. Nothing in that sense felt different but what did feel different was me, and it took me by surprise.

Traipsing around Liverpool for the best part of four hours, I realised how much of a battle it was and that my body wasn't as strong as it used to be.

And yes, that is part Fibromyalgia, Ankylosing Spondylitis, arthritis, lack of exercise, being overweight, and the fact I am getting older.

It didn't dampen my enjoyment but when I got home, I was physically and mentally exhausted and had to go to bed.

When I woke up a few hours later, I felt so disheartened, but it added to my resolve to become as fit and healthy as I possibly can.

What did I eat today?

Well, put it this way, I probably used a months' worth of Syns in one hour.

10 x Crispy duck pancakes, cucumber, all slathered in hoisin sauce. (No idea how to Syn this).

Copious slices of cheesecake, and sponge cake (Probably a trillion Syns, but SO worth it!).

Lime and Soda (Syn Free).

The morning after I woke with the lark and decided to cook a full roast dinner. Jon loves his food, and although it is quite the task just for two, I gladly did it.

Still, after my excursion to Liverpool, I struggled, wiped out, and the feeling didn't thrill me. In fact, it made me feel weaker and less of a person. The positive is, it lit a fire under my saggy old arse; to get rid of this weight and stop making excuses.

However, rather than stick to my resolve, I fell off the wagon and took a trip to the local shop.

Family Sized Wotsits – 15½ Syns.
Family Sized Aero – 15 Syns.
2 x Bags Spearmint Chews – 50 Syns.
Midget Gems – 20 Syns.
6 x SW HiFi Bars – 12 Syns.

Total - 112½ Syns. This is over half my weekly Syn allowance in one sitting. And I am certain I forgot other things that I shovelled in.

I need to get myself back into the swing of things, but there is not a chance I'll have a loss this week. But I'll take it on the chin and move on.
Right now, I don't mind admitting that I'm absolutely terrified of putting all the weight I've lost back on.
How do I make myself see sense?
The terror should outweigh the compulsion to stuff my face, and even typing this, it doesn't.
What will work?
Willpower and self-control, two words that are easy to type, but hard to put into practice.
Only one solution exists: THE DREADED GYM. I've been putting it off because of my neck, but it's another excuse. If I'm careful, I should be okay.
Anyway, I did it.
I joined, and although I am yet to step foot in the place, it felt good to do something pro-active, or perhaps you might think it as reactive action. Maybe it's a bit of both. Anyway, I can go and complete my induction whenever I want to, then begin using the equipment. I can also use the pool if I choose to—NEVER!
While I'd love to go swimming, there is no way I am stepping out of those changing rooms with my belly on show.

February 10
WEIGH-IN DAY

I have no idea if it is a loss, gain, or stay the same because I am poorly and don't even have the strength to get out of bed.
I cancelled work on my new co-write and slept the day away.
Aside from that, Jon's gout has come back full force in both feet.

What a nightmare!
I'm stuck on a hamster wheel of bad luck, and it weighs heavy on my mental game for shedding the stones I set for myself.

February 12 & 13

I'm feeling so much better, therefore back on plan. I have no idea what damage picking at anything and everything has done because I felt too poorly to cook. But I'll take the plunge on Friday.

A successful sports massage session with Ian, and I have noticed increased movement in my neck. That's the good news! The only downside was he slathered me in massage oil, which was rather enjoyable, but after the session was over, I slipped my T-shirt back on without thinking.

Once home, I sat on the edge of the bath and lowered myself down, leaned back and was launched into the water faster than the Jamaican bobsled team was catapulted around the run at the 1988 Winter Olympics.

To give you a mental picture, my legs shot up in the air, my head was submerged and when coming to a crashing halt at the other end of the bath, my backside had nearly swallowed the chain that the plug hangs from.

My bathroom looked like a scene from *The Poseidon Adventure* and was a stark reminder to wipe myself with a towel afterwards.

February 14
VALENTINE'S DAY

I can move my head.
I woke up without a stiff neck, but I could smell something unusual. After inspecting my various nooks and cranny's, wondering what it could be, I discovered massage oil behind my ears.

So back in the bath it was.

This time I gripped the sides like my life depended on it.

Jon is poorly, so we couldn't go out for a romantic meal, or to the cinema.

Stuck to plan, but it wasn't a romantic meal I cooked, but SW beef curry and rice. I don't like curry at all, and I'm not keen on rice because it often makes me sick, but I do quite like this recipe as it reminds me of Mulligatawny soup, so I can just about tolerate it.

"That was delicious." He always enjoys my cooking.

"I quite enjoyed it too." Until an hour later when I was reminded of why I shouldn't eat rice—I was sick as a dog.

But never mind, I waited a couple of hours and ate strawberries, banana, black grapes, and fat free natural yoghurt—delicious!

Jon left this message for me on my *Facebook* wall.

Happy Valentine's Day to you... You are my rock, Marco Lewis. You have looked after me this last year more than I could have ever expected while I am ill. You are 1 in 7.8 billion. I wouldn't change you for the world. Thank you for loving me the way you do. I love you xx

It meant more to me than any meal, or movie.

I needed no thank you for taking care of him because that is my job. Despite the ups and down of love, life, and our relationship, that will never change.

February 15

Is it only Wednesday?

It's hump day, and despite Jon still being immobile, and Valentine's Day being a damp squib, the past week has gone okay. Well, I say the week... at least from Monday.

I'm certain of another gain on Friday, but had I not reverted to plan, I dread to think...

Dinner was roast beef with every shred of fat cut off because Jon and I hate it (I gave my meat to the dogs) fry light roast potatoes, carrot, and turnip, Paxo stuffing, onion, & mushroom gravy.

Total Syns used: 3.

I've cooked so much this week, that I am sick of the sight of food. It doesn't help that I haven't stopped all week, from food shopping, walking the dogs, to running up and down the stairs taking Jon's meals up to him. I might have shifted a few extra pounds with the exercise.

Who knows?

Check back in on Friday with the good or bad news.

Ps. I still haven't done my gym induction but have looked into *Clubbercise* classes.

I like to think that I can dance, and I know that I do have rhythm, but I am understandably nervous trying something new in front of a room full of strangers. The only saving grace is that the room is in darkness save for glow sticks—I don't want to look like a big, shadowy, blob waving neon sticks about like I'm guiding a Boeing 767 into land.

Now, I'm struggling to find a class that works for me, and the one I'd initially found is no longer running.

When I find something that suits, it won't be my first foray into this kind of exercise.

Many years ago, I joined a local *Zumba* class with my aunty and assumed, because I learned all the routines to the various Steps' songs in my younger years, I'd take to it like a duck to water.

Wrong!

Mastering the routines was harder than I ever imagined it would be and what rhythm I possessed while dancing on those podiums in *The Escape* on Paradise Street, Liverpool, back in the day, had taken a vacation.

My Lycra-clad instructor had two speeds—fast, and supersonic—and would jump up and down on the makeshift stage like Zebedee from *The Magic Roundabout*.

As infuriatingly energetic as she was, it was her catchphrases that made the biggest impression, specifically this one...

"MOVE THOSE HIPS LIKE BIG FAT CHIPS," she would screech from her podium, while I laughed and struggled to keep up, puffing and panting like an old rhinoceros. I couldn't coordinate myself, and it took a few weeks to master the routines, only for them to suddenly change.

I didn't really care too much because I looked as daft as the others trying to learn it.

Looking back, joining when I did was a crazy idea because I'd not long recovered from pneumonia, having been admitted to intensive care for a week when I was in Goa, India, of all places.

It could only happen to me.

The plane landed at Goa Airport, and although thrilled to be back in the country that felt like home, I felt a little worse for wear, but put it down to the nine-hour flight, and the fact I'd only days before had major intestinal surgery. I was in the holiday spirit and raring to go.

Arriving at the resort, Lagoa Azul, about two hours later, I felt drained without a shred of energy. As this was my seventh visit, the hotel manager came out to welcome me back and noticed my death-like pallor. As it happened, a nurse from UK was checking in at the same time. Both were concerned. I assured them I'd be fine after a nap. The nurse kindly provided me with her room number and told me to find her if I didn't feel any better.

Five days later, and at my friend's urging, I finally emerged from the room into a waiting taxi to take me to the local hospital.

I was instantly taken for an X-Ray, then given the news that I was dying with terminal lung cancer.

"But I've never smoked," I protested, still in shock.

"That doesn't matter," the doctor replied. "We need to admit you immediately."

"Okay."

"Do you have insurance?"

"Yes."

"Good, but you will need to pay up front and then claim it back from them."

"Fine."

"Would you like a private room?"

"Yes, please." Feeling weak and tired, I couldn't be bothered with people in general, let alone what I imagined would be a mixed ward with people chattering in a language I couldn't understand.

I handed over my card and was instantly charged £500.

And that was that.

They wheeled me upstairs, no lifts, just sloped floors, to what I assumed would be a private room. I was pleasantly surprised to discover it was a private ward—white marble floors, white walls, white flowing curtains, and a 24/7 personal nurse to take care of me.

This was Goa's idea of private health care, and I approved.

Looking back, it was certainly luxurious, especially by Indian standards, which is not a slight on the country I love, and from what I'd seen of the horrific ward's downstairs. But I'd just been told death hovered ready to claim me, so I wasn't up to cartwheels, and worsening by the minute, the only thing I was interested in was sleep.

At exactly the same time, my mum was being treated for breast cancer, and although I was processing the news that I was going to die, I was terrified about something else far more important in my eyes.

"How am I going to tell my mum I'm dying of cancer?" I asked my friend, Lynda.

There was no right or wrong answer.

We'd come away for a two-week holiday in the sun, and I might just arrive home in a shipping crate.

"Don't tell my mum anything," I warned Lynda, worried the stress would cause a relapse. "Promise me."

"I swear, I won't."

As I had been admitted to a critical care unit, Lynda wasn't allowed to stay with me, and in all fairness, it was her first time in Goa. Luckily, she found it easy to make friends, so I knew she'd be okay. I felt terribly guilty though, but she couldn't have been nicer, and to this day, I have so much love for her, and credit her with saving my life. Had she not insisted I go to the hospital, she would have woken up the following morning to find me dead in the bed next to her. The doctor was quite clear when relaying that to us.

That night I drifted in and out of consciousness, and to this day, I can recall this next moment vividly.

I opened my eyes, surrounded by a white glow that hurt my eyes.

"Oh, my God, I've made it..." I don't follow any religion, nor do I believe in an omnipotent being arranging the goings on within the universe at his or her leisure. But those are the exact words I spoke. "I'm in Heaven."

I truly believed I'd died and felt at peace, knowing, against all the odds, I'd found my way to my idea of Heaven and was in some sort of cosmic waiting room.

That euphoric feeling didn't last for long.

A young Indian lady popped her head around the curtain and spoke in a high-pitched. "Are you paining, sir?"

"No, I'm not." Immediately crestfallen when I should have been relieved not to have shifted off this mortal coil.

Night had fallen and the lights in my private ward had been dimmed for my comfort, casting a glow through the curtains.

So much for Heaven.

Still alive, I can't remember a time I had felt so awful.

Anyway, the next morning, I was driven to another hospital, and recall the journey took about an hour, along bumpy roads that were akin to a white-knuckle ride.

Grossly overweight, the medical team, two extremely small, skinny, male orderlies, winched me into the MRI machine. They dripped with sweat from their efforts. Then, sandbags were placed on top of me to keep me as still as possible while the machine worked its magic.

"You are very fat," the doctor told me, just in case I'd forgotten.

"I know, but I'll be dead soon," I snapped.

"All here..." He rubbed my flabby stomach and surrounding areas. "Not good fat here." Then he begun a long-winded lecture about the dangers of men accumulating fat in the chest and stomach area.

He made me feel so much worse, if that was at all possible, and those irrational thoughts of being buried in a double wardrobe flittered back from negatives thoughts across the years.

Hoisted out of the machine by the same two orderlies then taken for a barrage of other scans, tests, and giving enough vials of AB negative to keep Dracula and his entourage happy for a month, it was back into the ambulance which was actually a small white van with a bed welded to its floor. I suffered the bumpy journey back, feeling almost seasick when I was helped back into my comfortable bed some hours later.

As it turned out, pneumonia, pleural effusion, and something else I can't remember the name of was diagnosed.

Thankfully, I didn't have final stage lung cancer. *Phew!*

I literally breathed a sigh of relief and almost hacked my badly damaged lungs up.

The doctor devised a treatment plan and took another £200 from my card for his trouble.

Later that afternoon, they hooked me up to all sorts of machines, but no matter what they did, my lungs refused to drain. The next morning, a team of doctors surrounded my bed, yammering away in a language I couldn't understand while I wondered what they were going to do to cure me.

I was losing valuable tanning time, but nothing could have prepared me for what came next.

"Right, I want you to sit on the edge of the bed," one of the doctors urged.

I was naked as the day I was born, and everything was on show. Exhausted, and frustrated to be in this mess, everything flapped about. Isn't it strange how shame flies out of the window when at one's worst. "What for?"

"Sit there and lift your arm and put your hand on top of your head."

Weird, I thought. And then I saw it. A long stainless-steel instrument that was reminiscent of a knitting needle, only thinner. "Where do you think you're sticking that?"

"We must drain your lung and will do a thoracentesis."

A what? I thought. But I got the gist. "You're going to drain my lung with that thing?"

"Yes, now, please lift your arm and put your hand on your head."

Exhausted and weak, I didn't have it within me to argue. "Can't you put me to sleep?"

"No, you could die."

One of the nurses shuffled around the bed in silence, and then I felt the familiar sting as she injected various spots around my back and side.

"This should numb the area—you should not feel any pain."

Words that should have brough comfort only alarmed me further, because I never heard a definitive, you will *not* feel any pain. Whatever sized needle they had used to inject the area with, I did feel excruciating, almost unbearable pain, and from the first insertion into my lung with this draining needle, I felt him wiggling it around inside of me.

I've never been stabbed, nor do I want to be, but from the moment the drain pierced my skin, that was my first thought. I can only describe it as air being drained from a balloon, but in reverse. There was a *whoosh*, followed by a thumping sensation, like I'd been hit side on by a bus, and to this day, I've never felt searing pain like it.

Once was torture, but the seven times he tried to drain the fluid from my lungs with not one trickle dripping into the kidney dish the nurse gripped was barbaric.

Perplexed, the doctor told me they would try the following day, so that night, nervous and knowing what to expect, I didn't sleep a wink.

I willed time to stop, then morning came, and I panicked as I saw him walk through the door of my ward. I was ready to refuse, not able to go through the procedure again, but I needn't have worried as they'd decided on an alternative course of treatment and hooked me up to another drip, assuring me it would help the fluid disperse naturally.

Thankfully, he was right. A few days later, with my lungs in better shape, I was discharged.

Wheeled out of my private ward and over a thousand pounds out of pocket, which I never got back from the crooked insurance company, I was unceremoniously dumped in the reception area to wait for a taxi, which I had to call myself.

While waiting, a lady rushed into the waiting area, sobbing, and three other men followed her. I assumed them to be family.

I couldn't understand everything they were saying, but broken English told me the lady was terribly distressed. She wailed and screamed like her life depended on it.

Then, the doors opened, and a patient was wheeled in on a gurney by two ambulance drivers and left smack bang in the middle of the floor, right in front of me, covered head to toe in a white sheet.

The family immediately surrounded the gurney., Then, the lady lifted the sheet off to reveal a young lad of no more than eighteen. Tears trickled down her cheeks. "He okay, he okay, wake up, wake up..."

My eyes were instantly trained on the poor guy lying on the gurney.

He was dead and by the blue tinge to his skin, had been for a while.

I tried to avert my eyes, but I was unnerved, not wanting to look, but compelled to.

Still, they seemed to refuse to accept he was gone and tapped his hands, wiggled his feet, clutched his face in their hands and when nothing roused him, they shook him gently, urging him to wake up.

"He will open his eyes soon," one of the men said.

As sad as this unfolding scene was, I remember thinking that they could light firecrackers in each nostril, and he still wouldn't wake up.

Even though my heart went out to them, I could feel my nerves jangling, roaring back to life, and laughter bubbling, so was desperate to escape.

Waiting for my taxi, I picked up what had happened. He'd been riding on a jet ski in the water off Baga Beach. He'd been going too fast and crashed it into a boat suffering extensive head injuries. From what I could see from my vantage point, the side of his head was caved in.

"Taxi for Marco." Finally free, I rushed out as fast as I could and hopped into the taxi. "Resort Lagoa Azul, please."

I wound the window down, relishing the fresh air against my skin.

Once back at the hotel, I decided to walk back to my room, via the pool area.

As I stepped past reception and down into the pool area, I spotted my friend in the pool and waved.

She shrieked and jumped up and down, waving and calling out my name.

"Is that him?" I heard other guests ask.

As I hated being the centre of attention, I immediately shrank into myself.

"Yeah, I told you he was real."

"Are you Marco?"

"Yes." I wondered what the kerfuffle was, but my friend relayed the full story to me later and I admit, I did find it funny.

Because nobody had seen me, those she had made friends with had wrongly believed her to be travelling alone. They whispered that I was a figment of her imagination and that she had created this elaborate story that I was ill in our room, too embarrassed to admit she was on holiday by herself.

My appearance shocked them, but at least they knew my friend wasn't a lunatic with an imaginary friend.

I remembered later... she did come to the room with somebody when I was poorly. I heard his voice, but I told her not to bring anybody in.

It amused me to no end when I realised that guy must have thought she'd thrown her voice, pretending to be me.

Months later, a few of the people she had befriended visited her, and we actually met properly.

So, after the eventful non-holiday, back to England I went, whiter than when I'd left... I was shaking my hips like big fat chips at *Zumba*, but because my lungs were still not fully healed. I did lose my puff quite a few times.

So, I explained my predicament to the instructor and decided to take a break mid-class.

It seemed she was a fan of *Living La Vida Loca* by Ricky Martin, and I hated it, and still do, with a passion. I would sit that one out every week and watch everyone else shimmy and shake to it, before wobbling back to the dancefloor for my favourite Bollywood routine, "SCREW IN THE LIGHTBULB, SCREW IN THE LIGHTBULB."

All was going well until the instructor introduced a new number with what I'd call a 'stompy' routine. I found it quite easy to master, although it was a good job we were doing it on the ground floor because there were a lot of heavyweights in our class.

My aunty didn't enjoy the new number quite so much, and after giving it too much welly this particular week, she hurt her foot and had to seek medical attention. As it turned out, she'd broken a bone in her foot.

"How did you do it?" Doctor asked.

"*Zumba*."

"Oh, not again. I see so many patients who have injured themselves at *Zumba*."

She never went back, and too cowardly to go alone, I stepped away as well.

MOVE THOSE HIPS LIKE BIG FAT CHIPS... I'm laughing at the memory, and the absurdity of her catchphrase.

Thinking back to India, perhaps I should have been a little more wary, especially after my first visit. While it was a revelation, both personally and spiritually, it certainly wasn't drama free.

With no expectations at all, and after a nine-hour flight, my friend, Mikey, and I landed at Goa International Airport, which seemed well organized, even though the police armed with rifles seemed a tad excessive. I tried to win a few of them over with a smile but most of them wore thunderous expressions so I decided my efforts were futile and quickly moved past them.

After being herded through customs, we found ourselves in the baggage claim area, and that's when the fun began.

I kept a tight grip of my suitcase, but as soon as I stepped through the doors, and into the sweltering heat, a swarm of men rushed toward me, trying to wrestle my case from me.

"Suitcase..." came the chorus of voices almost singing at us.

"I'm fine, thank you," I repeated, tugging the case back toward me, but still the grab and pull continued.

Mikey was a nervous wreck, so hid behind me.

"Suitcase, suitcase," they repeated.

"No, I'm fine," I tried to get past, with my friend still hiding behind me. Still, they blocked me. But I was made of stronger stuff and pushed through them. I turned to Mikey, sweating, tired, thirsty, and therefore not in the best of moods. "This is crazy." It seemed to reflect everything negative I'd seen on the television about the place.

Still, it was a brand-new adventure, and I wondered what all the fuss was about, but quickly realised their rush to help wasn't anything but an attempt to secure valuable pound coins from the English tourists flooding into the country to escape the miserable British winter season.

Desperate for a pound coin, or not, I wasn't about to surrender my case to a total stranger, so on the advice of my friend who had travelled before us, we decided against the coach, which looked like something rescued from the 1950's, and found the nearest taxi, eager to get to our destination, Arpura, as quickly as possible.

The journey to the village we were staying in was eventful, and very much in the vein of what I imagine a real-life Wacky Races contest to be like. I don't think speed limits exist in Goa, and if they do, they are ignored, plus the constant honking of horns is enough to drive anyone mad. A few years later, I went back with my mum, and she had an asthma attack in the back of the taxi, so scared was she by the speed the driver was zigzagging in and out of cars.

Anyway, I was parched from the heat and desperate for a cold drink. "Can you please stop at a shop?" I asked the taxi driver.

"Sure," he replied in perfect English. "There is a shop around the corner from your villa."

So, he stopped while I went into the shop and loaded up my bags with Mountain Dew, Lays crisps and other assorted goodies. I paid the lady at the till, then turned around, walked out of the shop, smack bang into an enormous elephant, and no I hadn't walked into a mirror before you wonder.

To say I was shocked was an understatement, I dropped my bags, then wondered how I was going to get past it. *Shoo*, and *excuse me*, didn't work, so I patted it gently on its rear, preparing to duck for cover if it took offence and swung its trunk at me... Thankfully, it idled out of the way, to reveal the taxi driver laughing hysterically, as was my friend.

"Your face, funny," the driver said, when I slinked into the backseat of the car. "Do you not have elephants in England?"

I wasn't in the mood to join in. "Yes, we do, but I don't often bump into them outside my local shop."

He chucked all the way to the villa, but shock aside, it was wonderful, if not a little scary, to see such a magnificent creature up close.

The next day, I'd already fallen in love with everything about the place, from the people to Baga Beach—I felt at home instantly.

The next two weeks were blissful, but not uneventful. After a few days by the pool, Mikey and I decided to venture further afield and walked to the main road to flag a Tuk Tuk. We waited for the next one to pull up, and as it slowed to a stop, the driver looked at me and waved his hand.

"No, no," he chunnered, waving me away. "You too fat, you too fat, you tip me over."

"Cheeky twat," I snapped, irritated, and embarrassed by his public shaming.

But he was right, and it was another example of my excess weight getting in the way of even the simplest of things like hiring a Tuk Tuk for a day out exploring. Eventually, we hired a taxi, but I wanted the experience of a Tuk Tuk—maybe when I reach target, I can go back without worrying about tipping it onto its side.

On our last night, I felt sad to be leaving and would happily have stayed for good. But Christmas was just around the corner. So, I washed my vests and hung them over the railings outside the front door to dry, deciding to finish packing after dinner to say goodbye to new-found friends. But fate had other plans.

I opened the front door to the villa, stepped one foot out, and all hell broke loose.

Pain like I've never experienced ricocheted up my legs and it took a few minutes to realise what I'd done.

Stepping into a pool of water from my drip-drying vests, I slipped and dropped into the splits. Now, I don't know many men in general who can do the splits comfortably, certainly not tipping the scales at twenty plus stone. So, I went down hard and fast until my plums were resting on the cold marble.

Once the initial wave of white-hot pain had subsided and I caught my breath, I felt foolish, then tried to move, and it was then another wave of pain creased me.

I took deep breaths, unsure what I was going to do, then Mikey appeared.

"What are you doing?"

I couldn't find my voice to answer him.

He stepped over me, and one look at my face, he realised I'd hurt myself and called an ambulance. For forty-five painful and embarrassing minutes I lay on the floor unable to move. By this time, a crowd of locals had gathered, making me feel even worse.

Once the ambulance arrived, in what looked like a tiny van, they were faced with the prospect of lifting me. Even with the smallest move, I screamed, but eventually they got me onto a stretcher, nearly giving themselves a hernia while navigating me into the tiny space.

Mikey sat in the back with me, and once settled, we both laughed at my clumsiness.

At the hospital, I was seen by a doctor who told me I would have to go for a MRI at another hospital. So, I was shoved into the back of the ambulance again, taken for the MRI, and then driven back to the first hospital to be told I had somehow broken a bone in my thigh and ruptured my quadriceps (I had never heard of them so will work on the assumption most others haven't and tell you what they are).

- A group of 4 muscles that come together just above your kneecap (patella) to form the patellar tendon.

- Often called the quads, this group of muscles is used to extend the leg at the knee and aids in walking, running, and jumping.

I had experienced pain before but never this agony, and alongside the injury to my quads, I had also damaged the inguinal ligament. This is a set of two narrow bands in the inguinal area of the body (the groin). The groin is the fold where the bottom of the abdomen meets the inner thighs.

The inguinal ligament connects the oblique muscles in the abdomen to the pelvis. The oblique muscles wrap the sides of the body, from the ribs to the pelvis. The pelvis is the part of the skeleton that connects the trunk (upper body) to the legs (lower body).

So, while I could feel the damage to my quads, that area of my body felt numb and when lifted by the nurses, the damaged leg swung like it was attached by a thin string. I was not in control of my limb or the muscles within.

The doctor told me it would take a while to heal, and I could not fly and should estimate six weeks until I could travel again. *Forget it*. Mikey had to be back at work and there was no way I was staying there injured on my own, and through Christmas.

There was a touch of comedy to the moment as I had been admitted and had to wait for orderlies to take me to my room—when they arrived, I soon discovered the hospital had no lift, so for me to get two floors up, I would be pushed up sloped floors.

Due to my height and weight, the orderlies struggled to push me, now lying flat on the bed, up the first ramp, and I was terrified they were going to let me go and the bed would take off down the sloped floor, sending me crashing into the wall.

Finally, they managed the first floor, but on the journey to the second, one of the orderlies lost his grip and started to scream that I was falling, so I did the only thing I could do and opened my arms as wide as humanly possible, literally using my hands as stoppers while the other orderly rushed around the bed to try and avert disaster.

I was yelling at the top of my lungs, wanting to jump off the gurney, but not daring to do it for fear of injuring myself all the more. "MIKE, HELP, THEY'LL LET ME GO…"

Mikey eventually stepped in but could barely breathe for laughing.

Once in the room, Mikey lay on the bed next to me and the doctor came in, thinking he was the patient. As a natural red head (dyed black), he hadn't considered the strength of the Indian sun, and although he had been using Factor 50, he said his legs were sore. It soon transpired that he had second degree burns that required treatment. So, by the end of the evening, the pair of us were in adjoining beds eating takeaway pizza.

I had no intention of staying in the hospital and did what I had to do to get on that plane, which was to pay the doctor (a fortune by their standards) for a letter clearing me for travel.

The next morning, I hired a wheelchair, checked in at the airport, suffered the humiliating body search whilst in the wheelchair and then wheeled across the tarmac to the plane. With crutches, scans, and x-rays in hand I was lifted onto the craft by four baggage handlers.

Thankfully, the pilot made an announcement that an injured passenger (me) had just boarded, and asked would anybody be kind enough to move to an alternative seat so I could lie down for the duration of the eleven-hour flight back to Manchester. Luck was on my side and people did move, and not only that, checked on me for the duration of the flight, which I thought was a kind gesture.

I was allowed to remain on board the craft in Bahrain and after a quick call to my parents to tell them of my woes, they would be there to pick me up from Manchester Airport.

They were there as agreed, and my dad drove me straight back home, then to the local hospital.

Once there, the doctor looked at my scans and x-rays, questioning when I arrived home.

"About two hours ago," I replied.

He was concerned and admitted me before sending me for more scans. When the results came back, he pointed to a large clot in my leg I had been unaware of and informed me that had it moved during the flight, it would have killed me. What could I say? If the worst had happened blame would have sat on my shoulders because I paid for the letter clearing me for travel.

A plaster cast from the top of my leg to my ankle was fitted and I was discharged from hospital two days later.

That was 23rd December, and the cast had to be changed every Tuesday morning at 8 am. Luckily, I lived in a basement apartment at the time and once in my apartment, I was fine. But my parents and friends lent a hand and did my shopping for me because I was basically useless. Fast forward to May the following year when I finally put my crutches in the cupboard, although it was three years before I fully recovered, hindered by the excess weight I was carrying, which had increased due to my lack of activity.

The following year I decided to return to Goa, this time alone, but stopped off first in Mumbai, then Nagpur to have a look around. Mumbai, or Bombay as it was once known, was a city I had always wanted to visit but turned out to be a disappointment due to the wall-to-wall traffic and unbearable noise pollution.

Nagpur, I knew nothing about, but I found myself there anyway. What an experience that was. Anyway, arriving back in Goa, I had the most amazing time and was invited to be the guest of honour at a Christening. As Goa is a Catholic country, I shouldn't have been surprised by the pomp, and while it wasn't my thing, I accepted. Had I been asked to attend such a service in England I would have refused because I am not religious, but I was made aware that to refuse would cause offence, so I threw my reservations aside and graciously accepted.

How nice to be asked, I thought, not realising that as the guest of honour, I would be sat on what was essentially a raised podium, a few feet above everyone else, with ladies filing past me offering me food from large silver trays.

For somebody who hates being the centre of attention, it took all that I had not to excuse myself and hide away. I must have looked ridiculous sitting there with copious mounds of food in front of me. Think Buddha on a makeshift plinth, and you won't be far wrong! So embarrassing, especially as a lot of the other Indian guests had arrived wearing Liverpool football shirts in tribute to me.

I had been asked where I was from and had said Liverpool because it is easier than explaining where I actually live so they automatically assumed I was a huge LFC supporter—nope, I can't stand football, but it was a thoughtful gesture, to which I played along.

By the end of the event, I was stuffed up to the eyeballs and swore never to accept an invite again.

But that is India, and my love for it remains. I cannot wait to return and hopefully Jon and me will be fighting fit when we do. I want to visit the Taj Mahal, and for us to experience the ultimate symbol of love together—something for my bucket list.

MARCO LEWIS

February 16

I woke up this morning with zero appetite, which is quite normal for me. However, if somebody presented me with a large slab of cake, I'd soon shovel it in.

Regardless, I got straight to it and went downstairs to cut up the chicken, so I could marinade it in natural yoghurt and various spices, for tonight's dinner—chicken and salad wraps with homemade dirty rice. I've already decided I won't have it but settled my mind on lentil soup. It's my go-to food when I can't be bothered eating, which also stops me from eating junk food.

Before dinner I'm working with Netta, my co-writer on *Act of Contrition*. So far, it's going really well, and we should be finished in the next two weeks.

Once work shuffled out of the way, I walked up to the hairdressers (Hello, Body Magic), got my haircut and beard trimmed. Plus, something happened with my eyebrows—they were once my favourite thing about me, but this morning, a few stragglers stuck out.

"Can you do my eyebrows me for, please"?

"Yes, I take them off for you." I don't know his name, but as he is from Kurdistan, his spoken English is broken at best.

"NO," I yelled, alarmed. "... not off, just trim them."

"You want trimmed?"

"Yes, trimmed, please don't shave them off." I was nervous at this point, imagining having to draw them on for weigh-in. I even made a noise, my interpretation of the sound the clippers make, hoping he would realise what I meant. God knows what he thought, but he did converse with his colleague. Whatever they were chatting about, I hoped my words weren't lost in translation.

My eyebrows are still there and a lot tidier.

Anyway, once the cutthroat shave had been finished and my beard shaped, I noticed that the turkey neck had crept back into existence which made me more determined to lose weight. But on the walk home I called a cosmetic surgery clinic to enquire about their procedures. I want a facelift, my neck tightened, and my eyes brows lifted. So, I shall hoof it over to Liverpool and see what the doctor can suggest. I know it's silly, but on the way home I felt self-conscious and kept rubbing at my neck, trying to smooth it back into place.

February 17
WEIGH-IN DAY

"Just a little pound..."

"On or off?" My hearing isn't the best, especially when Shelly speaks discreetly.

"On."

Yes, disappointment continued to plague me, even though I hadn't fully stuck to plan.

I can't grumble because if I had followed it to the letter, I would have had a loss.

The realist in me knows I need to pull my finger out of my backside, and buying myself an exercise bike tomorrow satisfies my goal-setting tendency for the moment.

ALSO, rather than pigging out on weigh-in day and the day after, I need to use my Syns and do the research.

What are the Syn values for my favourite goodies?

If I knew those values, perhaps I could treat myself every day, rather than shovel it all in over two days.

I am extremely disappointed with myself when I really have no right to be. *I* stuffed the chocolate and other goodies into my mouth, and never felt a shred of guilt in that moment. I hate myself for it, but the truth is like a child who says sorry after they've been caught up to no good. I know that had I stayed the same or had even a small loss, this last paragraph would not exist.

I am no different to an alcoholic or a cocaine addict waking up each day and claiming sobriety. Dealing with addiction is never the same on any given day and the reasons for falling off plan are never the same either. Still, it doesn't mean I feel any better about it.

February 18

Disappointment by yesterday's gain continued to roll about in my thoughts this morning. This defeated uneasiness switched the immediate gratification part of my brain to active, and me fancying a sandwich. I decided to walk the ten minutes to Hurst's bakery. Possibly distracted by the music pumping through my headphones, I took a wrong turn, and the actual journey took fifty minutes. I couldn't believe I'd done it but realised too late to correct myself. My sense of direction is usually flawless, but my inner compass drifted way off today. I ended up doubling back on myself. Eventually, I found my way, sweating, panting, thirsty, and with my shins in revolt thanks to fibro, I couldn't face the walk back so called a taxi. After waiting for twenty-five minutes, I called back to be told the taxi had been and gone.

"I've been waiting here since I booked it."

"Sorry, mate, but the driver said he waited outside the Acorn for five minutes."

"I didn't order a taxi from there." The Acorn is a local pub, and by this time I could have murdered a cold beer or three. Anyway, I relayed my location again.

"Oh, right, I'll get one round for you." He offered no apology.

When I arrived home about ninety minutes later, I'd lost my craving and ditched the sandwich in the fridge.

In a roundabout way, this day ended with a plus for progress on my *Body Magic* journey. These are awarded for various exercises completed over a given time period.

February 21

Today is Shrove Tuesday, the day before Ash Wednesday (the first day of Lent), observed in many Christian countries through participating in confession and absolution, the ritual burning of the previous year's Holy Week palms, finalising one's Lenten sacrifice, as well as the ritual eating of pancakes covered in sugar and lemon juice.

TRUTH: The only part of the above that has any relevance to my life is the eating of pancakes, and I devoured them with gusto.

So, you might have guessed that I have fallen off plan quite spectacularly, and for one simple reason; I am fed up with normal, healthy food consuming my life, and for those who might be confused, please allow me to explain.

If I'm not thinking about what to cook, I have to shop for it, cook it, then force myself to eat it.

I don't want to eat it and haven't done for many years.

I'm overweight because I cannot control myself with sweets, cakes, crisps etc, not because I overindulge in whatever normal, healthy food is.

As I've said before, I don't like butter, margarine, curry, kebabs, burgers, takeaways, or the usual foods that most readers would happily indulge in.

Yes, it is a matter of taste, but also because I don't have that specific hormone, ghrelin, in my body, the one that tells me I'm hungry. I would happily forego meals and stuff my face with goodies (or baddies, whichever way you want to look at it.)

Please allow me to be scientific for a moment and explain a few things...

What is ghrelin—the hunger hormone?

A hormone that causes me so many problems is the hunger-causing hormone and is produced or released in the stomach when it becomes empty. It's supposed to tell my brain when I am hungry, and to seek out food.

Think of it in these simple terms; the emptier the stomach, the more ghrelin is produced, hence more hunger.

As I have a ghrelin deficiency, I don't feel hungry at all, which means I have zero appetite.

Doctors have told me this can lead to eating disorders, being underweight (I wish!), and other health issues.

The absence of an appetite could also lead to me not having enough vitamins and nutrients that my body requires daily. This can lead to various physical and mental health issues.

Although there are some who would think being ghrelin deficient as a good thing, for me it is the opposite because it does have its advantages.

- Regulates Inflammation

A potent anti-inflammatory mediator and can provide treatment for inflammatory diseases and injuries. Ghrelin is needed for immune tolerance. It increases the anti-inflammatory cytokine IL-10.

- Help Fight Autoimmune Diseases

Ghrelin can help patients with rheumatoid arthritis, ulcerative colitis, multiple sclerosis, Parkinson's disease, Crohn's disease, cardiovascular disease, and inflammation from brain injury.

It protects the lungs, liver, kidneys, and other organs from toxic by-products of oxygen reactions and inflammation injury. It also protects the heart from inflammation and injury and improves heart function.

- Enhances Learning and Memory

Ghrelin can enter the long-term memory storage part of the brain through the blood.

- Influences the Growth Hormone

Ghrelin influences the release of growth hormone by activating the growth hormone secretagogue receptor (GHSR) which thereby increases growth hormone release.

- Enhances Dopamine Release

Ghrelin also amplifies dopamine action and enhances dopamine release in the hypothalamus, amygdala, and nucleus accumbens (pleasure centre). This dopamine release and amplification can increase physical activity and motivation.

Wake up... science lesson is now over...

My body does not produce this hunger hormone, and my disdain for food is a daily struggle.

There is no desire to eat any food, but I can eat sweets and chocolate in abundance, and out of habit, which is the worst thing I can do. My constant need to eat the latter is habit—I know this. Anything else, I really have to talk myself into.

This plan, although it works and I will never deny that, forces me to deal with something I have zero interest in, FOOD.

You could assume I have an eating disorder, and you would probably be right, but certainly not one that is common. I have spoken to specialists about it, but all they see is a fat person who claims not to like food.

I can almost hear them asking the question—*How can you be that fat and not like food?*

Because there is more to food than kebabs, curry, burgers, and toast with lashings of butter to name but a few calorie busting foods that I don't like...

How do I move forward?

I haven't figured that out and might never reach that understanding. Right now, what I do know is I want to be slim and healthy.

The issues I need to solve rotate through my mind more like blanket statements with no solutions in sight:

FOOD: I don't want to go shopping for it.
FOOD: I don't want to look at it.
FOOD: I don't want to cook it.
FOOD: I don't want to smell it.
FOOD: I don't want to eat it.
FOOD: I don't want anything to do with it.

In my wildest dreams, I wish somebody could invent a medication where I would never have to eat again, and that also means goodies.

My other half has a voracious appetite and demands regular meals. He likes everything I don't. As he is poorly right now, I cook for him and try to remain on plan.

As a rule, I usually do okay, but these last few days, my wiring seems to have malfunctioned. Even as I type this, I am trying to talk myself down and back onto plan despite knowing I have two family bags of roast beef Monster Munch, a family sized Aero and two bags of Haribo, mocking me from the bedside cabinet.

Is it supposed to be this difficult?

Yes, I think it is, and I keep telling myself not to be too hard on myself.

CHEWING THE FAT

When all is said and done, I am only HUMAN.

February 23

I've got an appointment at the Physiotherapy Department at Clatterbridge Hospital later today.

Today is my second visit to see this particular physiotherapist. I don't mind admitting that I am dreading it because the last time I saw him, he made me feel like I wasted his time.

I'm tempted to cancel it, but I won't. I'm well-armed. Three sessions with my sports massage therapist, and I know I have more movement in my neck.

Plus, he promised he would sort out blood tests after my last visit, and in time for this appointment. It didn't happen, which makes me wonder if I should ask to see somebody else.

Anyway, although I'm not his biggest fan, I will go in with a positive mental attitude and check in later.

So, it was a much more productive meeting with the physiotherapist who explained he had tried to call me twice to arrange the blood tests. He thinks the tests will either confirm or eliminate his prognosis based on what he observed about my case. I am not convinced, but he told me he is the expert, and I will give him the benefit of the doubt.

True to form, I did relay to him that I felt he didn't listen to me during our last session as well as the fact I felt any progress built up had stalled.

Because I felt like I was banging my head against a brick wall, I took matters into my own hands and hired a sports massage therapist.

Anyway, blood tests to determine inflammatory markers have been booked for next Monday, the results of which will be forwarded to the physiotherapist. Then, if need be, he can refer me back to a rheumatologist and continue physio at the same time. If I don't have these inflammatory markers in my blood, then he will devise a strict physiotherapy treatment plan based around the mechanics in my neck and spine.

I really can't be bothered with food today, but Jon must have a proper meal. So, I prioritised his wants and needs, but tailored the meal to something I would eat, if need be. Cooking it, I already know I don't want it. But it's either this or run to the shop and stock up on chocolate.

DINNER: Crinkle Cut Chips cooked in the air fryer: No idea on Syns (I ate about 3 of them).

10 x 100% fillet fish fingers: 12 Syns (6 eaten, the rest shared out between the dogs).

1 x small tin of marrowfat peas: Syn Free (I ate a couple of spoonsful).

6 x bags of prawn flavoured Skips: 21 Syns (No problem eating these).
Family sized Aero. 9½ Syns (Wolfed it down like my life depended on it).
And I know that won't stop there...
Syns: Through the roof and way off plan.

Because I barely ate any of the 'normal' food, I found the excuse to go to the shop and buy my typical cravings—it's so easy to convince myself off plan.

I wasn't at all hungry for obvious reasons, but no amount of trying to talk myself out of it worked. When it comes to sweets, crisps, etc, I am a bottomless pit, and as you have read above, proper food is hit and miss.

As per usual, I cooked far too much and threw the majority of it in the bin, which is unforgiveable, especially when there are people in this world who are starving or struggling to feed their families.

February 24
WEIGH-IN DAY

I'm not going because I can't face the shame of the scales. I know I need that kick up the bum to motivate me back to plan, and I also know weighing in is the only thing that can push me back on track.

No matter how hard I try to convince myself to go, I don't.

Go...

But...

It won't be that bad...

Later tonight, when I am in the throes of overeating, I will regret my decision. This is part of the constant circular battle I have with myself.

Logic speaks to me to do the right thing, and how to do it, but the illogical defiant, petulant side of me overpowers good sense and reasoning. When I am at this stage, no amount of talking to myself will convince me otherwise.

I should have gone to weigh-in.

February 27

It's a brand-new week, and after another crazy weekend of stuffing my face. I happily welcome a new week. Whatever damage binge eating did will reveal itself come Friday. Whatever the result, I didn't dare count the Syns.

Time to re-focus.

I've got an appointment for blood tests at Clatterbridge Hospital today.

Not keen on being faffed over, I am already thinking of how I can get out of it. "I can't be arsed going today, so I might reschedule."

"You've got to, Marco," Jon snapped.

"I hate needles."

"I know, but once it's done, it's done."

I hate it when he is the voice of reason.

Apparently, they will be looking for inflammatory and tumour markers alongside other things.

My therapist spoke in riddles, so I really didn't understand the hints he left for me to uncover, not that I took much notice anyway having seen far too many doctors and other medical professionals over the last couple of years.

Am I that typical man that who thinks he is invincible?

I think I have elements of that within me, not to mention absolute stubbornness and refusal to listen to anyone. It is my worst failing; I don't always know best.

Skirting about the issue and speaking in medical jargon I don't understand is never appreciated—say it or shut up!

What I did get was this; six separate tests have been requested. I'm dreading it because I am terrified of needles. Despite a full sleeve tattoo and various others dotted around my body the doctor's needles make me quake in my loafers.

I needn't have worried. The blood test didn't hurt, and the nurse was an angel. Just a small prick as the actress said to the bishop, and it was done. In all honesty, I'm certain that enough blood was taken to resurrect Dracula.

Now, the wait begins for the results.

February 28

I am as far off plan as I can get and am trying to talk myself back onto it. Little success has been had toward righting the ship.

What am I going to do?

I know I need to knock some sense into myself, but I don't know where to start. Maybe I can't do this alone as I thought I could. Perhaps I need to be surrounded by others fighting this same, annoying, tedious and mind-bending battle. So, I am toying with the idea of staying for class, but I am shy by nature, which isn't the only reason that stops me. Being too close to others after the pandemic is a factor, more for Jon than me. But the main reason is working on this book—I know there are people who stay for class that share their stories. I don't want to be influenced, nor would I like any of them to pick it up and think I had stolen parts of their life.

What I have done is drawn up a plan from Monday for the gym. A way to get myself back onto plan. I cannot put all the weight back on that I've worked so hard to lose.

- Treadmill—way back when, I used to burn off 1,000 calories per session.
- Exercise Bike—keen to give this a go.
- Weights—if somebody shows me how to use them, it will help tone my body as I lose weight.

Plans aside, I am really fed up with myself. No amount of chastising helps, and the truth of the matter boils down to my mantra; I AM ONLY HUMAN. I have probably said this a hundred times already, and if I haven't, I am certain that I will. Forgive me! But, while my humanity is a biological fact, I am a good person, with flaws, and those flaws cause riots, and oftentimes, war, within me. My size doesn't negate my heart, or many of my other qualities, and if I asked a handful of my friends, the outer package doesn't matter, and they truly accept me for me. However, I cannot accept me right now.

DAVE'S STORY

Sometimes, life gets in the way, and best laid plans fall to the wayside. Still, I was eager to sit down and get to know Dave a little better than the odd hello, and quick chat, at our weigh-in, and although it has taken quite a while, the stars finally aligned.

At fifty-two, recently divorced, and now single, father of one, Dave knows the struggle. He's been fighting it for most of his life, certainly from high school age... those delicate years where identities are forged and mean the most—carrying extra weight in an environment where other children can be cruel left its mark. "I've been big as far back as I can remember, certainly starting high school for sure. But I was chubby at primary school. I've never been skinny apart from when I got to my target."

Standing tall at six-foot-six, with a booming voice, most would see Dave as an imposing figure—true, but when all is said and done, he projects as incredibly intelligent, wise, kind, empathetic, self-aware—very much the gentle giant.

As a self-employed Housing and Tenants Advisor, he spends his days helping others.

That aside, he remains utterly devoted to his six-and-a-half-year-old daughter, Audrey—when she is good, in her doting father's eyes, she draws comparisons to the famed *My Fair Lady* actress, Audrey Hepburn, but when she isn't so angelic, Audrey II from wacky musical, *Little Shop of Horrors*. He speaks of her with a glint in his eye, but whatever the reason, she is his entire world, and that is plain to see.

We discuss the birth of Dave's weight issues, and while he emphasises no blame sits at any one person's door, his father, now ninety, born in 1934, lived through World War Two and through six years of horror.

As a broken world took its first steps towards a lasting peace, years of rationing, when food was scarce, came into force, and neither a cold, nor hot meal was guaranteed. Finding success in his chosen career, and with no financial worries, money ceased to be an issue for Dave's family, so an abundance of food was pushed his way—for those reading this, we can understand the reasoning and might have thought along the same lines, that living with the memory of having little to no food, he didn't want his child to suffer as he had.

"... because my dad was a child of the war and he lived through rationing, and then he became quite successful and wealthy, but don't forget that he had lived through almost famine... regardless, the feast and famine mentality kicks in when you've suddenly got the money, so every day for tea was meat, two veg and dessert, and he had the means to pay for it. Deep down in his psyche, he didn't know when the next famine would come."

It's understandable, after living through war and then watching the world rebuild itself.

"Rationing carried on well into the fifties, so it was through his childhood and youth, and he worked hard to become successful. When we got in from school it was a snack first and then dinner. Because dad worked long hours we had a later dinner."

Did his father struggle to keep his weight under control.

"Not really. But my dad was, and is a big guy, but nowhere near my sort of weight. He is six foot and is very hunched over now, but he was probably about nineteen stone and carried it well. He and my aunty were big, but my mum was very, very slim. She died when I was seventeen and never had weight problems."

Jumping forward, where and when did his weight loss journey begin?

"I joined *Slimming World* in 2013 and have been at this same class with Donna ever since. I couldn't leave, and I couldn't go to anyone but Donna anyway. I'm 28 stone now and weighing-in keeps me in check a little bit. Some weeks it's up, and some weeks it's down. If I hadn't kept coming back, I probably wouldn't be here now. I would put so much weight on, it would have been worse."

At his heaviest, Dave was approximately 32 stone, and at his lightest was 17 stone, 3 pounds.

"At my lowest I looked thin, but people got used to it. Saying that, even at my slimmest, I still felt overweight. Even with a loss, I think, that's good, but I still weigh this much."

I think those of us who have gained a lot of weight, and lost it, always see ourselves larger than we actually are, even if others don't.

"Right now, I wear a 5XL top and my waist is 52. The smallest top size I was in was 2XL, because I am broad. Doesn't matter about the front. My waist at lowest was 38 to 40 inches... I took pleasure in going to Tesco and buying something from there. It used to be High & Mighty, but it is so expensive and old fashioned. Then I went to Jacamo and I never, ever looked like Andrew Flintoff but at least you could buy the bigger size."

What is Dave's dream weight?

"I would like to be... about 16 stone."

We discuss what weight Dave should be according to the BMI scales.

"Between eleven, and eleven-and-a-half stone. It's absolutely ridiculous to think of myself as 11 stone."

Looking at Dave across the table, even I can see that such a low weight, especially for a man with his height and build, he would look gaunt. Like the rest of us, he has to be happy with what he sees in the mirror, and if that is outside of the BMI guidelines, so be it.

What food type is Dave's not-so-guilty pleasure?

"My major food downfall is pizza, any pizza."

Anything else?

"I'm more of a savoury person, so in terms of snacks, crisps, cheese and crackers. I do try and avoid bread, especially Tiger bread. I could go through a whole Tiger loaf in a day. That, or a cheese sandwich, any cheese, all cheese. I was on a Royal Caribbean Cruise once, and I discovered apple pie with a slice of cheddar cheese on top of it. It is absolutely gorgeous, because apple and cheese go together. It was actually on the dessert menu, and me being me, I'm the sort of person that if I see something I've never tried, I want to try it."

Where is Dave's mindset right now?

"At the moment, as soon as I open my eyes, I want to eat but I don't. I don't eat breakfast at the moment, and only sporadically. Lunch depends on how busy I am. Dinner would most often be a *Slimming World* meal—I hate cooking, so it's easier for me."

How does Dave view food?

"Food is my comfort and my addiction."

But like most of us, food can be our best friend and worst enemy—there is a fine line, and even that can be smudged at times.

Has there been any weight-related health issues?

"No official health implications. Losing weight helps me walk further but when I am heavier, I struggle with my knees. I haven't had any other problems yet... I am waiting for them. This might be part of my problem, but it never seems to have any effect on my health at all. And the other thing is, for instance, I've got to be at the weight I am for people to think I am overweight. Nobody turned around and saw me as overweight at 23 stone—they thought I was 17stone. I don't think anybody would look at me now and see 28 stone."

When does Dave think he will reach that point where he says, enough is enough?

"Well, I will be completely honest and admit I am only at that point now."

How have various weight issues over the years affected Dave's confidence—sitting with him now, I see no hint of shyness, or lack of confidence. But I am well aware of how people perform for others (I do), and there is the fact that we have spoken before this interview, so he isn't chatting to a complete stranger.

"The confidence is a strange one—I'm not confident. I'm very shy, but that doesn't work at my size because I can't hide. And I don't mean just the weight, but the height too. I've got a loud voice... part of putting the weight back on is because of my shyness."

I ask him to break that down, so it is clearer for me and the reader.

"If you are a larger size and you don't particularly fit in, you don't have to join in. So, it is almost my wall, and I've spoken to my consultant... after my nephew died there was covid, then after covid, I split up with my wife and spent a couple of years going through the divorce."

At his lightest, how was life?

"At my lightest I was very happy, and my wall was down. But my wall comes back up and it's not a result of gaining weight—the weight goes on as a result of the wall going up—it is my defence mechanism. People don't try to break down my wall in general because if you don't look right, people don't bother with you. Although I am going to contradict myself. If I go out in Liverpool at this size, guys come up to me, friendly, which they didn't when I was slimmer. But in the mainstay, nights out excluded, it's an easy way to hide. I don't ever try and keep people away, but I think it's almost making sure that the people who do approach me, they do want to know me, because it's not going to be casual. I'm very open and friendly, but the wall is almost a filter—if you don't think I'm good enough because I'm heavy, I don't want to know. I actually think there is so much behind my weight issues. I think part of mine is self-abuse because I don't feel that I am worthy."

Where does Dave feel comfortable to open up?

"I am shy everywhere aside from *Slimming World* and that is thanks to Donna and Shelly."

He admits to shying away from most people.

"It's difficult for people to get through to me. They can if they want to, but I never make the first move."

As previously mentioned, Dave is recently divorced, and while not wishing to pry into the specifics, I am interested in the dynamic between him and his ex-wife. Did addiction to food play any part in their separation. Did his ex-wife have her own weight problems to deal with.

"Emma struggled with her weight and joined *Slimming World* the week before me. I agreed to join if the scales went high enough, hoping they weren't."

Did Emma's issues impact you negatively?

"It was the opposite—she was the one who improved my eating habits. She has cerebral palsy and uses a wheelchair, so for her, the lack of exercise affected her weight, and she did absolutely brilliantly, as did I. But then, things hit me, but not her in the same way."

Sadly, things didn't work out between Dave and Emma. Did their shared journey affect the marriage negatively?

"Covid hit and my ex-wife's carer couldn't work, so I became her carer, as well as Aud's main carer. We drifted apart, and a lot of couple's have experienced the same thing—after children come along. I've talked to other dads at school and since the children came along, their relationship became strained too, but as hard as that was and is, I do have a good relationship with my in-laws still. During lockdown, because I had to be at home to take care of my wife and daughter, I was secret eating because that was my pleasure—Emma struggled to understand how I had gone back to old habits because we had done so very well. She was maintaining it. Me being me, I didn't even share with her the mentality behind the secret eating. I was struggling, but she wouldn't see it the way that I did and couldn't understand how it was happening—gaining weight. She didn't know. She did find out at one point and found my secret stash—it was in a high up cupboard in the kitchen that had cookery books in that nobody used."

What was Emma's reaction to that?

"Finding my secret stash, Emma took it as a breakdown of the trust—I didn't feel like I could tell her because I knew she would blame herself. It wasn't just that though, it comes back to no matter what other people think of me, I was lucky enough to get married, but it's gone horribly wrong—from my point of view, when we got pregnant it was through IVF, and a lot of hard work, the pregnancy was a lot of hard work for both of us, due to her condition, and me helping her so much due to that condition. I never entertained the idea of children because I didn't think it likely, and the dynamic was different to how I think my ex-wife imagined it. Our daughter has always been a daddy's girl, and my ex-wife struggled with that. We bonded because I was up all night with her as a baby."

His relationship with Audrey is pretty special, and he delights in talking about her. How has becoming a father changed his relationship with food? I wonder about his daughter's relationship with food.

"Audrey doesn't struggle with her weight, and I am more careful with her eating due to my own issues. But she has been to the dentist this week and had three fillings due to eating too many sweets—she hardly eats sweets at mine because I know how society looks at people, especially overweight children. Even as an adult, if you look right, you are going to have a better life than you would if you don't look right. And overweight doesn't look right."

I can't argue that point because he speaks the truth, as far as we see it anyway.

Does Dave cater more to Audrey's tastes, or does he find foods they can both enjoy together?

"When my daughter is with me, half the time, she either wants mashed potato or macaroni cheese, stuff which is okay for her in moderation, but no good for me. It's like I can't do the same thing for the pair of us. She is a fussy eater. She likes mashed potato for breakfast, and I don't have a problem with it. I went on holiday in Japan, and they have the biggest meal for breakfast—breaking the fast. It's not the way we work, but it does make sense. And if I can send her to school full on veg, I am happy to do that."

"Eating in between meals are partly my downfall, and Audrey's leftovers because she does not eat a full portion of anything, and I hate wasting food."

As a devoted father, does his own mortality cross his mind? Is that worry enough for Dave to change habits formed long ago?

"I need to be slimmer because I need to be here for my daughter. That is what is keeping me relatively stable at the moment. She loves swimming, but I'm too embarrassed to go. I didn't run in Aud's sports day because I knew I would come last, and because of the moobs. Next year, I want to run in that race for me, and for the banter with the other dads. So yes, I want to lose weight for her, but I'm not that selfless because I get so much pleasure from seeing her happy and enjoying herself that I enjoy my life and spending as much time as I can with my daughter. For every year that I am here, I only get her for half a year, so the more time I am here, the more time I have with her."

Dave is doing the best that he can, and while he is amazing father, I do feel he needs to place himself higher up that list of priorities too—he needs to be here for Audrey, but he also deserves to live a long, happy life, and actually live it.

What are his plans now that the divorce is out of the way?

"Divorce is finalised, and things are settling down, so when that is done that will be a massive weight off my mind. Then, I'm going to have all the positives of Aud when she is there, but not the negative of dealing with the bad stuff of a relationship ending."

She really is his world, but there are still concerns, not about his abilities as a father, but his physicality and how he is viewed.

"What makes me happy, is seeing her happy. And doing things with her. At the moment, all her friends love me, but as they get older, they are gonna see me as the fat dad."

Does that really matter?

"Part of it is our own perception—it's like, when Donna hugged me when I first started at her group... a couple of years later, I admitted how comfortable I felt—I'm thinking, who is this slim, attractive woman, it could be any woman, giving me a hug... a slim attractive woman is going to think, ugh... now she wasn't thinking that at all but my experienced prejudice because of my past reinforced that. I pretty much project the thoughts of, why would any of these people like me at this size?"

Does he think life is easier for the so-called slimmer, beautiful people?

"I had a previous job in a Head Office, and it was quite clear that the better looking, including smaller sized, were more successful. It didn't matter how well you know the job or how good at it you were, if you look a certain way you get a certain reaction. I am wary, and I wish I wasn't but that's how society is. I'm a pragmatist and a realist, and that is how society is."

He isn't the only person to think these thoughts. Right or wrong, we can only say how it affects us.

"I judge everyone else on who they are, not what they are. But myself and my thoughts of others judging me are on what I look like. I know they don't, but my first instinct is that."

As a single man, what does the future hold?

"Dating, what do you do? When you're going out—either food, or drink at our age. So, even though we can eat healthy no matter what, it's not weight friendly. When I am chatting online, it works really well—I've got a good personality, but when sat opposite... behind the screen, the personality is 100%. They've seen quite nice pictures of the face, close up, but face-to-face the personality doesn't change, but the visual is there. You want to hide certain things about yourself."

I've been there and know all the tricks of uploading pictures to online dating sites.

"I don't want to be by myself for the rest of my life—not being sexist, I think it's more difficult for overweight men to find somebody than an overweight woman would. There are a lot of men out there who like overweight women, not so much the other way around."

I have multiple views on this; when I had girlfriends, I can agree to an extent because those I met didn't seem to mind a bit of timber on a man, but when meeting guys, the pendulum swung the other way, and they wanted thin, unless the guy had a fetish for bigger blokes.

"A woman can't look at me at my size and find me attractive—I wonder if it's a bet that they have approached me."

I could easily try and persuade Dave that the opposite is true, but I would be lying if I didn't say I had those same insecurities.

"Relationships work best if you both think you're lucky to have the other one—why is she talking to me? There's something not right. Not to blow my own trumpet, I have had very attractive girlfriends. But I still don't understand—it's never been instant, but they've gotten to know me. I don't want to be by myself for the rest of my life. I'm happy living by myself and don't want to get re-married. I want someone. We all want someone."

I have no doubt that Dave will find his forever person.

Was there anything in his younger days, aside from his father providing a wealth of food, that he can think of that kickstarted the addiction to food?

"My mum died when I was seventeen and grief didn't form my addiction to food then, but it has done since. Just after I got down to my lowest weight, me and Emma went on a cruise with my dad. We got a call from my brother to say that my twenty-two-year-old nephew had been killed in a car crash on his way to work at Nando's on Easter Monday morning."

How recent was this?

"I was about forty-two when it happened and that really hit me. After my nephew died, eating was my comfort, but it wasn't immediate, almost gradual slipping back to old habits. My nephew, Johnny, was twenty-two and there were four hundred people at his funeral, and you think to yourself, if something like that can happen to someone like him, then what is the plan because if I'm honest, part of me thought it should have happened to me not him. I never build myself up. I will always put myself down. And it was like, he has clearly got so much to give, and he has been taken. I don't feel like I've got that much to give and I'm still here, so what is the point? It shouldn't be them; it should be somebody else. It's even more when it's somebody who is young because life is not supposed to work that way. Parents are not supposed to bury their children. I don't know how I would cope if anything happened to Aud."

Does Dave believe he is addicted to food?

"Probably pretty much everyone in this book has the addiction gene, and it's that gene which has caused my addiction to food. If not food, it would be something else. Going back, I worked at Littlewoods, and one of my best friends was a Muslim girl. And Ramadan was approaching. I gave it a go. And for somebody addicted to food, going a month without eating during daylight hours was tough. But when I had something positive to talk about, or going on, food generally takes a back seat. I still have it as celebratory, then it's back to the back seat. When I was ten, we were on holiday in Hong Kong because my dad was working there, and I had a pint of lager, and it didn't affect me at all. I can take or leave drink, and I can drink a lot if I want to. Did nothing for me. There is something that makes that certain thing your addiction, drink wasn't it, but food was. If we all had bog standard lives, we wouldn't be overweight, it's pointing out that these are the facts behind it. And maybe if people had been through it, they would have these same issues."

Where does Dave want to be this time next year?

"I focus on the reality that there is still a long way to go, but I'd like to be happy. I still want the same relationship with Aud. I also want to have a better relationship with me because at the end of the day, your weight and size aren't the only defining aspect of your life. I want to like me, and to see myself as my daughter sees me—the best thing since sliced bread. I want to like myself in twelve months and be well on the way to getting back to the weight I want to be. I won't be there because it's too much to lose in that space of time, but I want to be happy with myself. I don't care about anyone else. I want to be happy with myself."

Chatting with Dave has been a pleasure—he really is a thoroughly decent guy, not to mention a cracking dad to Audrey—the role he cherishes most.

Like most of us walking this seemingly endless road, he is far too hard on himself, but a lifetime of negative thinking can take another lifetime to shake off.

He deserves nothing but the best, and I wish him well on the next stage of his journey.

MY JOURNEY - MARCH 2023

March 2

I received a call from the doctor at Clatterbridge Hospital today.
"Five of your blood test results have come back clear from inflammatory markers."
"Thank goodness." I breathed a sigh of relief.
"The final one is more complicated so will take longer."
"Okay. Well, fingers crossed that one comes back clear as well."
"If all come back clear, and with no signs of inflammation or tumour, the physiotherapist can devise a treatment plan to help combat the condition with your neck."
Knowing one final hurdle stands in my way is exasperating, but I am at the mercy of this final test and must wait it out. But if this is clear too, I am hoping the physiotherapist begins his treatment in earnest. Physical fitness means everything to me, and regaining this will bring back an element of freedom that has been missing from my life for far too long.

March 4

I met up with my friend, Sandie, at 9 am and journeyed to Chester, for the first time in about twelve years. It was lovely catching up with her again, but the day once again highlighted how excess weight, Fibromyalgia, and a myriad of other medical ailments have rendered me an unfit slob, incapable even for a simple day out shopping. Add in new-ish trainers that I've only worn about three times that crushed my toes, and I spent too much time sitting down, on top of the copious mugs of tea, hot chocolate, lunch, and Victoria sponge breaks.
I struggled to do it, but refused to give in.
Arriving home around 3:15 pm, I sat on the sofa and actually fell asleep for about twenty minutes. I woke up with a start because my contact lenses suctioned to my eye—a little something forgotten when I drifted off. After feeding the dogs and cat, I shuffled upstairs to watch *Star Trek: Picard*, lay on

my bed and fell asleep until 7 pm. I was exhausted, wiped out, whatever you want to call it. But on top of that I was sad, hoping this was not how life was going to be going forward.

Is this my life now?
It can't be, and I won't let it.

March 5 & 6

Still in agony from my recent trip to Chester, I forced myself out of bed and walked to the gym for an induction on the cardio machines. Only a fifteen-minute journey at most on foot, I had to re-take control because while I could do nothing to cure Fibromyalgia, or rid myself of it, I could do something about my weight, therefore lessening its terrible hold on my body.

I feel like an old man.

Exercise done, I spent the rest of the day in bed, enjoying an early night. I woke up earlier than usual with every intention of going to the gym. Until I looked out of the window at the howling wind and rain.

"Stuff that," I said.

I really can't handle the cold. So, I didn't go, which disappoints me. But I did get back on plan, so the day wasn't a complete disaster. And I didn't sit about idle thinking about cake. Instead, I worked on a few books, but also looked through a book that a friend has been writing. I didn't think much of it—in fact, I found myself skipping parts because I became bored. That took up a lot of my day before I closed my PC down so I could sort dinner.

> Breakfast was bananas, strawberries, black grapes, tropical granola, and fat free natural yoghurt (5½ Syns), while lunch was skipped because I wasn't hungry.
>
> Dinner was a fancier affair, consisting of carrot, turnip, and fry light roast potatoes, Paxo stuffing (1½ Syns), onion and mushroom gravy (1½ Syns)

Total Syns: 8.

After dinner, I cleaned the kitchen then went back to writing. I have days like this—I can write for hours, until my bum is numb, and my fingers are sore, then nothing for weeks. Being in this mood keeps my mind focused, and off chocolate.

MARCO LEWIS

March 7

I woke up this morning and looked out of the window to clear, bright blue skies, which meant I finally found my way to the gym. Put out the bunting...

Arriving out of breath, I know it will get easier.

Truthfully, I was amazed I'd got there because I had to talk myself into going. Eventually, I did it, pleased that there were only about four people working out around me.

"Where is the locker room?"

The attendant remained silent and pointed to the back of the gym, which meant I had to walk past the area where the weightlifters usually congregated. I still had no idea where the locker room was situated.

Rude.

Thankfully, it was empty. Knowing myself well enough, its location will be an issue when the place is packed out. Already, I hate the idea that these muscle gods will laugh when they see me wobbling past.

Nothing to worry about today, apart from the fact I'd forgotten to bring my bottle of water.

I have been advised by my GP, physiotherapist, and sports massage therapist to start off slowly, and build up to a level that my body can tolerate.

So, that is exactly what I did, spending 30 minutes on the treadmill. I enjoyed it, switching intensity levels and inclines various times throughout. I huffed and puffed like a clapped-out old banger, but I felt better for it. My heart rate was well up, and sweat dripped off me, which apparently means that whatever I was doing was working.

The guy on the machine next to me could have been training for the London Marathon, while I plodded along beside him. But some exercise was better than none. I might get to a point where I can run again... I'd love that to be the case. But for a first time, it was an admirable effort, and I managed to burn 131.9 calories.

Next up was the exercise bike. I only managed fifteen minutes. I struggled with this from the first minute and lowered the intensity level. I used muscles I haven't given attention to in a long time. Listening to my body, I knew I'd had enough but my legs didn't hurt anywhere near as much as they had when I first started pedalling. I burned 73.2 calories, giving me a total of 205.1 for the session with 45 minutes of exercise time.

By the time I finished, sweat rolled off me, but I'm thrilled with my effort. Even with such a short, low intensity workout, I knew my body wasn't happy. But I will do as the experts advised and build myself up slowly and hope to increase the duration of my workout and calories burned week on week.

Fibromyalgia and my other ailments mean I'm never going to become the next Sir Mo Farah. But slowly, slowly catchy monkey is the order of the day—in other words, I might take longer to get to where I want to be, but less haste means I will eventually get there.

Not bad for a first session, and tomorrow I shall try and increase the minutes.

I told myself that walking into the gym was my first win, so staying and exercising was a bonus.

The people seemed welcoming enough. I'm not in my comfort zone, yet, and never at ease when surrounded by the so-called beautiful people. They make me feel less than I am. I needn't have worried because the only attention I got was from an older Chinese lady wearing what looked a fluffy brown toilet roll holder on her head.

As well as the gym, I need to start using my weighted hula hoop again but might wait until the weather is nicer, so I can take it outside. I have used it indoors, but the first time wasn't a success as I knocked the candle off the table, sending it flying across the room. But only last week, my cousin, Nicola, used hers for the first time and the weighted ball snapped off and crashed into her television screen, leaving a ball shaped hole in it. Of course, I laughed, but I won't tempt fate by using mine indoors.

I walked home and prepared food.

Once again, breakfast was bananas, strawberries, black Grapes, tropical granola, and fat free natural Yoghurt (5½ Syns), and tonight's planned meal is Syn Free chicken curry and rice. As I've said before, I am not a fan of curry at all, but this recipe doesn't have that sickly taste I dislike so much, so it is tolerable.

March 8

I had a dreadful night's sleep and woke up in agony. It's apparent that what I did at the gym yesterday, which wasn't a lot, was too much. So, I couldn't go today, but am miserable that after only one session, my body waged war on me.

Even though my arms are sore, and I feel like I've been kicked in the back, I refuse to give up and plan another session tomorrow.

Despite the pain and my body in revolt, I cooked and stuck to plan.

I'm a creature of habit so it was bananas, strawberries, black grapes, tropical granola, and fat free natural yoghurt (5½ Syns) for breakfast.

Lunch was skipped because I wasn't hungry, and dinner was 4 x slices of Hovis bread (5 Syns), minced beef and onion (1 Syn), fry light roast potatoes (Syn Free), carrots and peas (Syn Free).

I walked the dogs after dinner. Then I sat at my desk to do some much-needed work on my new crime fiction book.

March 9

After another night of disturbed sleep, I woke up in agony, knowing the gym was not happening again. I hate that I am not fit enough to go, but I have to listen to my body.

So rather than loll about in bed, I got up and went downstairs intending to find something productive to do. Perhaps tidy the garden ready for Spring. I opened the back door to a blanket of deep snow and was instantly relieved that I couldn't go to the gym. I'm not a fan of walking anywhere in the snow, especially when it turns to ice. I live in fear of falling over in public.

It's weigh-in day tomorrow, so I am aiming to get up at 8 am and go before I face the scales. It might help shift a few of the pounds I know I have put on.

However, I can't avoid the snow completely today as I have an appointment to see my sports massage therapist at four thirty this afternoon. I was tempted to cancel, but as my lower back is now giving me trouble, the timing couldn't be more perfect.

Am I falling apart?

Although I don't have the hunger hormone to spur me to eat, I already know I don't feel like food, so as I type this at 1 pm, nothing has passed my lips, aside from water.

I arrived for my sports massage, and spoke to Ian, advising that my neck had felt a lot less stiff and restricted, but that I'd had a sore back on my lower left side, and that there was a throbbing in my left bum cheek (gluteus maximus as he referred to it—who knew—I always thought he was a character from the Gladiator movie).

He went to work straight away.

During these sessions, I am usually naked from the waist up, but I have learned not to worry about it where Ian is concerned because he sees my body as a doctor does, like a piece of meat, and is not affected or offended by the sight of an overweight person.

The ambience in the room is one of relaxation and calm, helped by the music playing in the background—this time, *Eternal Flame* by The Bangles and

It's a Sin by the Pet Shop Boys, followed by countless 80's classics. As a child of this fabulous decade, it's always a thumbs up from me.

As he worked on a previously unexplored part of my body, I had to pull my gym leggings down past my backside, while he massaged this area. Having my bum cheek massaged and pounded vigorously, he even used his elbows, admittedly a first for me, I found it relaxing enough and was on the brink of drifting off until I heard a strange sound—*pop pop*—I opened my eyes, wondering what the noise was.

"What was that?"

"What was what?"

Then I realised it wasn't a sound per se. The *pop pop* was my backside waking up during the rigorous massage. Mortifyingly, I'd passed wind... I wanted the ground to swallow me whole.

"Oh, nothing, I thought I heard something."

"I didn't hear anything." Either my bottom burp was drowned out by Europe's *The Final Countdown,* or he was ultra discreet. I'm certain it's the latter.

So, I closed my eyes again and drifted off.

I experienced a weightlessness and felt calmer than I've felt in weeks. I fell asleep. For my therapist, this was seen as the ultimate compliment; that I was so relaxed I let myself go.

My back felt a lot better. After the session, I walked home but noticed the speed and determination in which I made the journey.

I made a quick detour to my local Chinese restaurant. Jon fancied chicken fried rice and curry sauce. Once home, I served his meal, then jumped back on the diet and re-heated the leftovers from the previous night; minced beef and onion (1 Syn), 2 x slices of Hovis bread (HEXB – for breads and cereals). As a creature of habit, and my dislike of having to eat, I really should try other foods before boredom sets in.

Surprisingly, I shovelled down bananas, strawberries, black Grapes, tropical granola, and fat free natural yoghurt (5½ Syns) before bed, washed down with Coke Zero and water.

Total Syns used today = 6½ out of 30. I need to start using my healthy extras.

March 10

WEIGH-IN DAY

I woke up with a sore back, again, and took two anti-inflammatories. Before I set foot out of bed, I knew I wasn't going to chance the gym.

Never trusting weather reports, I looked out of my window, and to my dismay, the weather forecast was spot on. Storm Larisa had arrived and brought the biting winter back with it.

Ugh! As far as the eye could see were blankets of crisp, white snow. Admittedly, it was a pleasant sight to behold, but instantly forgetting the view; how was I going to get to class so I could get weighed?

Cars were not getting in or out of my road, and as my house is halfway up a hill, I considered not going. But I'd been back on plan since the start of the week, and even managed one session at the gym as well as the marathon hike around Chester last Saturday. Eager to know how much I'd piled on, I was determined to get there, so I could get my brain in gear and focus on continued damage limitation.

So, even though I was terrified of falling, I braved the elements. The cold was biting, but I'd slipped into my teddy bear fleece hoodie, not caring that I resembled Bungle from *Rainbow*. I took it slow, and at times felt like I was tip toeing rather than walking. But I made it!

Stepping onto the scales, I warned the lovely lady who's name I need to ask, that I'd been off plan for a while, but had recently gotten back on. I braced myself for the bad news, "Go on, I know I've gained so hit me with it."

I am certain there are times the ladies weighing me, and others are exasperated because we are so hard on ourselves. "You haven't gained—you've stayed the same."

"The same?" I had convinced myself it was going to be a gain, had to be, so hearing anything else took a moment to register. "Really." I hadn't been weighed for three weeks, so this was major news!

"Yes, well done."

"I can't believe it." I stepped down off the scales, overjoyed inside, buoyant even, because getting back on plan had allowed me to regain ground and lessen the damage.

After a quick chat with Donna, I walked home. My frigid steps from the scales back to home changed with a bigger spring and maybe a more confident swagger. I gave myself a pat on the back.

I am adamant that come rain, hail, sleet, snow, or hurricane, I will get to that gym on Monday morning. I want to give my back time to heal, then I will get myself into a regular routine.

I WILL DO THIS!

March 13

After a heavy weekend, and falling off plan, again, I am pain free and back at the gym this morning.

With no appetite, or desire to eat, I tell myself to eat some fruit, my preferred food, at least before setting off. I know what I am doing, and how to look after my body in positive ways. I just wish I could shut out the negative impulses.

The torturous wind and freezing temperatures almost made me turn around, but I persevered, cursing myself all the way for being so stupid as to join in the first place.

Even at this early hour, I soon discovered every locker occupied. I couldn't leave my ruck sack unattended because it had my medication, credit cards, phone, and other items, so I waited twenty minutes. I held to my personal promise, determined not to skip today and head home. Lesson: buy a gym bag and take the bare essentials, then I don't have to worry.

Treadmill Duration: 30 Minutes. The blowing air conditioning caught my attention as it created an arctic air system my way on this already cold day. I ignored its initial taunt as I knew I'd be sweating within minutes and would praise its existence as perspiration soaked through my clothes. My heartrate rose as my steps increased one after another and compared to some of the other people there, catwalk ready, I must have looked a fright. I caught my reflection in the glass and my face glowed a bright red. Still, I calmed my nerves knowing my purpose—work out, as the end game for me had two components. My overall health required I lose weight and get fit, end of story.

Treadmill Calories Burned: 155.2, which is pleasing as it is an increase from last week's 131.9.

Exercise Bike Duration: 25 Minutes. I didn't enjoy this last week and feel that I am stuck on a hamster wheel of routine. I know what I need to do, and what I must do. Working out helps to tone my legs and improve on my overall strength. Still doesn't mean I am not at a point where I wish I was doing anything other than this.

I sat down and placed my feet on the pedals, got comfy, and pumped my legs at a decent rhythm. After ten minutes, my wondering mind clued me in to the fact I'd left my locker key on the treadmill. A little panicked, I stopped peddling, hopped off the bike, forgetting to photograph my progress, retrieved the key, and started again. I didn't find it as difficult as last week and increased the effort level. A little ego boost in my mind and it felt like a pretty big win.

Exercise Bike Calories Burned: 100.7.

My total exercise time of 55 minutes yielded a calorie burn of 255.9.

The gym overlooks the swimming pool. The little ripples from other swimmers silently invited me to plunge right in, but I wouldn't have the confidence to walk out of the changing rooms with my belly on show, even though I see plenty of people with differing shapes and sizes bobbing about in the water. I'm a people watcher by nature, so I instantly noticed those individuals who never emerged out of the water past their shoulders. I imagined their dash to cover up in a towel before rushing off to the locker rooms once their time elapsed. I knew it's what I'd have done. Maybe after a couple more stone dropped from my frame, I may feel braver. Swimming without shame checked another box on my list of goals. No argument existed that didn't support swimming as a great way to get fit and stay that way. Plus, it put less stress on my joints. And, as mind numbingly tedious as the gym can be, I do get that buzz from it, but also, knowing how it eases the fibro symptoms makes it worthwhile. An hour pain-free makes all the difference to my day.

Back home after today's success, breakfast should be on my mind. Not too surprised that hunger evaded me. I asked Jon if he fancied a cheese and onion omelette with bacon, but he admitted his stomach didn't call to him either. So, that suited me; if he wasn't having anything, neither would I.

On the menu tonight for Jon, after missing breakfast and lunch, was sausage, onion, and mushroom casserole with mashed potatoes and garden peas. Nothing would ever convince me to eat that, and as I couldn't face food anyway, I gladly ate nothing.

Admittedly, skipping food and meals has become a terrible habit. I am burning calories, but not refuelling my body as it needs. Being healthy is *not* about being thin and looking good in a new pair of jeans.

I have a duty of care to my entire self, both inside and out. There is little point looking good if everything on the inside wages a war.

March 14

I woke up this morning and before I'd managed to get out of bed, I'd thought up countless excuses not to go to the gym.

Too tired.

Too sore.

Can't be bothered.

I finally wrestled with my conscience, silenced my inner saboteur, and walked there. During the walk, and battling the gale force wind, I argued with myself. On one shoulder sat the Devil of terrible moods haunting me while the angel reminded me how great yesterday boosted my ego. Thankfully, with my inner self warring its own battle, the gym appeared fairly empty this morning.

Thirty minutes I spent on the treadmill and in all honesty, I really struggled with this today. Though I wanted to beat yesterday's target, I quickly realised today a new goal couldn't be met. I tried various speeds, and inclines, high and low, but my body refused to play ball. I did manage to do the full thirty minutes, but relief struck me when the machine slowed to a stop. Still, I managed to burn 135.9 calories, which is less than yesterday's 155.2.

I fared a little better on the exercise bike. Completing thirty minutes, I think I've found my groove because I can sit down and rest my back as I peddle. At times the stationary aspect bores me, but I found the time passed by relatively quickly. I watched the swimmers in the pool below and was surprised to complete the full thirty minutes and even upped the intensity level to 10. My legs fought me a bit and with heavy pushes it felt more like I needed to move a truck than push a simple pedal. I couldn't keep up such high intensity for the whole workout. I did what I could and hopefully my efforts helped build up the strength in my legs. This might be the way forward for me cardio wise, especially when fibro flares up.

Distance cycled was 5.57 miles, burning 185.7 calories. I was so surprised by the result because if you told me that I had to walk five plus miles, I'd laugh and refuse. The hour spent there was painless and necessary. I managed to burn 321.6 calories.

Not in the mood to eat, I diverted to Tesco's on the way home and picked up supplies because Jon does like to eat.

Brunch was bananas, strawberries, black grapes, mango, tropical granola, and fat free natural yoghurt (5½ Syns).

Dinner was a healthy option; chicken and vegetable orzo (Syn Free), 5 x sunflower oil sprays (½ Syn).

In-Betweens were not so healthy; 3 x bags of Quavers (16½ Syns), Diet Pepsi, water.

Total Syns: 22½.

March 15

I didn't turn the TV off until nearly 4 am, then I awoke at nine to go to the gym, fully recalling the strangest dream.

I rarely dream, and if I do, I tend to only remember the wild and wacky ones.

How funny that real life shapes what we see in our sleep?

Anyway, in my dream, at the gym, I worked out on the exercise bike gazing down at the pool. Young fathers teaching their kids to swim filled the water when suddenly, a loud bang erupted and I catapulted from the bike through the glass, landing in the pool below. Dazed and confused, I looked up and the entire gym area vanished. The place lit up in a mess of debris and carnage; all around me lay bodies of those who survived and those trying to make their way out of the pool.

Is the carnage I witnessed a representation of how I feel inside? I'm no expert on dream analysis, so I can't say for certain.

But the explosion and being catapulted through the glass into the pool wasn't the strangest part. I waded uninjured despite people floating dead around me. I had no concern for those people, only my rucksack which I'd stored in the lockers upstairs. Bizarre I know, but the mind works in strange ways. If anyone can interpret, feel free to message me via *Facebook*. I woke up as I exited the gym with my rucksack over my shoulder, not giving the devastation inside another thought, then headed home.

My thoughts kept re-playing through the dream as I shifted out of bed. I shook my head in an attempt to change the direction and instead found myself back in the loop of the usual struggle of not wanting to go to the gym. The rubbish of the disturbing dream would not overcome my progress, so I decided to walk there. My body ached from the past few days, so I knew the session wasn't going to be as successful as yesterday's.

I avoided the treadmill today and went straight to the exercise bike. I knew I didn't have the strength to stand for any prolonged length of time, so this seemed the ideal solution. Once again to my fortunate surprise, the gym remained relatively empty so the added pressure to rush didn't overwhelm my reticent mood.

I managed twenty-five minutes on the exercise bike and though I struggled, I gave it as much as I could. The intensity level averaged out at 5 throughout. I did increase it at various points but couldn't keep up the pace, so lowered it back to 5 again.

I managed to cycle 4.57 miles and burn 147.6 calories which is lower than yesterday's 185.7. Despite feeling rough, I think I did well.

I'd initially set my program for half an hour but stopped five minutes short. I sat for a few minutes, panting, out of breath, sweating, focusing on regulating my heartbeat. Once I felt calmer, I drank some water, then guilt kicked crept over my shoulder. I told myself I could do more, so went for a second blast.

Then, I managed another 2.09 miles in thirteen minutes with 63.8 calories burned. I gave it my all but knew I'd reached my limit and stopped.

I won't lie and say I wasn't disappointed, but my GP previously warned me about this exact situation. I couldn't push myself too far or too hard. The end result would leave me bedbound for weeks, which would only put me right back to the beginning. I kept telling myself to slow down, but I've never been the most patient person and am easily frustrated with myself.

Today's total is 6.66 miles in 38 minutes, which is up from 5.57. Total calories burned is 249.5.

I came out of the gym and two students from the college opposite walked past me scoffing down Cadbury's Mini Eggs—strange but true, I never had the urge to rush to the shop and buy some. That's progress, but I'm self-aware enough to know that might not be the case tomorrow.

I walked home along the same cinder path I used when I was in primary school. But slower, and steadier than in my younger days. Still, my legs trudged along like lead weights. I didn't push it and had to take a breather quite a few times. My last stop was at the school I went to from the age of four to nine—I stared at the building, remembering how happy those early memories of life made me. My gorgeous and funny best friend, from then, to this day, Sarah, and I, had some magical times within those walls. While the reflection of years long since passed brought back a warmth in my heart of those carefree days, I didn't stand around reminiscing too long in case nosey neighbours reported a man in a fluffy teddy bear hoodie hanging around outside the school gates.

Once home, I ate my breakfast of fresh fruit, tropical granola with natural yoghurt and prepared the vegetables for tonight's dinner.

I tried and failed to ignore the fact my house sat in shambles. I needed to hoover the stairs, landing, and living room, mop throughout, dust, put things away, sort out the shed, de-clutter. It's never-ending and it does need doing. I turned a blind eye, my energy left behind at the gym, while hoping that tomorrow would be a better day.

The chores wouldn't wait forever though as this weekend my mother-in-law planned a visit for Mother's Day. I volunteered to cook, so the house needed to be ship-shape for her arrival, not that she would care if it looked like Stig of the Dump had moved in. But Jon and I were houseproud and would hate to be viewed as messy. If I'd thought it through, I could have booked my cleaner to come. In pain or not, I refused to rely on her, so I asked her to do the jobs I either disliked or couldn't do such as cleaning out the fridge or worse still, the oven. Life is too short to clean an oven and the £15 an hour well spent.

I called the pain management clinic as I had been waiting for an appointment for the last eighteen months. A lovely lady on the other end of the line told me she had not seen my referral in the system, despite my GP showing it to me on the screen during my last visit. I told the lady that I also had a letter from the rheumatology department at Arrowe Park Hospital confirming my Fibromyalgia diagnosis and that he discharged me to pain management services. Very strange, but she assured me she would get to the bottom of it. I hoped so, because standard medication did not ease the pain at all. My body repeatedly told me it was at that point where the consideration for stronger options had become necessary.

Dinner was baby potatoes and Brussel sprouts (Syn Free). I did prepare smoked Haddock and was looking forward to it. To my absolute horror, the first bite presented me with a bone, so I threw it in the bin. If I must eat flesh, it can't resemble an animal, so that means no bones, claws, tails, skin, faces, hooves, or eyes. So, dinner was a damp squib, and I felt unsatisfied and instantly started craving chocolate. I didn't cave which shows what I am capable of when I put my mind to it. In the past I would have given in, but I know that I do have the power to change my own mind, I just have to remember to exert that power.

Later on, I enjoyed two bowls of multi-grain Cheerios (7 Syns for the second bowl) with two servings of milk. Healthy extras used.

It might not have been the best idea, especially after a plate full of sprouts... I might be playing *The Symphony No. 5* out of my backside later, but I swept the board and ate six portions of fruit and vegetables.

Total Syns: 12½.

I am engaged, finding the plan easy, but also encouraged by the power of exercise. I might not have broken any world records this week, but I've done more exercise than I have in years.

That's got to be a good thing, right?

March 17

WEIGH-IN DAY

On plan, but my appetite still evades me. My body groans at the idea of hitting the gym. Whether it is doing me more harm than good continues plaguing my deepest thoughts. I had a restless night as my legs twitched and trembled refusing to stay still. It's one of the more annoying fibro symptoms, and when it starts, it drives me bonkers. So, today I gave it a miss, just to allow my body time to settle, but even as I type this I really want to go. I won't give up but would become more attuned to what my body tells me—so, I convince myself on a new plan of gym days every Monday through Thursday, which gives me three days of allowing my body to recover. I am not going to worry so much about targets and will do only what I can do without wiping myself out.

Gym issue settled, today brought about new mental struggles. *I really don't want to do anything or see anyone.* I cancelled my dentist appointment because the thought of having a stranger's fingers in my mouth rolled my stomach. If truth be told, I'd rather have an operation than visit the dentist, and this phobia has existed since childhood when Dr Gent (Nickname 'The Butcher' by my aunty Terri) climbed on top of me to extract a tooth. I've hated dentists ever since, not least because they always insist on engaging me in conversation when they've stuffed my mouth of latex-coated fingers and stainless-steel instruments.

Weigh-in didn't happen, and not because I hid away, but because my muscles ached from head to toe, and the short five-to-ten-minute walk to group overwhelmed my protesting body.

Serious cravings for *Jacob's Cornish Wafers* with cheddar cheese, pickled onions, and chutney ramped up within my desires, but my new mindset and strength from several weeks of successfully executing the plan had me resisting temptation. It would push me way over my Syn allowance for the week. Thank goodness for the sliver of logical determination left in the back of my mind.

March 20

Ever heard the phrase, going hell for leather? Yes, well, that's me. *Ugh!*

I gorged as though eating food was coming into prohibition, and all the wrong kinds. One success for the day came when I cleaned the house and even hired a *Rug Doctor* to scrub the living room carpet, rug, stairs, landing, and my office carpet. I was knackered and will never use one of those contraptions ever again because my hallway resembled a paddling pool. My arms ache, but I'm thrilled this chore can be checked off my list of things to do.

Tidy house. Tidy mind. Body in revolt.

From Friday to this morning, I ate 15 Cadbury's Crème Eggs (135 Syns), 12 bags of assorted Monster Munch (66 Syns), a whole box of Pink & Whites (22½ Syns), 8 Scones (No idea on Syns), 10 McDonalds Chicken Nuggets (15 Syns), and so much more that I cannot truthfully list everything.

What am I doing?

Having fun, yes.

Piling weight on, definitely!

Breakfast was skipped again, while lunch was cheese on toast (Syns = your guess is as good as mine). Dinner was minced beef and onion (1½ Syns). In-Betweens, I went crazy; Cadbury's Crème Eggs (18 Syns), a bag of liquorice (No idea on Syns), 2 x family sized Roast Beef Monster Munch (11 Syns), Tropical Skittles, and I don't think that was everything, or all Syns accounted for.

This rollercoaster of guilt remains never-ending and mentally exhausting. The amount of space taken up in my brain with the constant thought of what to eat, what not to eat, admonishing myself when I fall off plan, but still beating myself to death when I do stick to plan. It's an ugly cycle.

Right now, I swing on a fragile pendulum, swaying from a state of normal to a state of absolute chaos. There seems to be no happy medium.

Not knowing where I currently stand weight wise doesn't help either.

My inner saboteur works overtime steepling his fingers, planning devious ways for derailing my progress.

March 21

I woke with the lark, and brilliant blue skies with no sign of rain. With trainers tied and my bag packed the time came to head back to the gym. I won't lie; I am in pain, my fibro is currently engaged in an active spurt, but it feels good to regain an element of control in my life.

Exercise Bike Duration: 26 Minutes. I started on this today, and quickly found my rhythm, increasing the effort level up to a personal high of 13, before lowering it to a steadier 5. Calories burned clocks in at 158.3.

Distance: 5.04 miles.

Treadmill Duration: 16 Minutes. Although I was proof-listening, and loving, the audiobook of my very first co-write with Netta, *DI Dylan Monroe Investigates: One - Avaline Saddlebags*, I was quickly bored with this type of exercise and couldn't wait to get off. Calories burned: 55.9. Distance: 0.56 miles. This is a piss-poor result, and I do need to make more effort, especially walking on an incline.

Another session on the exercise bike yielded okay results. 26 Minutes. (Again!) I continued listening to the audiobook, and even though I am one of the writers, I found myself laughing because the narrator, Jordan Hale, nailed the characters, especially the waspish drag queen, Betty Swallocks. I had to remind myself that I was in a packed-out gym and people would wonder what had amused me.

Calories Burned: 162.4. Distance: 5.03 miles.

Total exercise time was 1 hour and 8 minutes with 404 calories burned. I imagined this figure to be much less, but it seems to add up nicely, especially when using the exercise bike.

Surprised to note miles covered was 10.63. Yes, I am sitting down on the exercise bike and only seeing the same old view, but it's the exercise that matters. I am going to focus on increasing the miles I am cycling in the hope of building up the strength in my lower body.

I'm going to try and stick to fruit and Syn Free foods as much as possible, and not only because I want to try and claw back, but because bloating has me miserable. The thought of healthy food causes nausea. Jon thinks I am on the verge of giving up all meat and becoming vegan—he could be right although I would miss bacon on the odd occasion. I would survive, but do Cadbury's do vegan Crème Eggs, I wonder?

Breakfast was a healthier choice of bananas, strawberries, black grapes, tropical granola, and fat free natural yoghurt (2½ Syns). Dinner, I completely ballsed up here and went off plan with crispy duck and pancakes from the local Chinese restaurant. I'm too scared to Syn what I ate. I didn't eat all the duck because I'm not big on meat but happily scoffed the rest. There was cucumber and some other grass-like stuff included which I troughed, so that's good, right?

March 22

No amount of rain, hail, sleet, or snow could keep me from the gym today after crashing headfirst into the wall last night by going off plan.

I stuck to plan for my first meal of the day with mushrooms (cooked in Fry Light, so Syn Free), canned tomatoes, scrambled eggs (dash of Milk - HEXA).

I decided to give the treadmill a miss today and focus on the bike. I varied levels from 5 to 10, but averaged level 7. Distance: 5.29 miles in 28 minutes, burning off 176.6 calories.

I had to take a break to adjust my shorts, but also to take a breather. During this second session I watched a show on BBC iPlayer, which helped pass the time. I do find the gym terribly boring sometimes so anything to take my mind away from what I'm doing is a plus.

Exercise Bike Duration: 17 Minutes. (Again!). Calories burned: 98.2. Distance: 3.02 miles.

And another break, this time because sweat was rolling off me.

Exercise Bike Duration: 19 Minutes. I'd had enough of tugging at my clothes so cut this short. Calories burned: 59.2. Distance: 1.84 miles.

Exercise time was 1 hour and 4 minutes with calories burned totalling 334, which is down from 404.

Miles covered is 10.15. This was a little lower than yesterday and though I wanted to hit fifteen miles, I could have done much more. But my chosen shorts were driving me mad, rubbing me in the wrong place and giving me bollock splinters. I have ordered a cup to wear underneath my shorts, so this doesn't happen again. Ten miles is still quite an achievement, so I celebrated with a trip to the local café and spent ninety minutes gossiping with an old friend who happened to be in there at the same time.

I wasn't hungry, so missed lunch. Dinner was canned tomatoes, omelette (Syn Free), 2 x slices of Hovis Nimble toasted bread (HEXB) and 5 x Sunflower Oil Sprays (½ Syn). In-Betweens was a sensible choice of milk (HEXA), bananas, strawberries, black grapes, tropical granola, and fat free natural yoghurt (5½Syns).

I felt better for going to the gym. Fibromyalgia comes with a myriad of problems; painful tender points, deep muscle pain, and fatigue, so exercise isn't the first thought that springs to mind. Nor was it recommended when I was first diagnosed.

Yet, in such a short space of time, the medical world has decided otherwise; maybe just what the doctor ordered.

Whether it's daily walking, stretching, swimming, yoga, tai chi or Pilates, low-impact exercise programs can help keep me fit and may help reduce pain as well.

Personally, the advantages became apparent fairly quickly.

- Burning calories and making weight control easier
- Giving range-of-motion to painful muscles and joints
- Improving my outlook on life
- Improving my quality of sleep
- Improving my sense of well-being
- Increasing my aerobic capacity
- Improving my cardiovascular health
- Increasing my energy
- Stimulating the secretion of endorphins or "happy hormones"
- Strengthening my bones
- Strengthening my muscles
- Relieving constant pain

CHEWING THE FAT

March 23

HAPPY ANNIVERSARY TO US!

Jon and I have been together for 11 years, and while we have had more ups and downs than The Big One at Blackpool Pleasure Beach, we have stuck together because love is love, and when all is said and done, what relationship is perfect?

I adore him, and want to knock him out, most days, in equal measures, but he has been my strength since the day we met, and though we are as different as chalk and cheese, he guards my heart.

So, to begin my special day, the gym beckons, and even though it's pouring down outside, I decide it best I shuffle my way there.

Exercise Bike Duration: 30 Minutes. I varied levels from 5 to 13, but averaged level 7. Calories burned: 190.8.

In the absence of bollock protection, I had to take a break to adjust my shorts, but also to take a breather.

Exercise Bike Duration: 14 Minutes. Calories burned: 78.6. Distance: 2.45 miles.

Sweat poured out of me—gross, stopping me in my tracks. But I won't be beaten.

Exercise Bike Duration: 18 Minutes. I'd had enough of tugging at my clothes so cut this short. Calories burned: 100.2. Distance: 3.17 miles.

Total exercise time was 1 hour and 2 minutes with 369.6 calories burned, which is a slight improvement from 334.

Miles covered was 11.32. I wanted to try for fifteen, but I was exhausted. I am thrilled with my progress, especially as I have cycled 32.1 miles since Monday.

Still, my day is nowhere near over.

More writing today from 12:30 pm to 2 pm, and we've finished the new book, *Act of Contrition*—exciting! Now we have one more read through from start to finish before sending it out to beta readers, who will scour it for spelling errors and storyline blips.

Had another Sports Massage session at 4:30 pm, and my body is protesting even as I type this.

Breakfast was Cheerios, semi-skimmed milk. Healthy extras used. I skipped lunch and ate popcorn chicken (13 Syns) for dinner. In-betweens; 54g bag of Quavers (14½ Syns – Crikey!), Diet Pepsi, water.

March 24
WEIGH-IN DAY.

After a disturbed sleep, because the sports massage left my muscles screaming, I awakened before my alarm which rarely happens.

I got straight to my morning routine, teeth, hair, lenses in, then to the toilet, trying to expel as much as I could. Weigh-in day, and typically so, my body refused to rid itself which didn't bode well for my arch nemesis—the scale.

My heart pounded heavy within my chest, knowing not a pound would be shed—just my luck!

So, rather than dither until the 11 am class, I decided to face the music anyway and attended the earlier one.

I walked slowly to class and for the first time in a few weeks, felt stiff and doddery. The reluctant pace mirrored my anxiety bouncing around like a tennis ball escaping from the menacing beating from the rackets. I danced around on the scales in the same way, trying every which way to avoid one step upon the evil traitor.

My eyes blinked rapidly at the unexpected sight before them—2 pounds OFF.

I'm really chuffed with this loss because of the fifteen crème eggs I scoffed. And yes, I know I have hammered it at the gym, but nothing pointed my untrusting mind to believe a loss might be on the cards for me. This surprise brightened the start of my day.

Suddenly, the possibility existed that I could make a bigger dent because summer loomed close behind.

Jon and I planned an outing to the Refreshment Rooms for a belated anniversary celebration lunch. Decisions plagued my thoughts after the scales tipped my direction earlier.

Do I throw caution to the wind and have cake, or knuckle down?

Only time would tell.

March 27

Some good news happened this morning as I received an appointment from pain management services. It seems the mistake was on their end, and they hadn't acted on the referral, so they booked me an appointment in May. At least I don't have to go to the bottom of the list, and with a bit of luck, they will be able to prescribe things my GP can't.

I started the day with my usual fruit and natural yoghurt, then head for the gym, thrilled by the change to the shape of my legs—less chunky and more defined. Vain, yes, but that alone makes these gym sessions worthwhile, especially after a struggle-free roam around town for three hours on Saturday. The miles I am covering on the exercise bike must be strengthening them. I am pleased with myself which sets me up for a great workout.

Total exercise time today was 57 Minutes. Calories burned was 369.7.

I wanted to do more but refused to overdo it and set myself up to fail once more. There is nothing wrong with building up slowly. My end goal is to cycle fifteen miles per day. Oddly, I leave without a guilty conscience and that's a small win.

Dinner was Quorn Bolognese (2 Syns), but I was stuffed after eating this. I'm not really a fan of pasta, but I did enjoy the sauce, although I did overserve myself.

My brother was kind enough to come and fit my six new garden lights—I've had them for ages but am useless with anything DIY related. Summer is looming, and I'm reminded that I want to look my best.

After he left, I faced the spider-cluttered out-building and proceeded to paint the trellis ready for the Jasmine to be planted. Already five pm, I could have picked a better time. It was only due to fading light that I stopped, but I did manage to touch up a few other parts of the fence as well.

Pleased with the progress, I walked around the garden a few times once the sun slid over the horizon, watching as each light popped on and illuminated my garden. I can't wait for the warmer nights when I can sit out here with the music on and fire pit lit.

March 28

I opened my eyes and wished I hadn't.

The sky poured down fat, cold drops of rain, so any idea I had of working out was quickly abandoned.

"Sod it," I mumbled, turning over and going back to sleep.

The next time my lids flutter open, the digital clocked screamed at me, highlighting in bold numbers, 11:22.

"Ugh," I groaned in the silence of nearly mid-day.

In no time at all, I found myself pumping my legs on the bike at the gym like my life depended on it. Guilt swept through my veins once the realisation struck me from my bed. I refused to fail, and nothing stood in my way of sticking to the plan this week.

Determination fuelled me. If you've ever seen a water feature, picture the human variety—me—sweat rolled off me. I dabbed myself with my towel... it reminded me of that old Meatloaf video, where he's sweating profusely and wiping his face with a red handkerchief. I can't sing a note in tune by the way, but the amount of perspiration, you'd think I'd just performed a two-hour set at Wembley.

Exercise Bike Duration: 57 Minutes. I varied levels from 5 to 25, but averaged level 7. At level 25, I felt like I was trying to move a JCB... my thighs burned and while it felt good, there was no chance that I could maintain it. Calories Burned: 398.8. Distance: 11.63 miles.

Total exercise time was 57 minutes with 398.8 calories burned.

I wanted to try for more, but I'd arranged to meet Jon at a local Bistro for food, so I was literally on the clock. Even after eleven miles, I beat him there, walking at top speed. Concern laced my brow when I noticed how sluggish his gate became on our five-minute walk home. His complexion and body language portrayed his unwell situation. He needed to lose weight and try to regain his health. Some of his habits caught up with him, causing his diabetes to fluctuate far too often.

I worry about him, but he isn't the type to be forced to do anything and will dig his heels in if he thinks he is being managed. So, I approach it in a sneaky way and make him think it is his idea.

"It's been ages since you last saw the doctor."

"So?" He is instantly suspicious as to where the conversation is heading.

"You probably need to go and get your blood pressure looked at." I know this is one thing that plagues his mind.

"Yeah, I'll call them when we get in."

Manipulation and I are not usually bedfellows, but life happens, and sometimes I have to do things I really don't want to do. It's a sacrifice worth making for the man I love.

He is seeing his GP next Monday but must have bloods taken before then. I hope something will finally be done to put him on the right track.

After dinner of Cheerios (14 Syns) & milk, I walked the dogs afterwards. But as they are 16 and 15 respectively, it is only ten to fifteen minutes at most. I am certain they would go for much longer, but I am aware of their ages and on the vet's advice, don't want to tire them out.

March 29

My routine was thrown out first thing because Jon wanted me to go to the doctor's surgery with him as he had blood tests booked. Knowing his anxieties could push him into cancelling, I accompanied him. I was quite happy in the waiting area, but he insisted on dragging me into the exam room with him.

Coward that I am, I covered my eyes when they took his blood—not because I have a fear of it, only of seeing things pierce the skin. I write horror, crime, and supernatural novels, but I can't stand anything gory, and in the absence of a pillow to shield my eyes, my fingers would have to do.

Anyway, once that was done and after an impromptu trip to ASDA, where I managed to avoid the 'bad' aisles, we grabbed what Jon needed, and on the way home, he dropped me off at the cinder path that leads to the gym. I smiled and looked forward to this workout.

Yes, I went and smashed it in two sets. When I was finished, I must admit that my legs felt like jelly, and stiffer than usual. I did really push myself, but I felt fine five minutes later during the walk home.

After 58 minutes, I managed 12.52 miles with 437 calories burned. My levels ranged from 5 to 20, but I averaged level 9.

Lunch was lettuce and red onion (Syn Free), 4 x Hovis bread (HEXB + 5 Syns) with Colman's English mustard (1 Syn). Dinner was baby potatoes and Bolognese (Syn Free). In between I had 4 x HiFi peanut bars (12 Syns).

Jon was shattered from having not slept the night before, so I volunteered to walk the dogs again.

My energy levels, lifted by the successful workout had me inspired to settle down in front of the PC to write. I slipped my *AirPods* in my ears and started my playlist because I can't write listening to my own thoughts. Although today's thoughts had me in a better mood, and I jumped into my characters mindset in no time with the music lyrics fuelling my creativity.

March 30

Lazy mornings happen, and although I set my alarm for the gym, I didn't go because the stiffness in my neck agonised me, and I could barely move it. *This is a nightmare.* I'm learning to listen to my body. I took two tablets and hoped the pain would subside, and I would regain more movement. It hasn't yet, but I do feel guilty missing the gym, even though it was for the best of reasons.

Breakfast was a mushroom omelette – disgusting!

I'm seeing my friend, Jacqui, at 4:30 pm. It's not anything important—more to do with vanity than practicality—an open evening at a clinic so I can explore options for refreshing my skin, and perhaps a mini face, neck, and eye lift with bag removal too. I'm squeamish, so I hope I don't have to sit through any surgical videos.

I ate before leaving. Dinner was Cheerios with semi-skimmed milk, using my healthy extras.

While I was nervous because I knew I would be surrounded by strangers, I forced myself to go. Walking through the door was unnerving enough but then I noticed that I was the only guy there, surrounded by about fifty other women. But I soon settled in, and after avoiding the trays of cakes and goodies, plus the multitude of sweets in jars on offer, I walked about the place, watching the various treatments being advertised carried out on willing volunteers.

Mortified that I was chosen as a guinea pig of sorts and offered a free Crystal Clear Microdermabrasion treatment, I tried to think of excuses not to go through with it. I hoped they would be too busy when it came to it. Nope! Most people would be thrilled by this, and though I was happy and genuinely appreciative of the opportunity, having this treatment in full view of strangers horrified me.

I was given the bumph to read; Crystal Clear Microdermabrasion offers a safe, controlled method of skin exfoliation allowing superficial peeling of the Stratum Corneum reducing its thickness through mechanical abrasion of the dead skin cells. By placing the hand piece on to the skin and covering the micro-switch, a flow of crystals will impinge directly on to the skin surface. The speed of the crystals together with their abrasive nature can gently remove the epidermal cells layer by layer. Used crystals and dead skin cells are drawn away through the vacuum action.

Okay! I played along because I've had this treatment done before, about fifteen years ago. But I was a lot younger and had fantastic skin with elasticity aplenty.

So, the time came, and I settled onto the bed, holding my stomach in as much as possible, suddenly surrounded by women eager to see how it was done. A mask was placed on my face—Michael Myers from *Halloween* was my first thought before I closed my eyes, trying to pretend I wasn't the focus of attention, or that so many strangers had their eyes on me.

I don't know how long the treatment lasted because I did eventually relax, but I held my breath for long periods of time, terrified my belly would look huge with me lying flat on my back.

Once finished, I did notice how fresh my skin looked afterwards, and tomorrow should see even better results. The therapist, Melissa, was efficient, kind, and friendly, and despite my reservations and embarrassment I thoroughly enjoyed it.

While there, I was asked if I had ever considered Botox.

"No way, I hate needles."

But I did consider having a go until another beautician took a closer look at my skin. "Scrunch your face up please."

"What for?"

"So I can see what your skin is like."

"Okay." I did as she asked.

She approached for a closer inspection. "Sorry, Marco, but you're not a good candidate for Botox."

Not that I was remotely considering it, being told I couldn't have it, then I wanted it. "How come?"

"Because your skin is in great condition. Do you mind if I ask how old you are?"

"Almost forty-nine," I replied.

"Well, you certainly don't look it, and your skin looks wonderful."

I was chuffed to say the least.

We left the open evening early. Once home, I avoided the dining room because an inviting pile of easter eggs and Cadbury's Crème Eggs taunted me from the table. Those had all been set out and ready for me to dish out to family and friends.

Those sweet treats called, "We're in here, come and eat us!"

While the addictive side of me pushed to give into the temptation, the stronger changing man headed to bed instead. Jon and I watched *The Great Celebrity Bake Off in aid of* Stand Up to Cancer. It's perhaps the wrong show to tune into, and I almost jumped out of bed and flew downstairs. Cake was worth stepping off plan for, but I didn't.

Will I ever not desire cake?

March 31
WEIGH-IN DAY

After a crappy off-plan weekend, I'm terrified of stepping onto the scales, and the temptation to swerve weigh-in resonated strong inside me. I kept telling myself it wouldn't be as bad as my mind conjured, and while I knew I'd been to the gym three days this week and remained on plan from Monday to Friday, I wasn't sure I'd done enough to counteract what I shovelled in last weekend.

The good news... following yesterday's microdermabrasion treatment, my skin glowed. But there was more to come.

"Three off. Well done," Shelly told me.

"That's great." I smiled.

The bad news... I fell off plan, again, which means I needed to hammer the gym next week. I needed to get into the next stone bracket, and I currently sit only six pounds away from that.

SARAH-JANE'S STORY

Sarah-Jane walks through the door—glamour personified, yet appearing timid, head bowed, with her hands shoved deep in her pockets. She stops at the bar and orders a drink, then turns, having sensed that I noticed her. I smile. But she struggles to meet my eyes. I nod and approach her, aware that I could be considered an imposing figure, towering above her—she is on edge, so maybe that's it? I'm not sure because we have only ever conversed over social media.

"Hi Sarah-Jane."

"Hi, Marco." I needn't have worried as she shakes my hand and flashes a smile back at me with a grip that conveys strength, and confidence.

"It is lovely to meet you. Thank you for coming."

"Lovely to meet you too."

As I have tried numerous times to book a date to have this chat, I had thought she might make an excuse at the last minute, but I am pleased to see her—I know how hard speaking on record is for her because she doesn't consider anything she has done to be worthy of inclusion. I happen to think otherwise but please judge for yourself.

I pay for her drink and allow her to lead me to where she will feel most comfortable.

She takes her seat, and sips at her drink.

"Are you ready to begin?" She nods, so I place the *Dictaphone* on the table between us. "How are you this morning?"

"I'm so nervous, well terrified really." Sitting opposite me, wringing her hands together, her legs shake, a tell-tale sign her anxieties are rising.

"What are you nervous about?"

"This interview."

Instantly I try to put her at ease, not wanting this experience to be an unpleasant one. "Please don't think of this as an interview, but more an informal chat between friends who share a common bond."

"Being fat?"

She is direct, but I prefer that trait in a person. "Well, one of us is, and it definitely isn't you." To paint a clear picture of what I see, Sarah-Jane has long auburn hair, a flawless, China-doll-like complexion, is what would be considered slim, and about five-feet tall, if that—and from what I know of her, she turns forty in October, but you could knock ten years off that number as she looks remarkably fresh faced. There are no tell-tale signs of yo-yo dieting.

"If I had to describe you, Marco, fat wouldn't be the word I would use." And instantly, we're on that merry-go-round of politeness.

"I've been bigger, which is why we're here to talk."

"This is the smallest I've ever been."

"Do you mind if I ask what you weigh now?" I always dread asking that question, especially of a lady, but it forms an integral part of this book. Our weight, good or bad, is what brings us here.

She shifts uncomfortably in her seat, and I half expect a refusal, which is of course, is her right, and I wouldn't push it. "Eight stone dead." According to the BMI, Sarah-Jane sits in the healthy weight category.

"And what was your heaviest weight?" I pause, waiting for protective walls to surround her.

Quite instantly, she answers. "Fourteen stone, eleven pounds when I decided I had to do something. Especially after my doctor told me my BMI was, I think forty-something at that point."

Why does that BMI figure seem to stick with so many people? Do doctors hammer it home to scare their patients? I understand why it is used, but I still think the method is outdated and needs a serious overhaul, considering changing times, and the varieties of foods and drink that are readily available now. "So, you've lost nearly seven stone."

"Yes, near to that, but it wasn't easy."

"Do you mind if I ask you how you did it?"

"Surgery. To start with anyway."

I'd have no inkling she had resorted to surgery because she had never volunteered that information previously. "Bariatric surgery?"

"Yes, when I was twenty-two."

"Was it a gastric bypass, gastric sleeve, or a gastric band?"

"Full bypass—I don't do things by halves, and I didn't like the idea of having the band filled and drained—something had to stop me in my tracks, so I decided the bypass was the one for me."

I tell her of my experiences, similar, yet different from hers, but it gives us more common ground. "Okay, did you regain the weight you had lost soon after the procedure, or was it a gradual increase?"

"As soon as I was allowed to eat properly, which I think was six weeks post-surgery, I realised I could eat past it, cream cakes, crisps, kebabs, and before long, I was consuming meals the same size as I was before, throwing up, then going back for more—I had an eating disorder before surgery, and then afterwards, what was supposed to make me normal, I became bulimic, bingeing, vomiting, then carrying on until I was crying in agony as the stomach cramps kicked in. Then I started to lose my back teeth due to acid rotting them from constant vomiting."

"How did being stuck in that cycle again feel?"

"Truthfully, I wanted to kill myself, and thought, what's the point living like this." She looks into my eyes and doesn't flinch. "I couldn't see an end to it and didn't want to live the rest of my life feeling guilty and obsessing over foods."

Obsessing over food can drive a person to distraction, and I'm certain we have all felt hopeless at some point. "I'm sorry to hear that."

"Stupidly, I pinned my hopes on the bypass and paid sixteen grand for it because the NHS doctors told me I'd be dead in six to twelve months. But terrifying me, then on the other hand telling me that I had to wait three years, and that was after attending their weight loss program, which including counselling me past my desire to eat—I got into huge debt to pay for something that didn't cure me. But it wasn't supposed to cure me, was it, only teach me."

Her words take me right back to my spookily similar scenario. If only we could learn lessons so easily. I certainly didn't. "Yes, I think it is meant to make you smarter when it comes to food, but the brain is a tricky piece of machinery."

"I was the same as a kid, tell me not to do something and I had to do it. Self-sabotage, that's what it was—I was the master of it. Stubborn too, and not learning lessons from past mistakes. I thought, I'll start a diet tomorrow, which then became next week, or Monday, then in time for summer, then Christmas, then New Year, and before long those new years rolled into years. I could have put a stop to it sooner, but being told, you're too fat, I just stuck two fingers up at anybody in authority, teachers, doctors... I knew better, or so I thought. Stupid, I know that now."

"Are you still in debt?"

"No, and that's only because my dad died and left me money, so I paid off my mortgage and my debts." Tears fill her eyes.

I don't want this process to upset her. "Do you want to take a minute?"

"No, no, I'm fine, really."

"I've lost a parent too and know how awful it is."

"Losing Dad made me realise I had to change."

"Did your dad struggle with his weight?"

"No, never, but my mum was massive and had struggled since she was a kid."

"And what about now?"

"We did it together."

"Lost weight...?"

"Sorry, yes. I had the surgery, ate past it, Dad died, and I realised that I was in charge of my destiny, not a surgeon asking for thousands to fix me, and that if I didn't have the mindset to change myself, nothing I did was going to work."

"So, what did you and your mum do?"

"We joined *Weight Watchers*. But it took a long time to pluck up the courage to walk through those doors."

I explain I had been a member for a long time, and that while I initially thrived, I failed because my heart wasn't in it. "How was that experience?"

"Amazing, I loved it, and my leader, Wendy, was fantastic, even though she was on the hefty side herself."

"How much did you lose at *Weight Watchers*?"

"Six stone the first go around, which I found surprisingly easy because my heart was in it."

I was half-expecting her to tell me it had taken numerous attempts to lose that incredible amount of weight. "So, you joined more than once?"

"I can't remember how many times I joined, lost weight, then something or other got in the way and I piled it all back on, and more."

"What was the headfirst-into-the-brick wall point for you?"

"Mum had a massive heart attack, and I walked into that awful, sterile room, horrified to find her hooked up to beeping machines, struggling to breathe. I had a flashforward to myself lying in that same bed, puffing, and panting, trying to tell my kids that I would be okay. I was terrified that she was going to die and kept telling myself if she did, I would be an orphan, which for a grown woman is bloody stupid."

"It's not stupid at all. How is your mum now?"

"She's doing fine and has her weight under control and even gave up smoking."

"I'm pleased to hear that, for her health and your peace of mind."

"Seeing her vulnerable and frail like an old woman lit a fire under my arse because we enabled one another."

"Enabled? Can you expand on that a little please, just so I and the readers can understand your mindset?"

"I mean, if I was having a crappy day, which was often, she would encourage me to indulge because she needed an excuse to indulge too. We were like crack addicts egging each other on."

"I get that totally, but food addiction is still an addiction. It doesn't matter how slimmer people paint us—we're not just fatties who can't control our impulses—we need help, just like an alcoholic or a drug addict does." No matter how many different people I speak to, one thing bonds us all—the ability to concoct any excuse to indulge, but Sarah-Jane is wise beyond her years and sees addiction for what it is—like cancer, it does not discriminate. "So, seeing your mum basically at death's door was the wake up call you needed?"

"Yes, and no. And while I did well for a while, that little voice still whispered at me to just shovel it in and worry about it later."

"I still have that voice nagging at me and wish I could turn it off."

"You never will, and that's the truth."

"I've come to terms with that."

"Even now I can still hear it, and sitting here talking to you, I know there is a café, and a shop over the road filled with everything that I used to think makes me happy." She is self-aware enough to realise that food doesn't make her happy. That is a big step for any of us to grasp. "But I think of my kids and don't want them to bury me until I'm an old woman, and it's my time to go."

"How long has your weight been stable for this time?"

"About ten years, but that means nothing, and you can ask any person who is on a diet or goes to fat club—it's never a done deal no matter how long you've been stable for. I still have to go to meetings, just like an alcoholic goes to AA—to keep me on the right path because I could walk out of here and something could snap inside me, and I'd race straight to that shop over there and spend twenty quid filling a bag with everything I love, take it home and scoff the lot."

"I know exactly what you mean. I will always struggle."

"Yes, you will, but it's easier to lose a re-gained stone than ten, if you know what I mean."

"I get it totally. But for the readers, how did you manage stability?"

"I joined *Weight Watchers*, then I left and joined *Slimming World* because I was too ashamed to go back to my old leader, not that she would have judged me."

"I've been there too."

"But then I realised that I had to find a way to do it myself, without backup because backup wasn't always going to be there. Yes, I still went to meetings, but then lockdown happened, and I panicked because I couldn't bubble with my mum, so I was alone with my kids who didn't struggle with their weight and had no concept of what I was going through. Talking on the phone or Zoom meetings did nothing to help—I needed face-to-face contact."

"It was hard for a lot of people, not least those people with addiction problems."

"So, it was my test, could I go it alone?"

"And...?"

"Despite thinking otherwise, I did do it, not that there wasn't a flood of tears and tantrums, there was, but nobody is more surprised than me."

"How?"

She appears sheepish. "In my mind's eye, I imagined emerging from lockdown and seeing people again, and them noticing a slimmer healthier me, and that spurred me on."

"So, it was like your own version of Extreme Makeover?"

She laughs and her face lights up. "God, I remember that programme and used to dream about being in their place, so yes, kind of, well, actually, yes it was just like that without the plastic surgery."

"And how did it go, that big reveal?"

"I went to see my mum first, and she was so amazed that she sobbed, and typical her, she heaped praise on me, and I finally saw the hard work I had put in. Although I had used the tools provided by *Weight Watchers* and *Slimming World* and creating my own eating plan to a fashion, I still did it on my own."

"I'm amazed you were able to do it that way. I'm not sure I would have had the willpower during that time to be so strict with myself."

"So was I, but don't sell yourself short because you've lost a lot of weight."

"Thank you. I know I shouldn't put myself down but for bigger people it seems to be a default setting."

"I have a friend who used to be severely overweight, and he refused to pay any organisation, didn't agree with corporation diets as he called them, so he bought a diet book, discovered what he was and wasn't supposed to consume fats wise and tailored his eating to that. He did it, and if he could, so could I—he was known as Fat Paul, how bad is that? Never Paul, always Fat Paul. People are so cruel." Her mind wanders for a moment. "But I want to stress and please include this in the book, it *was* and still is what I learned from *Weight Watchers* and *Slimming World* combined that gave me the courage to try myself."

"I won't redact anything you tell me, unless you ask me to, because this is your story to tell."

"That's what I was worried about, that you would make me look like a raving nutcase."

"Far from it—your story is yours to tell, just as mine is. I will print whatever you say to me word for word if that is what you want."

"I just want people who aren't big or who have never experienced what it is to be fat or struggle with their weight to understand that we are human beings with feelings. We don't need to be laughed at, approved of, or pitied even, just understood that we make mistakes like other people, and that while you're standing there with your cigarette in your hand, sniggering at the fat girl, or snorting lines of coke in the toilets of a nightclub, or chugging back vodka every night in the pub, take a long, hard look in the mirror because you have an addiction too..." Her tone changes and is laced with bitterness. "... it's just yours is deemed more acceptable by society. Fat isn't cool, pretty, or healthy, I know that, but neither are smelly clothes that stink of cigarette smoke, nor is a purple nose from guzzling too much booze, losing your house through gambling debts, and a nose missing the septum isn't a good look either—don't you see, we all have our failings but when one addiction is deemed the lesser of many evils, it's wrong. Society is screwed because it sets these ridiculous parameters. Rather than help, let's mock and hiss at the fatty squeezing into the plane seat, but let's all laugh at the fun drunk, or the life and soul of the party coke head. It makes me so mad. Addiction is all consuming and one is as crushing as the other, and I make no apologies for this, but mine is harder to navigate because food is everywhere I turn."

"That is a very honest answer."

"Yeah, but it might not be a popular one."

"Maybe not with some people who read this, but nobody, including me, is going to win overall approval. This book is about truths, not living in a dream world. Accountability is the key word here."

"I just get so bothered by it—fatty, stop eating, simple. No, it's not that easy because there is always a reason for it. I got fat because my mum thought feeding me was showing me love. I knew she loved me, so I didn't need excess food to prove it. But from a young age, I fell into that cycle that she set me on. I didn't do that with my kids because I knew enough about my own misery not to push them down that same road. Instead, I instilled in them from an early age, a healthy, balanced breakfast, lunch, dinner, a bit of supper if you fancy it, then you're done, and you don't need any more. There was no fridge or cupboard raiding allowed in my house. They did have sweets, of course, just like most kids, but they weren't given to show love, to praise them, or to bribe them to do something. Sweets were treated as occasional treats, and not a food group. I had my own stash under my bed, not that they ever saw it. I parented hypocritically; I admit it and still feel terrible about it."

"I don't have children, but don't most parents do that to a certain degree? You don't want them to make those same mistakes, right?"

"Right. And as much as I hated fruit when I was younger, and even when struggling for money when they were growing up, I always had it in the house. So when they wanted something sweet, they had a banana, or a pear, or a bowl of grapes or strawberries. They do eat sweets and crisps, but only now and again. Chocolate didn't become all-consuming or a must-have. I did that for them, and not to control them, but to save them from the misery of food obsession and addiction." Her eyes glaze over. "What is that old saying..."

"Eat to live, not live to eat." I could be wrong.

"Yes, they eat to live, whereas I was always lived to eat."

That phrase pops up quite often during these interviews. "And now?"

"I am definitely in *their* camp, and I have never felt better—still, that desire to consume as much as I can lives inside me. When I am fed up, I resort to my default setting—chocolate, *Cadbury's* fruit and nut, the family size—my favourite, but then I think, fresh fruit and fat free Quark or Cottage Cheese will satisfy me. It usually does the trick, sometimes it doesn't, and I need what I need. But then I get my head together and know that gaining it all back isn't worth two minutes of pleasure. Then again, nowadays, there are so many things we can have if we fancy something naughty."

She still sees herself as overweight, even though you would be hard pressed to find an ounce of fat on her. I don't correct her, because like me, her mindset has taken decades to set in place and it won't shift in a hurry and might never shift to a place where she is accepting of a true perception of herself. "Regardless, don't sell your efforts short. You did it, got to target and have managed something many of us struggle with still. You have maintained and exist in a place you can be happy occupying."

She smiles as the brief anger and vestiges of self-hatred dissipates. "Yes, I did, didn't I."

"Was it easy, hard, as expected... tell me?"

"Anything worth doing is difficult and to be honest, counting and weighing everything almost made me lose my mind, but locked down and furloughed, what else could I devote my time to, aside from me? I dieted, exercised, ran up and down the stairs like I had cabin fever—I even did the garden, and I hate, hate, hated gardening more than anything—worms, and creepy crawlies terrify me. Now, my garden looks like a show garden, but it was all that, even stuff I hated doing that took my mind off wanting to while away the boring days with sweets and crisps. It would have been so easy putting my feet up, stuffing cakes while watching daytime television."

"You're amazing, I hope you know that!"

"Hardly, but I wanted to be thin more than I wanted to be fat, and that was my mantra if you like—put this in big capitals—I WANT TO BE THIN MORE THAN I WANT TO BE FAT—I wanted to be, and to feel healthy—perhaps I should have it tattooed somewhere but my mum would go mad." She laughs again, and her face lights up with joy. "... she hates tattoos..."

"You are an inspiration to me and will be to so many others."

"I really want to be, and not to stroke my ego because I don't have one, but as a poster girl to say if *I* can do it so can you, and trust me, I was a lost cause as far as doctors were concerned—I was the fat, jolly girl in the pub, knocking back pints like a fella, just because I could."

"So, there has been quite a change, not only in your appearance, but behaviourally too?" I note that she is sipping pink gin and diet lemonade from what most would call a ladylike glass.

"No more pints for me—it was just greediness, and food replaced something else I was missing."

"What was missing?"

"A sense of purpose."

"But you have children?" I know this will spark a reaction, and she will give it to me both barrels. It's the type of truth I seek.

"But I am more than a womb, just like you are more than a sperm donor."

"True." I fall silent and wait for her to divulge more.

"I love my kids more than life itself, but I wanted a career, and I had a good one. Then I had my babies—my ex-husband was as much use as a fart in the wind, so I lost myself in being mummy, and when I dared to look, wanting to find myself again..." She pauses, reflecting on what it was she had lost. "... I couldn't find the girl I was and all I could see was a fat, ugly, shapeless thing staring back at me."

"So, losing weight helped you find you again."

"I always struggled with my weight, but getting married, then having my kids so close together, I ceased to be Sarah-Jane. Instead, I was reduced to playing roles—wife, mother, cook, and bottle washer, invisible, so I took comfort *again* in everything that was bad for me. I can only blame myself."

"So, what is different now?"

"Me."

"Just you?"

"That's all it took, to remember, just me."

"Interesting." I'm reminded that I'm not the only one who ceased to be— addiction robs you of life, instead replacing it with a half-life.

"We forget who we are and what we're capable of. I did, you did, you already told me as much over the phone which is why I agreed to do this—you get me, you get what the struggle is like for us and millions of others, but at the same time, you get the fact it is *you* who has done the damage and *you* who has to put it right."

"You are a very wise lady, Sarah-Jane."

"Don't get me wrong, Marco, I am as blind as the next person until something hits me head on, and it took staring death in the face through my mums eyes for me to see that I have one life and once this one is over, everything I worked for, and achieved came down to the fact I died because I was fat and couldn't control myself—no way did I want that on my tombstone—*Here Lies Sarah-Jane. Dead because she was a greedy, fat pig.*"

Her words slap me about the face, and I don't know why I have the sudden urge to laugh. Perhaps her thoughts mirror my own, and her caustic descriptions remind me of me. There is lingering pain behind her words, and I know how easy it is to project that into the world before the world can project its opinions of you onto you first. "I don't know what to say."

"All I can say is, try, try, try, and if you want it hard enough, there is a way. It might be surgery that works, and that is fine, it might be the gym, it might be yoga, the Atkins Diet, living on cabbage soup, or *Weight Watchers* or *Slimming World*, whatever, if it works, great. Oh, yes, I forgot this one diet I signed myself up for, *LighterLife* that involved only shakes. They were thick, chalky, disgusting and made me sick. I lost eighteen pounds that first week, but I was terrified of those shakes knowing one mouthful would make me gag—I had to stop, not to mention it cost about sixty quid per week to buy the shakes, and I wasn't pleased with the weekly pee tests either."

I also did *LighterLife* too, and for a time it worked for me. For the same reason, I dreaded mealtimes. I thought the cost was daylight robbery too, and survived on the bars, before I realised it wouldn't work long term for me. I refused to do the pee tests, regardless of them wanting to know if I was in ketosis or not. "You had an epiphany of sorts; would you agree with that?"

"Yes, I did, but for me, it was a combination of two well-known weight management groups in competition with one another that worked, and the realisation that I want to live—it's a powerful realisation, choosing life, and that is what I did because I was eating myself to death."

"On a scale of 1 to 10, how happy are you now?"

"I'd say a solid eight."

"Not a ten?"

She laughs again, as though I've muttered words of madness. "Never. Who is happy all of the time? Are you?"

"God, no. I'm not a miserable person by nature but—"

"There you go then," she interrupts. "My life isn't perfect, but whose is? I could look like Jennifer Lopez and have ten million quid in the bank; doesn't mean I'm going to be doing cartwheels, does it?"

"True."

"Life is what you make it, Marco, and for me, the key to my happiness, aside from my kids, was finding me again and part of that was shedding the weight that held me prisoner for too long."

"Is that how you felt? That it kept you prisoner?"

"I was captive to fat, as you are now. It won't always be that way—sorry if that bothers you, but with an addiction, the addict is the prisoner always struggling to break free."

"You did it."

"Yes, but addiction is still addiction. Breaking free isn't the end because you always have to maintain the loss, or it creeps back on. But like I said before, that is easier than looking at yourself in the mirror knowing there is ten stone to lose."

"I hate the word—addiction, but it is what it is."

"Get on board with it. The sooner you do, the sooner you have another tool at your disposal. Knowledge is power, Marco, and you might think that sounds cheesy, but it is the best weapon you will ever have."

"I feel like I am constantly learning something new about myself."

"You are, and so am I, but we're not the only ones where addiction is concerned. I have a friend who gave up smoking six years ago and just started up again. I asked him why and he said he missed it. How can any person miss smoking? To me it's a disgusting habit. But if I turn the tables on myself, do I miss nights on the sofa with a bag full of chocolate? Yes, I do, and to the smoker, or the alcoholic, or the drug addict, or the person craving sex, me shovelling endless bags of crisps down my throat might be disgusting to them. Horses for courses as they say—we all have something, and I am under no illusion that I am cured. There is no cure for my addiction, not for any addiction. But it can be managed successfully and if anybody knows that I definitely do."

"How?" That's the million-pound question.

"I can only answer for myself, but through experiencing the ups and down of my weight issues, I somehow managed to learn enough to realise how to manage it, and to accept myself on any given day as best I can."

As our chat draws to a close, a haunted look settles in Sarah-Jane's eyes. The same look I have seen many times while working on this book, and I get it; this experience, no matter where we are with it, never leaves. It is called addiction, and it is waiting to strike back. She knows it, I know it, and so do you. "Thank you for sharing your story, Sarah-Jane."

"It's been a pleasure—you're doing a wonderful thing; do you know that?"

"I think this book will help a lot of people who are struggling. Not only that; it will allow others to see us for what we are—people who aren't perfect, and that doesn't make us bad people, just flawed."

"You're right."

"Opening the dialogue is what is needed, and I am proud to have been a small part of your work."

MY JOURNEY - APRIL 2023

April 3

After an okay weekend of jollying around the town centre, painting planters, and food shopping, I had an epiphany of sorts—despite my dad and two brothers being in the construction and interior design business, DIY is not in my DNA. But that's no surprise to those who have seen me struggle to put a fuse in a plug. That aside, wandering around clothes shops, not thinking about Syns, or anything weight related, I realised that I am master of my own destiny and therefore allowed to just be me for one day without berating myself for it. From this time last year, I had done incredibly well.

Monday morning arrived with blue skies, so I walked to the gym and back, after cycling 10.73 miles in 52 minutes and burning 376 calories. Yes, it is lower than yesterday's 437, but I worked at varying levels—from 7 to 15, and averaged level 8. However, I should, and could, have done a lot better.

The warmth of the sun shining inspired me, but my own sabotage nagged at me, and I cut my exercise short. I felt self-conscious surrounded by the beautiful people. I wanted to use the leg press, but never got around to it. Still, I managed ten plus miles, so I won't be too hard on myself.

I treated myself to a pot of tea in the local Bistro on the way home, and as I am having a roast, minus the meat, for dinner, I didn't dare to eat because I wouldn't want anything else.

When I got home, Jon reminded me that he had an appointment with his GP, so I walked there and back with him. I didn't struggle at all; the gym sessions must be helping.

My house sits in total disarray because I am having my sitting room redecorated. Fingers crossed the work will be finished today. I CAN'T STAND THE MESS! The floor fitters are coming to measure up later this afternoon and with a bit of luck, after I've finished my writing session. Netta and I still haven't finished reading through our latest book and need to get that done this week so it can be sent to the Beta readers.

My to-do list grows ever longer by the day. I seem to cross one thing off and ten extra things appear. And the more I have to do, the less time I have to focus on food, and while that is a positive, there is a negative because I will avoid cooking which then sends me running to the shop—there's my excuse to go wild in the aisles and shovel anything in that is loaded with calories.

Breakfast was skipped just because, while dinner was as planned, using only 3 Syns. In-betweens was a pot of tea with whole milk and a nectarine.

April 4

It's Groundhog Day, no, not really, but it certainly feels like it because routine has taken over every single aspect of my life. First stop is the gym, again. It's not that I don't want to go, I need to go, but willing myself to walk there is the issue. But I do it anyway. You might wonder why I grumble about it—routine is fine, but the things I have to do all seem to centre around something I don't want to think about—food. It rules my life in entirely negative ways.

FOOD, FOOD, FOOD...

I try to think positively about it but fail every time. I must eat to live, so I do it, although it brings no sense of enjoyment or fulfilment.

To my astonishment, I cycled 14.37 miles, up from 10.73, in seventy minutes, burning a massive 485 calories on an average of level 8.

Although my session lifted my earlier wishy-washy attitude, to say my thighs burned would be an understatement. I pushed myself harder than ever, and even I was surprised how far I got. Elation from success surged through my veins and provided me with a huge high—who would have thought it? Not certain I could do that daily, but after falling off plan, every minute of exercise helps.

Dinner was basically a re-hash of yesterday, but only using 1½ Syns. I have no desire to eat anything because I really do not enjoy the taste or consistency of food. Aside from the missing hormone, it is also a reason I am reluctant to eat. In-betweens were slightly more enjoyable—4 x Asda Low Fat Smooth Strawberry Yogurt (14 Syns). Truthfully, I didn't want them either, but as I had only used 1½ Syns today, while fighting the urge to eat something sweet, I chose them, knowing they would quiet the whisper. Plus, the frugal side of me knew they would pass their use by date, so it was a case of eat them now or throw them in the bin. Eating them did save me from myself. A valuable lesson: something as easy as eating yoghurt can stop me in my tracks when I want to bury my face in a box of chocolates.

April 5

I can't be arsed going to the gym today.
After yesterday's mammoth trek on the exercise bike, I told myself a day off was warranted. But I went anyway and although I didn't match or better what I did yesterday, I still did very well and whiled away the time watching *Long Lost Family: What Happened Next*, trying not to cry as families were reunited after decades apart.

13.03 miles were covered today in 61 minutes, burning 436.1 calories on an average level of 8.

I knew I could have done more, but my thighs burned like the blaze of a three-alarm fire, and continue to smoulder, over an hour later. Listening to my body, I told myself to stop, but I have set myself a target to do at least ten miles per day, and anything over that is a bonus. I'm doing well considering my physical and medical problems. This quest to lose weight has taken me into strange waters.

Do I love exercise, or do I hate it?
I think it is a bit of both, and while I am there, I seem to enjoy it. Although, I find myself clock watching. To combat this, I cover the screen with my towel, so I don't focus on the countdown. Another bonus was a quiet gym. I much prefer it when I'm not surrounded by others.

Lunch was a healthy option of fruit, granola, and fat free natural yoghurt (2½ Syns).

Dinner was SW Beef Curry & Baby Potatoes (Syn Free)

In-Betweens consisted of 2 x HiFi Peanut Butter Bars, 2 x HiFi Salted Caramel Bars (6 Syns), Builders Tea, Sweeteners & Semi Skimmed Milk, Diet Pepsi, Bananas, Black Grapes, Tropical Granola & Fat Free Natural Yoghurt (2½ Syns). Healthy extras used.

I was lucky enough to be treated to a facial, including exfoliation, from Jon, and whilst doing that, I took off my top, and he commented on how much weight I'd lost.

"What are you after?" I asked, suspicious about the impromptu but welcome offer.

"Nothing."

"Hmm. You're being unusually nice to me."

"Well if you don't want it, just say so."

"I do." I'm not turning down a pampering session from anyone. Now if I could get him to scratch my back, shins, and tickle my head, I'd be in Heaven.

To my surprise, he said I looked a little flatter above the gunt area. Thank you very much!

His compliment meant a lot to me, but as I wander about the house naked every single day, I silently question why he hasn't noticed before?

I'm being dreadfully unfair because he has noticed, and perhaps my response is me still not being used to receiving compliments from anyone, not even my life partner.

My house is still a mess, but not as bad as it was—the decorating is nearly finished, and then work will start on the hallway, again. Tidy house, tidy mind is very much my motto and as my house and its contents sit askew, so are my thought patterns. I need order and discipline in at least one part of my life, and while I know that my diet is not topping that list right now, nor do I have full control, I can exert that when I close my front door, at least where tidiness is concerned. Without that, I find I cannot settle, which doesn't bode well for keeping any other part of my life in check.

It's nearly 1 am, and my gym clothes are in the tumble dryer. I've got loads on my mind, thinking about a career change and perhaps going back to working for a big company rather than writing. But it's a big decision and would mean getting used to the 9 to 5 again.

Decisions, decisions, decisions.

Stuff it, I'll think some more tomorrow. Right now. I'm going to bed—my workout gear should be dry when I wake up.

April 6
WEIGH-IN DAY

Good Friday brings weigh-in a day early this week, and today *is* that day!

My alarm pulled me from a peaceful slumber at 8:30 am, and I finally managed to drag my tired, old carcass out of bed an hour later. I really didn't want to go to the gym and ummed and ahhhed for a while, but I went, later than usual, which threw my day out.

11.13 miles cycled in 53 minutes, which is less than yesterday, but still over my agreement to myself of 10 per day. Although I could have done more, I was bored from the start and just wanted to get out of there. Still, I achieved over ten miles which is my daily goal—I do feel slimmer. Calories burned was 384.3 on an average level of 9.

I'm aiming to weigh-in later this afternoon, but Jon and I have errands to run first, starting with a stop off in the local Bistro. It seems I am never away from there, but I feel so comfortable, I don't worry about eating in front of strangers. The lady that owns it, Anne-Marie, is a joy, as is her chef, Sandra. Both are lovely and complementary, not to mention encouraging, that it is almost a home from home.

Breakfast is mushrooms, beans, tomatoes, scrambled egg (Fry Light & Syn Free), 2 x dry wholemeal toast (HEXB + 5½ Syns), builders tea with semi-skimmed milk (HEXA) & sweeteners.

After eating at the bistro, I dropped Jon off at home then went to get my hair cut and beard trimmed. As I was already out, I went for a session on the sunbed, then food shopping, before heading home, itchy, and sweaty.

I'm still planning on going for weigh in, but I want to catch up on some TV first.

Dinner was Cheerios (14 Syns), skimmed milk (HEXA). I fell asleep while watching the TV, so any plans I had went out of the window.

So, I missed weigh-in, but I'm not down about it. In fact, I'm feeling positive that I have lost weight because I do feel smaller in my person. I know especially at my weight saying this might seem strange, but the gym must be doing some good. Looking at my legs in the bath last night, they've never been fat, okay, my calves and thighs were a little wobbly, but I can definitely see positive changes. Once my lower half is in order and I have more strength and stamina, I can start on the top half—I'll need a miracle.

Inevitably, I will be asked the question, "So, where were you last week?"

I won't lie about why I haven't been there; I never do.

Jon has mentioned moving back to Prestatyn again, but having lived there twice, and despite being a great place to visit, I was miserable. It really wasn't the place for me to settle in permanently.

"I won't ever move back there but if you want to go, feel free." I resent feeling cornered, or that I am expected to do something just because.

"Fine, I will."

"Bye then."

"My family are there, Marco."

"And mine are here, Jon."

"You barely see your family."

"And yours are only 45 minutes down the road, how often do you see them?"

It is the usual argument, with no side tipped to emerge victorious.

I won't be railroaded into moving anywhere, but it is obvious we see ourselves in different places.

Could we survive living in different towns? I don't think so. It's sad, and the last thing that I want, but what can I do?

His immediate family are there so I understand his needs totally and would never hold it against him, but mine are here, as are my friends, and while I am not tethered to any of them, I feel at home here because I was born here, whereas he was born in Stockport.

Whatever happens, I hope that if he does want to leave and we do split, there is no animosity, and we can part as friends... say goodbye and walk away with a clean break.

The conversation did make me think more about quitting writing, especially as his mum is my writing partner and friend. It would be too awkward continuing our partnership and friendship if Jon and I weren't together.

April 9
EASTER SUNDAY

It's Easter Sunday, or Cadbury's Crème Egg Day. *Yum!* Despite the Syns, I can see the positives. The only negative is that after today, I'll have to wait until New Years Day to buy more. Unless I do the rounds and stock up now. Hmm, what to do? Naughty I know, but courtesy of Jon, I already have a box of 10 mixed crème eggs, and 3 big Easter Eggs—2 x Cadbury's Mini Eggs and 1 x Cadbury's Flake waiting for me... I have a penchant for one brand of chocolate, guess which one... Haha! I can't wait to tuck into them, but I aim to exercise restraint, which shouldn't be too difficult judging by how good I was last year. If they are in the house, I crave them less and can leave them alone, but when I don't have any, I WANT them and must have them. Am I the only person with this mindset?

April 10

I'm at a loss today because the bank holiday has thrown off my routine. Usually, I am up and heading to the gym, but it is closed. However, I am back on plan, again. I have come too far to undo all of my hard work. I like myself more, which might be a bold admission, although true.

Not one flake of chocolate passed my lips yesterday, but how long can I hold off? As long as possible. I know I have the Syns available but once I open one, it will be downhill from there. I can't exercise portion control and put the rest in the fridge, you must be joking.

I am missing not working out and looking forward to tomorrow. I will hammer it this week and maybe treat myself.

Lunch was a healthy affair, consisting of fresh fruit, tropical granola & fat free natural yoghurt (2½ Syns). Lunch was baby potatoes, rocket / mixed leaf salad, boiled eggs. (Syn Free).

CHEWING THE FAT

April 11

Jon is going to visit family in Wales today until Saturday and while I will miss him, there is the bonus of not having to cook. He loves proper meals, and I would be happy never to cook again, but in preparation, I made a huge pan of soup yesterday and will eat that over the next few days. Don't get me wrong, my preference is for cakes, chocolate and sweets, but common sense and the desire to win pushes me to eat healthily.

Stock from boiled ham, potatoes, onions, cannellini beans, carrots, leeks, sweet potato, courgette, lentils, barley, split Peas, stock cubes... well, that was the plan.

I went to the gym, and absolutely smashed it, and the great thing about it was, not being able to go yesterday made me realise how much I actually enjoy it.

15.21 miles cycled, in 70 minutes, burning 533 calories on level 10. I am finding it easier as the days go by, even with breaks in between sessions, and have noticed more change in the shape of my legs. I wonder how much I could achieve if I went seven days a week—a pipe dream fibro will never allow.

And then I went and ruined it by eating crème eggs and bruschetta, not together I might add. But there is little point me feeling guilty. I did it, time to move on. I might not have done that much damage, especially after my mega-workout session. Still. I'm bummed but trying to shake it off.

The dogs were groomed today, so they look cuter than ever. Both are sulking because Jon is away, but they can sleep on my bed tonight, which should keep them sweet. I'm under no illusions that when Jon walks back through the door, I won't see them for dust.

April 13

After yesterday's pig out session, I had plans to go to the gym, but after a sleepless night with the dogs snoring, I woke up looking and feeling like I'd just been resurrected from death. Still, I was determined to go, before the heaven's opened and it peed down.

I missed my physiotherapist appointment because I slept through my alarm, so had to call them with an excuse—thankfully they have rescheduled me for the 17th May which just happens to be the day my new flooring is being fitted, so that will be a busy day I'm already dreading.

Add into the fact that my house is still a mess because the decorator has left the job half finished, so I am not in the best of moods, well, furious and ready to scream if I'm honest. I've had to secure the services of another decorator, so not only have I paid the other to do the work, I am also having to pay to have it finished which will add another £300 to the bill.

If the day couldn't get any worse, I had a huge row with a family member who refuses to grow up and accept responsibility. Then Jon brought up the one subject that can cause all-out war between us.

"I'm not happy here, Marco."

"So, go back to the Pearl of Prestatyn then." At my most snarky, I know that I am being unreasonable to his feelings and speaking childish words that will spark a reaction. But the only thing that will seemingly make him feel better is for me to agree to move. Over my dead body!

I don't get it. He tells me he isn't happy, but shouldn't he be happy wherever I am? I would say so, but judging by his recent comments, said in the heat of the moment or not, this relationship is only viable to him if he lives in North Wales.

Maybe I should be happy wherever Jon is, in fact, I know I should be, but our lives are very different. I am not the stay-at-home-type, whereas he is a home-bird, and yes, his health issues do leave him housebound a lot of the time, so I go out and do all that is needed, so he doesn't have to.

I ask myself the same question; why should I leave my world behind only for him to live the same old routine?

I know he loves his family—wonderful, but it's not enough for me to uproot my life, especially as I can't see his parent's staying in North Wales forever. One day, they will move away, probably to sunnier climes, and we're left behind to do what, or would I be expected to move again?

I've had the odd conversations with his mum about this, and she says that him being in Prestatyn means they would be able to take him out and spend more time with him. Fab, but what about me? I don't want to spend my days lolloping or visiting different family members to fill my time when not writing. I know Jon's world would open a lot more because he would be out of the house, but I'd be stuck twiddling my thumbs while he enjoys days out with his mum and gran. I am never not invited, far from it, they have always welcomed me and I love them dearly, but it's not the life for me.

It seems the same old argument comes around on the same old loop. He says he will be happier there, and that might be true, but I know that I won't be. I do believe his family want to be closer to him, and I understand it, but they could always move here. Stubbornness is one of my worst traits, especially if I have weighed up all the options and mainly negatives win. So how do we move forward and find a compromise? I haven't found the answer yet, but he has to do what he thinks is right for him. I really don't care, but I know I am fed up with the never-ending stress being laid at my door. At nearly 49, I don't need or want the hassle. It's not like anyone takes care of my mind.

Angry and stressed, I scoffed two crème eggs, and while I know I have more downstairs, I am trying not to eat my way through a range of emotions.

Two hours later and I am still hopping mad, but I stuck to my guns and left the chocolate and served myself a bowl of homemade soup. I made far too much so passed the neighbours some too.

April 16

"Oh, God, I feel shocking," I grumbled to Jon.
"Go back to bed then."
"I can't." I hate wasting my day in bed.
"You're doing too much, Marco." He often accused me of this.

My body vibrated with pain, leaving me feeling like I'd been dug up, then walloped with the shovel. My neck, shoulders and pelvis hurt, and it's not because I have been hammering it at the gym, because I haven't been since Tuesday—I'm just generally tired and my fibro is on the march again.

Jon came home yesterday, but whenever he's away I don't seem to sleep the same. So, I think I have just been in a deep sleep and not moved, hence why my body is stiff.

A part of me wishes he hadn't bothered to come back because I find myself in Groundhog Day again, moving to bloody Prestatyn—hell will freeze over first.

Angry and ready to throttle him, I'm seething and not so quietly either.

With my day ruined and my mood murderous, I forgot to factor in one thing; his impending hospital appointment could be the cause of his antagonistic behaviour.

Hmm, I wonder... he isn't the type to tell me that he is stressed. His bark, worse than his bite should be enough of a hint.

Still I'm livid at being on the receiving end of it, whatever the underlying reason. The result is, I've binge eaten my way through my feelings.

April 17

After a terrible week, and missing the gym, I made sure I went first thing.

15.19 miles cycled in 70 minutes on level 9, burning 550 calories. I did slightly less than my last session, but only just. I really didn't think I'd stay for the two sets because I am still annoyed, and I couldn't be bothered. But once I'd completed the first set, I thought I may as well carry on. I told myself I wouldn't finish the second set, but I did, and I was pleasantly surprised by the results. It wasn't really a struggle either and I seem to have found a good rhythm despite missing the last six days.

Once home, I prepared tonight's dinner. Jon will have cottage pie, and as I can't stand mashed potato, I will have roast potatoes done with Fry Light, and whatever else I fancy.

At midday, Jon threw a spanner in the works because he had forgotten to put his tracksuit bottoms in the washing machine.

"Have you washed my tracksuit bottoms?"

"No. You didn't ask me to."

"I'm not going then." Anxiety talks, so I don't rise to it.

"We're leaving for your appointment in two and a half hours... they've been sat in a bag since Saturday... so what is it that you want me to do?" There is little point arguing.

"Forget it, Marco."

"I'll wash them now."

"They won't be ready." Any excuse not to have to go. We are all guilty of this. But not on my watch, not today—even if I have to iron the bloody tracksuit bottoms dry, he is going.

"We'll see, but you *are* going, Jon."

With Cinderella duties tended to, I got ready to take him to Clatterbridge Hospital, even though it was the last thing I wanted to do because he had been a pig, and right now I can't stand the sight of him. I know his anxiety has been his voice of late, and I get it, but I still wanted to kick his teeth in. Anyway, being the better person, I swallowed down my anger because today is his final cancer check—I'm terrified in case they find something while the camera is up there, but pleased he is being seen religiously as promised by the oncologist last year. The sadist in me is thrilled he is having something rammed up his pee hole because after him being so awful to me, I want to bury my size twelves where the sun doesn't shine. Fingers crossed all is okay.

I hate cancer with every fibre of my being. It robbed me of my mum, three of my grandparents, my dad currently has terminal prostate cancer that has metastasized to other parts of his body, a thought that never leaves my mind, and on Thursday, my sister told me she had found a lump in her breast. I had to stop myself from crying when she told me—my mum died of breast cancer, and that broke me. But losing Tammy, my only sister, no, I refuse to contemplate that.

She hadn't told anyone and had been worrying, which was exactly what my mum did, and that decision cost her her life. I am still mad with my mum for that, so would rather Tammy be forearmed.

"Have you booked in to see your GP?"

"No, I'm too scared—I hate showing my boobs."

"Don't be silly, you're just a piece of meat to them." Easy to say I know.

"I can never get an appointment at my doctors anyway."

"Tammy, I don't want you to die, and if it is something horrible, you need to know—you have kids and grandkids to think of too."

She made excuse after excuse, but I am not backward in coming forward and excuses don't wash with me. So, while she was driving, I called her doctors surgery, and as usual, a haughty receptionist tried to throw obstacles in my way.

Sorry, no. I wasn't prepared to give in.

"Can she come in now?"

"No, we're about an hour from home."

"Well, I don't have anything."

"Well," I snapped, my tone bordering on hostile, "my sister has found a lump in her breast, so I want an appointment for her with a lady doctor as soon as possible." I would drag the snooty cow down from her high horse with a thud but tried the polite route first.

"Hang on," she huffed, "I'll see what I can do."

"Fine."

Tammy cringed at my abruptness.

The gatekeeper came back to the call a few minutes later, offering an appointment for the following day. "I didn't know I could book appointments for things like this."

Well, if you didn't, you should have made it your business to know. I wanted to say it, but I took the appointment as the win. "Thank you."

"Did you get one?" Tammy asked.

"Of course I did, tomorrow at 9:25."

"I'm nervous now."

"How did you manage to get one so soon?"

"You know what I'm like, Tam, so make sure you go."

I did offer to go with her, but she said declined.

I text her twice that morning to remind her to go for the examination. The doctor did find lumps in both boobs and said it is probably just 'lumpy breasts' but discovering that our mum died of breast cancer at 61, she has been referred to the breast clinic, just to be on the safe side.

She confided in her daughter, Holly, who was understandably angry at being kept in the dark. She will accompany my sister to the breast clinic.

The universe better prepare itself for one hell of a kickback if it inflicts cancer upon my sister. But for now, I am telling myself all is well, and lumpy boobs it is.

Back at the hospital, I had to go inside the usually restricted waiting area with Jon because his anxiety shot through the roof, and the forty-five-minute wait did nothing to alleviate his fears. Despite wearing a teddy bear fleece hoody, my nipples stuck out like football studs because it was bitterly cold in the waiting room. I thought it was just me, but one of the nurses walked in and said, "It's freezing in here."

Jon was called in, and ten minutes later reappeared, looking a little pale. I had played every awful scenario in my mind, and how I would act given bad news.

"Are you okay?"

"That was awful."

"What was?"

"Having the camera shoved up there—the water they used to flush me felt quite relaxing, and the camera didn't hurt when it first went in, but then the doctor shoved it past the muscle, and I nearly grabbed him..."

My knees snapped together like a Venus fly trap. *Stuff that!*

"Oh, God."

"It really hurt."

I've chewed my fingernails down to stumps... But that's not the important part.

"How did it go?"

"All clear."

It was the best news we could receive, and to be on the safe side, even though this was designated Jon's final check, it has been decided that he must have a check every twelve months for the next five years... I'd be worrying already about repeating the procedure, but he will deal with it when it comes.

We called in to see a friend before going home, one Jon hadn't seen for ten years. It was nice, and there wasn't a shred of awkwardness... back home Sally had left me two presents near the back door as revenge for daring to go out without her. There is a dog flap, but she will only use it to come in from the outside, not the other way. Strange dog that she is, I love her with my whole heart, even though I was hanging over the sink ralphing after having to pick up her number two's.

Dinner was nice, roast potatoes (Fry Light), mince beef & onion with carrots, mushrooms & gravy (1 Syn), and now I just want to go to bed. But I still have laundry and writing to do. In-betweens was 1 x 70g bag of Cheese & Onion Disco's (18½ Syns – I can't believe it! They were NOT worth it).

April 18

Awake at 5:40 am, so I thought I'd get up and go to the gym early. Then I remembered that it doesn't open until 7:30 am. To pass the time, I lay on the bed and watched re-runs of *Neighbours* on *Amazon Freevee*. Bugger it, I fell asleep again, waking at 9 and then I headed to the gym.

Distance: 16.03 miles in 71 minutes. My thighs yelled at me to stop, but determined to beat yesterday's total, I pushed myself. I even started a third session, wanting to hit twenty miles but then thought better of it—my GP's warning echoes in my head, that if I push it too far, I will hurt myself and be forced to stop for weeks, ruining the progress I've made thus far. It isn't worth the risk and derailing my efforts. Exercise Bike Calories Burned: 584. Levels: 7 to 13, but averaged level 10.

One thing I have noticed is that the exercise is rapidly diminishing my desire to eat, and I struggle to force myself at the best of times. I find that for many hours afterwards, the thought of food is worse than ever. As I've mentioned before I don't have that hormone that tells me I am hungry, but I know I have to. Since starting at the gym, I talk myself into eating more and more.

Good news, my legs are looking slimmer with a more defined shape. They are also less flabby at the top, so something is working. My top half still looks like jelly, but I will deal with that later.

After a quick pit stop at the bistro for a pot of tea, it's back home to work on the final read through for *Act of Contrition*. It seems to be dragging on, and if truth be told I am bored rigid with the whole thing, but as Jon was with his mum last week, I knew we wouldn't get any reading done.

Hopefully, we will finish it this week and get it off to the beta readers. I can't see there being any more after this. I'm bored of it already and hate this part of the process, so the sooner I can offload it, and move on, the better for me.

As it turned out, we did well, and only have one hundred pages left to read.

After work, I raced to get my hair cut and beard trimmed. My turkey neck looked worse than ever, leaving me more determined to find something surgical to fix it. Looking fresher, I went for a sunbed—twelve minutes, and my backside and heels were on fire. I know it's considered unhealthy to use a sunbed, but I look so much better with a bit of colour, and in the absence of sunshine or a holiday, it's the next best thing.

Back home, I begrudgingly started preparing dinner. I am having the same as last night. Jon is having something totally different from me—Holland's cheese & onion pie, and cauliflower cheese—yuk! He's feeling sore today, well, after having the camera shoved down his pee hole, I am not surprised.

My dinner was roast potatoes (Fry Light), carrots, mushrooms & gravy (1 Syn). In-betweens was 1 x 40g bag of Kings cheese & onion crisps (6½ Syns). 4 x wholemeal bread, lettuce, Coleman's English mustard (HEXB + 6 Syns), builders tea with semi-skimmed Milk (HEXA) & sweeteners.

April 20

I was in such a deep sleep that my alarm barely registered. But I forced myself out of bed and walked to the gym.

Combining my workout from yesterday and today, I have cycled 22.18 miles. The heat in the gym and the arrival of a gang of girls who seemed to spend their time flirting with another group of guys meant their volume superseded the music pumping from my ear buds, sending me veering off course.

One of the worst symptoms of fibro for me is hypersensitivity to different noises coming at me at once—I put music on to drown out my surroundings, enabling me to work out, but so loud were they, I heard their din over everything else, leaving me disorientated and agitated.

Then to make matters worse they seemed to migrate to where the exercise bikes were, which made me feel closed in and claustrophobic.

Calories burned: 963.2.

Food is the last thing on my mind. I don't want to eat and have only had fruit.

"You should eat more," Jon reminds me.

"I don't fancy it."

"You never do."

"And I never will." He is right but I won't force myself.

April 21
WEIGH-IN DAY

I am dreading it and although I usually attend the 11 am weigh-in, I am out of the door for 9.

After missing it these last two weeks and missing the gym for six days over that period, I am anticipating a gain, But I have worked like a trojan since Monday in the gym... it's time to send a prayer to whoever is listening.

I am desperate to get into the next stone bracket because it puts me in the final stage of hitting target.

Stepping onto the scales, I never look and anxiously wait.

"3½ off."

YES!

Okay, spread over three weeks it's not a lot, but I've been off plan for most of that time.

Now I have two and a half pounds until I am in the next stone bracket, which also happens to be within my target range. Sixteen and a half pounds and I hit target. I am closer than I have ever been, I just have to get there.

April 22 & 23

Guess what? I'm off plan, but nowhere near as bad as I usually am at this stage of the weekend. *You have no self-control, Marco.*

Oh well, back to the gym to try and undo some of the damage.

Aside from that, today is a good day because I have booked to go and see ABBA in London again on 4th August.

This time, Jon is staying at home on dog-sitting duty, and I am going with my friend.

I'm already excited and have my outfit planned—slim into the trousers I've bought, and I'm not too far off from that point. What I don't want is to have to jam myself into them because I've gotten quite used to clothes no longer hurting me.

I'm reminded of something... many years ago, well before I started writing, I had decided to walk to work, so cut through the town centre. As I wasn't concentrating, I dropped my phone and instinctively bent over to pick it up, horrified to hear a tearing sound echoing through the rapidly busying, town centre. I knew instantly what had happened—I'd ripped the arse out of my suit trousers, but not just the arse, the tear went right down one leg. Mortified, and on the clock, I shrugged out of my hoodie, tied it around my waist and hot footed it to the nearest clothes shop—Burton—hoping I would find something that would fit me. I did, but I was late for work. Still, I was thankful nobody witnessed what happened, or at least I hope they didn't.

I bet I'm not the only person this has happened to.

April 24

I was wide awake before my alarm this morning, so got up and walked to the gym.

The weather is bright and sunny, but cold, so I've got my winter fluffy hoody on, which swamps me now. It could probably accommodate Jon and me and falls just above my knees. I've decided that I look stupid in it, which is why people probably stare at me. I need to unpack my other zip-up hoodies.

I'm feeling quite cheery as I walk along and find myself listening to the Initial Talk remix of *Solid Gold* by Delta Goodrem on repeat. I'm away with the fairies, as my mum used to say, and so engrossed with people watching, I haven't noticed the song has been playing on a loop for fifteen minutes. Nor do I notice the car as I step into the road without looking. I've always said I refuse to be buried in a double wardrobe, but I'm not ready to shuffle off this mortal coil yet, so need to take more care when crossing roads.

Today brough a productive session, and thankfully the place was emptier and quieter than it had been last Thursday.

Distance cycled was 14.08 miles. I actually could have done more, but I started to get bored as the Table Manners podcast that I was listening to came to an end. Also, I wanted to try some of the other equipment while the place was empty. Calories burned: 517.7. Levels: 7 to 10, but I averaged level 10.

I finally worked up the courage to try the seated leg press and managed 150 presses.

I found this quite easy and less intense than I imagined it to be. Once I figured out how to work it, and guessed what weight to set it at, I tried all three positions. I need to increase the weight as I managed to do all three with ease. But I will ask the instructor tomorrow to point me in the right direction.

The one thing about this is, I don't know if it burns calories, or how to measure anything, but I suppose any results will be seen in the shape and strength of my leg muscles.

I had every intention of cooking, until Jon and I went out to buy plants for the back garden. And I fell off plan within minutes. But it is what it is, I won't feel guilty, and I will get back on plan tomorrow.

April 25

I struggled to get out of bed. But the sun shone, and I refused to waste the day lying in my pit.

Still, I felt weary and out of sorts. *It's all the junk food you ate last night.* That wouldn't be beyond the realm of possibility—I need to do some research.

Breakfast was 2 x 115g Lemon Muller fat free Greek style yoghurt pot (1 Syn).

Anyway, I walked to the gym, arriving about an hour later than I'd like. I suffer from hay fever and have done since my 30th birthday, but this morning it was particularly bad. By the time I arrived at the leisure centre, my eyes and nose were streaming, and my face was bright red. Taking a tablet, I waited ten minutes then got to it.

Aside from the sneezing fits earlier on, today was a great day because I hit a new personal best. I'm unbelievably proud of myself, not least because I thought I'd have to abandon exercising a few miles in.

Why?

Whenever I'm working out, I have music or a podcast playing, otherwise boredom takes hold quickly, and the surrounding noise from other people affects me.

Today was no exception but through the ear buds I could hear, "Wooop, woooop, wooooooh," so I paused the music and turned around to look, but I couldn't fathom where the noise was coming from. So, I resumed exercising and then I heard it again, but this time it felt like a herd of elephants had stampeded past me.

I decided to ignore whatever it was, but then I heard it again, "Wooop, woooop, wooooooh," and was distracted enough to pause my workout.

As I turned, I watched a man rush past the exercise bike I was sitting on, making the noise I'd been hearing.

It was then that I realised, after seeing an explosion of ticks, that he had Tourette's syndrome. *Okay*, I thought to myself, cracking on with pedalling, but every time he approached and ticked, he made that same noise.

Now, I have nothing against any person with any form of different ability, and as it happens, one of my ex-partners suffered horribly from Tourette's and could tick quite violently, leaving him in agony, but it always set my nerves on edge.

I know myself well enough to know when I'm about to lose it.

Years ago, my ex, Matt, and I, were socialising in the Northern Quarter in Manchester, and it was his turn to go to the bar. I sat chatting with friends, and as I turned, I saw Matt approaching our table with a tray of drinks. At the worst possible time, he suffered a tick and threw the tray, drinks included, everywhere. Glasses shattered against the floor, making a right din. As I've mentioned before, the ridiculous always makes me laugh, and anything Carry On-style sets me off in hysterics. Of course, I wanted to help Matt, but I couldn't move for laughing. By this time, the whole bar had fallen silent because it was quite obvious that he was having an episode, with only me making the racket. I tried to calm myself down but kept replaying the moment in my mind's eye, which sent me into uncontrollable hysterics. Tears were running down my cheeks, but I couldn't reign myself in for what seemed like an eternity, by which time the DJ had resumed the music and people were getting on with their own business, shooting filthy looks my way. At various times throughout the night, I would burst into impromptu laughter as I relived him flinging the tray. True to form, Matt found it funny too, as he always did, but I always dreaded him having an episode in public, not because I was embarrassed by him, more because I had such little self-control over myself.

Today could have gone the same way, and the more noises this guy made, the more I suppressed the laughter bubbling inside. Thankfully, he left, and I settled down. I know I will have to leave the gym if he comes again because I would hate anybody, especially him, to think I was laughing at him.

I managed to cycle 16.54 miles on level 10. I didn't struggle at all with this today, and could have done much more, but I was nervous in case the guy came back, so I came off and moved to the leg press. Still, it is a personal best... now onto the next one. I would love to hit twenty miles per day, but I know this won't always be possible. But I'll take today as a win, and after stuffing my face last night with goodies, I need all the help I can get. Calories burned: 603.9, which is an improvement on last time.

Seated Leg Press – 150 presses. (Feet Positioned High, Feet Positioned Together / Low & Feet Positioned Apart) – This was easy, until I got to the gluteal exercise, and I felt it pulling right up the backs of my legs and past my bum cheeks. I'm sure it will get easier, but if it stops my bum cheeks from dragging along the floor behind me—no pain, no gain.

Total exercise time = 78 minutes.

Back on plan and I've been well behaved. Still, it's only 6:22 pm. There is plenty of time to screw up. But I won't.

As I had a late breakfast, I didn't bother with lunch. Instead, I got cracking preparing dinner.

Dinner was chicken casserole with onions, carrots, mushrooms, leeks, mange tout, red pepper, green beans, courgettes, potatoes, stock pots, stock cubes, Fry Light (Syn Free), gravy powder (1 Syn), Schwartz Chicken Provincial mix (3 Syns).

In-betweens was fresh fruit, tropical granola & fat free natural yoghurt (5½Syns), builders tea with skimmed milk (HEXA) & sweeteners.

By my reckoning, I've used 9½ Syns, but this is good because I've eaten lots today and had way more than my five a day (I've had 12), which included plenty of speed foods.

For the rest of the night, I am going to do some work on a new book I've been working on, as well as tinkering on this one. I also need to start planning the interviews for those people who wish to include their own story in this.

April 26 & 27

It's only Wednesday and I'm bored. But needs must so I walk to the gym.

Cycled 14.07 miles on level 10. I wanted to do more but boredom took hold, so I moved onto the next thing. Calories burned: 518.2.

Seated Leg Press – 160 presses. I was pressing heavier weights, and crikey did I feel it, especially in my backside.

Total exercise time = 75 minutes.

Food not too bad today, and I clocked in at 29 Syns, which is a lot for me. But I did eat eight meringues at 2½ Syns a pop—I enjoyed every single one but need to work extra hard at the gym tomorrow.

As soon as I opened my eyes, I knew the gym wasn't happening. Miles cycled and calories burned = sod all.

"You're pushing yourself too hard," Jon reminded me.

"I'm fine."

"No, you're not." He was right, but I wouldn't admit that.

The creases in my elbows and back of my knees are very sore, as are my thigh muscles. Yes, I could be accused of not listening to people, but I am listening to my body on this occasion, especially as I am supposed to be going to Liverpool tomorrow on a shopping trip.

April 28
WEIGH-IN DAY

Here I go again!

Well, I missed the scales.

Instead, I went shopping earlier than planned to Liverpool and started with hot chocolate topped with walnut cream. I'm too scared to count the Syns because the cream alone would push me right over the edge.

Add in the sweet and sour vegetables, garlic green beans, naan bread, and two slices of banoffee gateaux accompanied by a handful of gummy bears, and I was screwed.

I did walk around Liverpool for two hours, so that's got to help, right?

I will go back next week and tell the truth, I always do.

"Where were you last week?" Donna will ask.

"Shopping," I will reply, and they will laugh. I can't be bothered making excuses.

MAGGIE JANE'S STORY

Our paths are yet to cross, but after many conversations not related to weight, and good belly laughs, over the past eighteen months, I had conjured a mental image of fifty-four-year-old, Maggie. Is it right, or wrong? I don't know, but I have promised that we will meet during her planned trip to this part of the world in the not-so-distant future.

Happily married for thirty years and currently residing in California, USA, she is a devoted mother to her three children, plus three fur babies who are vying for her attention during our conversation.

Maggie lives with the struggles of carrying excess weight, but unlike many of those featured in this book, she has never been a member of any weight loss group. Negative experiences conveyed to me of her experience with one well-known organisation will leave you in no doubt of her feelings on them.

In one of our extended phone conversations, she shared, "Before returning to education, I worked in a video production/post-production house. We had many clients who were leaders in large exercise and weight loss programs. Over time, it became clear that these corporate clients, through their PR firms and advertising, cared little for the health of their clients. They were more focused on profits than genuine well-being. I noticed that these companies preferred the yo-yo dieter, benefiting from clients who continued to gain and lose weight without learning to change their relationship with food. Their programs didn't address the mindset needed for long-term change.

"They promoted drastic calorie cuts and company developed prepackaged foods, pulling clients out of the real world to achieve quick results. These methods disrupted natural metabolism, leading to rapid weight loss but eventual regain, often with additional pounds. This cycle not only hurt clients physically but also financially. Watching these corporations' profit while clients suffered turned me away from such fraudulent companies."

Currently a US size 10/12 and weighing 180lbs, Maggie would be considered overweight according to the Body Mass Index. But as many of us agree, this index is an outdated model that demands an urgent overhaul. Yes, as a species, we do tend to be bigger or curvier than our 1950's counterparts, yet medical professionals cling to this index for dear life. Previously tipping the scales at two-hundred and twenty-five pounds, she confesses, "My ideal weight would be one hundred and fifty pounds."

This isn't the typical path I experienced along my search for answers to this all too typical dilemma and I asked her, "What caused your weight gain?"

She responds candidly, "Overeating was never my issue. Between ages twenty and twenty-five, I weighed as little as 125 pounds at 5'8", but life took its toll. I have a slow metabolism, unlike my brother, who has always maintained a perfect physique without counting calories. At fifty-one, my thyroid rebelled, leading to its removal. Despite continuing to exercise and eat less, I gained 40 pounds in six weeks post-surgery. Nearly two years later, I'm 12 pounds away from my pre-surgery weight, thanks to a new medication that helps manage my hormones. Unfortunately, many people don't understand that circumstances beyond our control can impact weight gain and loss."

I appreciate her honesty and ask, "Besides health issues, are there any other problems caused by being overweight?"

She sighs, "I haven't faced additional health issues related to my weight. The thyroid problem arose after my brother was diagnosed with cancer, prompting family testing, but it wasn't connected to my weight."

As Maggie and I spent a long time getting to know one another through DMs and phone calls I didn't hesitate to hit her with another loaded question, "What do you see when you look in the mirror?"

She takes a moment and then in her genuine manner says in earnest, "Some days I see what my husband sees, and some days I see a little snout with an oink rattling around in my head!"

Maggie is certainly no different to those of us who see a skewed, and if truth be told, unfair version of ourselves in the mirror, so her answer isn't the least bit surprising. Although her weight issues are still an issue, thanks to a rigorous exercise regime and medical intervention, she stays in great shape and looks fantastic. But how does she see herself now?

"I fluctuate between feeling sexy and frumpy, depending on the day. I haven't gone through menopause yet, which contributes to these feelings. My husband thinks I'm beautiful every day, but it takes time to reshape my self-image, influenced by societal norms that label anything above a size 4 as obese. The beauty standards have shifted since the 1950s, creating unrealistic expectations for those of us with curves. Ultimately, I know I'm a kind and caring person with a solid support system."

Maggie and I discuss many things, but I'm always curious what others do to keep nourished and strong while trying to manage the weight.

"I eat healthy—no sugars, no grains, no extras! It's a life choice to keep balance between mother nature and ageing and the way a body processes carbs and sugars into glucose levels and high blood pressure issues. However, I also exercise daily by speed walking 5 – 7 miles and doing yoga."

You may think, as I do, that Maggie is a warrior with iron-clad determination. But there must be one food that is her Kryptonite... "Cheese... I love cheese! It is my biggest weakness. I have to be careful because it is loaded with calories!"

As we continue discussing all things I nudged her one more time about her hopes for the future.

She said, "I hope my medication continues to work, allowing me to lose this last bit of weight. My family supports everything I do, which is essential for avoiding negative self-perception."

With her family's unwavering support, I wrap up this interview with her final thoughts about her ultimate goal.

"I want to maintain a healthy weight without obsessively counting calories or exercising, and simply live content knowing I'm doing my best for myself."

MY JOURNEY - MAY 2023

May 1

I rolled out of bed, feeling refreshed and ready for the start of a new week, so I walked to the gym to find the gates locked. BLEEP, BLEEP, BLEEP, BLEEP, BLEEP... Mad with myself because I hadn't thought to check if it was open on a Bank Holiday, I peered through the gates. Instead, I went shopping and bought loads of healthy stuff; chicken, 5% mince, vegetables, fruit, and not-so-healthy strawberry meringues. Having started the day with the best of intentions I hoovered the meringues, two family bags of roast beef Monster Munch, Tropical Skittles, and jelly sweets. Am I ever going to get to target? Not if I continue to sabotage myself I won't.

May 2

I've been on and off plan since last week but made a concerted effort to go back to the gym today, after checking it is open. Cycled 17.17 miles which is a personal best. To say I am thrilled is an understatement and proves what I can do when I set my mind to it. I did have to stop at seven miles because the little plastic thing that fits on to the end of my ear bud detached itself and worked its way down my ear. I tried to loosen it with my little finger which only pushed it in further, so I went back to my locker, and retrieved a pen from my rucksack. I jammed that down my ear, and into the plastic thing, and after about five minutes of trying, pulled it out. It was lodged pretty far down, and I had visions of having to go to A&E. Panic over, I went back to the bike and carried on. Calories burned: 643. Levels: 7 to 10, but I averaged level 10.

Seated Leg Press – 160 presses. I think working too hard on this last week was the cause of a lot of the pain I was in, so while I did the same as last time and wanted to do more, I didn't. This I will need to be careful on—I'll build up slowly and incorporate other things into my workout.

Workout time = 86 minutes.

I walked home and ate lunch. Half of honeydew melon (Syn Free), tea with semi-skimmed milk.

Then I got in the bath to soothe my protesting joints.

I don't have a clue what I am going to have for dinner, but I will leave that to Jon. Posting in the group, I came across a promo code for the JD Seasonings and ordered twenty of those—I can't be the only person fed up with cooking and eating the same meals. At 4:30 pm I had a sports massage, which was perfect timing because I cannot turn my neck to the right.

Ian noticed as soon as I walked in and got to work.

It HURT LIKE HELL, but I knew it was because he was trying to 'free' my neck. An hour later, I had some movement, and even though it's sore now and tender to the touch, any improvement is better than nothing.

"Go online and buy yourself a wheat bag."

"What's one of them?"

"It's like a snake. You heat it up in the microwave, then wrap it around your neck and/or shoulders."

"I'm willing to try anything." So I ordered one as soon as I got home. It should arrive tomorrow, so I shall give it a go, and hope it has some positive effect.

About 10:30 pm, I fancied something to eat, so rather than run to the shop, I settled on bananas, strawberries, black grapes, tropical granola & fat free natural yoghurt (5½Syns), washed down with more tea. I also polished off 8 strawberry meringues at 3½ Syns a pop.

While in the kitchen I prepared tomorrow's dinner.

May 3

With two days of appointments to combat, my mind is unsettled. Out of bed at the ungodly hour of 7 am because I have my first with the Pain Management clinic—I've only been waiting about twenty months so it should be interesting what they advise and prescribe.

Sitting in the waiting room, I felt disorientated due to the bright lights, then I nearly jumped out of my chair as a siren blared sending my hands to cover my ears.

"Don't worry, sir, it's just a weekly test." The receptionist rushed over to advise.

"Frightened the life out of me," I roared, over the continuing din.

"It will ring for sixty seconds then stop."

Hypersensitivity is a bummer, as is hypervigilance, so when I walked into my therapist's room for the first time, I felt like I'd been jolted from my body, and agitated.

"Are you okay, Marco? You seem a little spaced out."

"I'm fine now," I lied. "I just felt a little out of it when the alarm started ringing, and it's so bright in here, I can't focus."

Dave pulled the blinds down, which made it a little easier.

A productive first meeting left me feeling positive, although I had no idea what to expect next, he couldn't have been more helpful.

"You have to learn to pace yourself, Marco."

"I try but there's always so much to do."

"You're going to crash and burn if you don't slow down."

"I know, and my doctor has told me the same thing, but I never seem to stop."

As I've mentioned before, I was one of those people that foolishly believed that Fibromyalgia was 'all in the mind' but after speaking to Dave, and telling him my previous thoughts, and how my mindset has changed, I felt validated; that I wasn't losing my mind, and that I do have a condition I'd readily denied before.

"What medication are you on?"

"All sorts, but I don't like taking it because it makes me feel nauseous the following day."

"Okay, well, I'm going to refer you to the clinic pharmacist, and they might trial you on a different medication."

"I'm willing to try anything."

"So far, this new medication only works for one out of eight people but could help you regulate your sleep pattern."

"That would be good."

"I'll also schedule another appointment to go through some relaxation techniques with you."

Oh, no! I imagine myself lying there and counting crème eggs, but he assures me nothing of the sort. "What does it involve?"

"Listening to music, or relaxation podcasts."

"I once tried a rainforest podcast, and while it was soothing, it didn't help me sleep because I was up and down peeing all night."

He has also referred me to an organisation called THIS WAY UP. I'd never heard of it before; they are a not-for-profit initiative of St Vincent's Hospital and the University of New South Wales in Australia written under the supervision of Professor Gavin Andrews AO, MD.

As it is online based, I have my login details, and although I don't know much about it yet, Dave spoke highly of it. So, I am willing to give anything a try if it helps.

"Exercise is essential, Marco."

"I try and go to the gym as often as possible."

"Continue using the exercise bike or use other machines that are considered low impact."

"The more exercise I do, the less I hurt."

"It is vitally important for people that suffer from your condition to remain as active as possible. But remember what I said about boom and bust."

Dave wants me to start with the CHRONIC PAIN PROGRAM, which has been designed to give me the practical skills to better manage chronic pain, in order to improve my quality of life. It contains eight lessons which I can complete in my own time. Dave can also login to this via a portal and see my progress—no pressure there!

I left the meeting on a high—aside from my GP, somebody had listened to me and understood.

Afterwards, I headed to the gym as I have a lot of lost time to make up.

Amazing! I cycled 20.08 miles on level 10. It took me about eight weeks to build to it, but I finally managed to hit my target. I'm not sure if, or when, I'll ever be able to reach it again—I did it, and I felt exhilarated. Calories Burned: 740.3

Seated Leg Press – 160 presses. I varied my routine today and focused more on the higher position, which made my bum ache as it was working those particular muscles.

Total workout time – 105 minutes.

I walked home and finished off the honeydew melon. (Syn Free).

While I should have been writing, I couldn't be bothered so sat down and watched re-runs of *Neighbours* all afternoon, until it was time to cook.

Dinner amounted to 7 Syns, but 6 of that was for cooking oil, while in-betweens was 5½.

My day was quite successful, and I finished it with something that might surprise you—I applied to become a SW consultant. What am I thinking? That I could excel in the role perhaps. I won't know anything else until they contact me.

I'll forget about that for now as tomorrow's dentist appointment is on my mind.

MARCO LEWIS

May 4

I woke with a feeling of dread.

Nicole, my new dentist, seems nice. But she is that rare breed of professional I simply do not trust because of past experiences.

"I'm terrified of dentists." I see no reason not to be honest with her.

"Don't worry, Marco. I'll look after you. I just need to have a look at the information that you provided." She checked my medical history and medications and laughed. "I think something has gone wrong."

"Oh?"

"You have your medications listed as sprouts, diet Pepsi, and somebody called Jonathan." For some unknown reason, my phone had overwritten the information on the form.

I found it quite funny. "Jon is more of a pain than any medication."

She laughed. "How many of each are you taking?"

"All three twice daily," which made her laugh all the more.

So, I slid into the chair and opened my mouth.

"Ah, I see," she replied.

"Can you fix it?" I asked. One full veneer has popped off and the other is snapped, leaving my teeth resembling toe separators. While I'm waiting for the new veneers to be crafted, I shall be practicing ventriloquism, the art of speaking with one's mouth closed. My next appointment, to have the new veneers fitted, is in two weeks, so I better be a quick study.

Now it's over and done with, I'm glad I went. Nicole is a joy. And while the deed is never as bad as the thought, I still didn't enjoy being in the chair.

She did say something that made me chuckle... "You do have a very active tongue, Marco." My mind immediately conjured an image of Kenneth Williams from the Carry-On movies... I was itching to reply, "Ooh, Matron," but as she had her index finger holding my tongue down, I let it pass.

When I'd finished, she explained what treatments were needed so I have appointments booked over the next four weeks which doesn't thrill me but I'm paranoid about my teeth so will do what needs to be done.

Turkey teeth are beckoning. I just have to organise a new passport and get over there. And while I know it's controversial and will no doubt encourage Simon Cowell comparisons, I don't care.

I'm still on plan and decided to be adventurous—I followed a recipe which is always lethal, needless to say the chicken was still raw, so I had to take it away, put it back in, which meant the potatoes, green beans and cous cous went cold.

Eventually, I just ate the potatoes, while Jon waited for the chicken and abandoned the rest.

To say I am peeved at botching dinner up is an understatement. I am tempted to tuck into my last easter egg, but I won't. I'll have fruit and natural yoghurt later instead.

May 6

The last few days have been awful and spent in pain due to a flare up. I never made it to weigh-in yesterday although I really wanted to see where I was up to. But every part of me hurt, so I stayed in bed.

Today is King Charles III, and Queen Camilla's, coronation, so I forced myself up to watch it. I found the service extremely moving, and I know there are those amongst us who don't believe in a monarchy. They are entitled their opinion, but I am of the opinion that they do a lot of good for the UK and the Commonwealth, not to mention the countless millions they bring into the economy. Aside from that, *nobody* does pageantry and pomp better than the British. A proud day indeed!

May 12
WEIGH-IN DAY

After missing weigh-in the last two weeks and being on and off plan, I went to get weighed today.

"Five on." Shelly dropped her voice.

My heart sank. "Okay." What else could I say? *I'm so disappointed in myself.* I think it but don't say it.

"It's a new week, Marco." There is always a smile.

"I know."

With others to weigh and didn't need my life story, or excuses.

Distance cycled this week is 39.68 miles on level 10. It has been a struggle, but I have tried to battle through the pain and the ever-increasing fatigue that seems to have come from nowhere, and fast. I did what I could. Calories burned is 1,503.92.

Seated Leg Press – 130 presses. I really felt the burn in my muscles this week and can see the change of shape to my upper thigh. I will keep going, and although I did want to do more. I had to admit defeat. Still, it was better than nothing.

Weekly workout time: 169 Minutes

I was quite deflated by the gain, but seeing my physiotherapist, he reminded me that the gain could partially be muscle mass gain, and unhealthy eating, too. I really didn't think of it like that, but I won't hang on to that hope. He did send me this via text...

Gaining weight after working out is likely due to muscle fibre inflammation, muscle glycogen and water weight gain, and over time, muscle mass gain. If weight loss is your goal, seeing an increase on the scale when you've been making an effort to exercise can be frustrating. However, it is a normal, common occurrence that is likely temporary.

Target is now further away from my grasp, but I am determined to get there.

May 15

Today is a new day. It's time to re-focus and put the past behind me and crack on. Last week was a disaster health wise, and the weight gain. I'm not going to dwell on it, but I did try my new trousers on last night—I bought them for ABBA Voyage on 4th August, and I am determined to comfortably fit into them, and fasten them.

Distance: 15.41 miles on level 12. Calories burned was 604.

I really wanted to do more, but the temperature in the gym ruled it out. I took a picture of myself while cycling and sent it to Jon.

"Why don't you smile?"

"Because I'm exercising and sweating, what's to smile about?"

"You're quite handsome when you smile..."

Quite handsome... bloody cheek. I know what he means. But I am not a natural smiler, especially when I am in the middle of major dental work.

Total exercise time: 60 minutes.

I skipped breakfast but popped into my local café for a pot of tea and a gossip.

Dinner was roast beef, mint sauce (1 Syn), roast potatoes, carrot & turnip, leeks, mushy peas, stock pots, Fry Light (Syn Free) and gravy powder (1 Syn). In-betweens was fresh fruit and yoghurt (Syn Free).

May 16 & 17

Tired and sluggish yet still on plan, I don't feel like doing anything—from cooking, to walking, to going to the gym. Still, I pushed myself and achieved good results the past few days.

Distance cycled is 31.45 miles in two hours on level 10. Calories burned is 1247.

While I was surprised at my achievements, I did more than I should have done. I'm worried my body is about to revolt. Still... *Go, Marco.* I am at that point where not going to the gym bothers me. How odd!

May 24

I've had quite the time since last checking in and have had a massive fibro flare up. Every part of my body hurts, from the creases in my elbows, to my neck, to my toes. Add in the unbearable burning sensation all over my body, I am in a mess. I've scratched the backs of my legs in my sleep with my toenails and cut them to ribbons.

It's my own fault... Dave's words haunt me... *boom and bust*. Both him and my GP warned me it could happen if I pushed my body beyond its capabilities. But today is a new day, and I am on plan, and have been since Monday, and have been back to the gym.

Great news! I achieved my Silver Body Magic Award from SW, so I am chuffed. Working towards Gold now—I will do it.

Distance cycled today was 12.14 miles in 50 minutes on level 13.

I feel like I haven't stopped eating today. But I haven't even used 1 Syn, and that's not through calculation, just the way things happened.

Lunch was poached eggs, mushroom & beans (Syn Free), and a cup of team with milk (HEXA).

Dinner was SW curry sauce and rice (Syn Free), 2 x Warburtons wholemeal bread (HEXB) with honeydew melon (Syn Free).

Even though I've had a few days being on plan, I still feel so far away from where I need to be and totally disheartened. I need to alter my state of mind and get back into it. Strange as it may seem, I am looking forward to weigh-in on Friday. Hopefully I will have had a small loss, but even if it's a gain, I will suck it up and keep going.

May 26

WEIGH-IN DAY

Today is one of those days—I have so much to fit in, and things that cannot be cancelled, but little time to do it all in.

So, I don't want to miss weigh-in and decide to go to the early class. I arrive at 7:45 am, totally baffled at how many people are there so early. There are queues to get weighed and every chair is full waiting for Donna to start the class.

I must admit, I felt immediately uneasy because I didn't recognise any of the faces, bar one, so I was a stranger in their midst too. I felt all eyes were on me, and I might have been imagining it, but I couldn't wait to get out of there.

Donna was busy talking to another member, and the lady weighing me I didn't recognise. I'm so distracted by the volume of people around me that I took no notice when she spoke to me and immediately started talking about something else.

Then, something clicked in my head.

"How much?"

"Seven, off," she replied.

"Off?" I was convinced it would be a gain, and if not, a tiny loss of maybe half a pound.

"Yes, well done."

So, I was overjoyed and am now only half a pound away from my next stone bracket, and more importantly, I am only 1 stone and half a pound away from my agreed target.

May 30

I spent the weekend sunbathing and stuffing my face. What's new? But I am back on plan, and officially give up trying to stay on it permanently because I just can't do it.

I had a phone call from a lady who works for SW. She was calling regarding my enquiry about becoming a consultant. I'd totally forgotten about it. She apologised for the delay and advised her manager had been off, so she was catching up on calls. I couldn't talk to her properly, but she is calling me back on Wednesday evening for a proper chat—I will let you all know.

Anyway, that's the last Bank Holiday until August, so back to the gym today.

Once there, I feel at peace. But I hadn't missed the sweltering heat inside, and it wasn't long before my T-shirt clung to me. As usual, I was looking down on the swimming pool wishing I was floating in the water. Perhaps I should bite the bullet and go for a swim.

I cycled 13.05 miles on level 13, burning off 531 calories. The sun was shining, and there wasn't a cloud in the sky, so I felt antsy being inside on such a glorious day. I focused on getting up to ten, so was pleased with my result.

I managed to do thirty on the seated leg press, a poor attempt, but I did what I could before my legs began to throb. I'm learning to listen to my body more, and while I wanted to do more, I stepped away.

Total workout time was 53 minutes.

Lunch was omelette, mushroom, beans, Fry Light (Syn Free), 2 x slices of Warburtons wholemeal bread (HEXB).

After lunch I lazed about in the garden, then at 4 pm, I had another sports massage. Then I headed home. Jon had cooked, so even better.

May 31

I achieved nothing of worth today. I didn't even go to the gym because I was sore after my sports massage. So, I spent the day watching TV, waiting for the sun to come out so I could head into the garden. By the time it did, I was too tired to be bothered.

Stuck to plan again and had an interesting telephone conversation with the lady from SW regarding training to be a consultant. It's not going to be an easy road, and nor should it be. Nothing worth having ever is. And while I will go to the fact finders meeting, this part of my journey might be something that waits further down the road for me.

Why?

Quite simply… how can I lead and motivate a group of people when I haven't reached my own goal? I don't think I could stand and face a room if I hadn't. It would be like a smoker coaching a person to quit—come back and tell me that once you've done it!

Standing in front of a class hoping to inspire others to follow your success will only work if people believe in you, and what you're saying, and until I've mastered my own failings and stood on those scales to be told that I have done it, I can't in all conscience proceed.

So many times over the years I've heard tittle tattling from members of various weight loss classes,

How can she lead this group when she's overweight?

Or.

I wouldn't be inspired by an overweight leader.

For some of those reading, you might disagree with both statements, but I can agree to an extent. I want to lead by example, but also remain a member, while ensuring my own journey remains on track. I fear that if I was successful in my mission to be a consultant that I would slowly cease to be a member, and my travels would grind to a halt. I can't lose that small amount of control

I'm holding onto because I am three and a half stones down and to regain it would not only be heart breaking, but confidence-shattering.

From our chat, it seemed that the lady from SW and I are strikingly similar in many ways, from our mindset to sharing a sweet tooth to the fact we won't sacrifice everything that we enjoy simply to lose weight. I cannot and won't do it, and it seems, nor can she. While her story is not mine to tell, I was inspired by it, and she made me feel that bit more human in my approach to reaching my goal.

I WILL get there, just as she did, but it might take me a little longer, and while I know for certain that I could have reached it by now, if it takes me another two years, so be it.
That's not a bad thing because I've already come such a long way—thanks for the motivation!

LEIGH'S STORY

To say fifty-year-old Leigh has been on a rollercoaster for the better part of the last decade is an understatement. But like many of us living with similar issues, it's a ride that seems to have no end in sight.

Although locked in that torturous and vicious circle, he has seen many successes because he is a prime example that will power, and perseverance wins the day. Victory, in part, is his.

Presented with a framed photograph, it is hard to reconcile the man sitting before me with the man in the picture. But they *are* one and the same—the man in the photograph shows Leigh as he was at the latter end of the 1990's.

So, before we delve into his life over the last ten years, allow me to offer some context as to the man he was then.

Fiercely athletic, his achievements would put many, including mine, to shame. As I was never the sporty type, I shudder to imagine how much hard work and dedication it took to compete in even one of the competitions below, let alone all of them.

Liverpool 10k – 1996 + 1997
BUPA Great North Run - 1997
London Marathon – 1997 + 1998
Great North Run – 1997 + 1998
Liverpool Echo Half Marathon - 1997
Waterloo 15k – 1997 + 1998 + 1999
Liverpool Tunnel 10k – 1997
Hoylake 10k – 1997
East Cheshire Half Marathon – 1997

Impressive, right, and while Leigh might think back to that time and wish he was still physically capable of such mammoth runs, praise is deserved because he actually competed in them all and has the medals to prove it. Nobody, and nothing, can take those achievements away from him.

Fast forward to 2017, where Leigh's weight loss journey begins

Concerned, his GP had referred him to the local NHS Weight Management Programme, which supports adults living with obesity. It is a twelve-week behavioural and lifestyle programme that is designed to encourage healthier living.

Alongside this vital programme, Leigh was offered a twelve-week referral to his local *Slimming World* group. Accepting the support he remembers weighing in at thirty-four stone, five pounds.

Sitting no more than a foot away from me, he looks extremely well, and for the life of me, I can't imagine such a number because I have no concept of weight in other people.

I simply see Leigh as he is now.

At 6ft 1, he is a fine figure of a man, hovering in that world of successful weight loss and dreaming of the day he gets to where he believes content lies. Thirteen stone, a number unlucky for some, but that is his magic number, where piece of mind exists. It might seem a distant dream, but good things come to those who work hard for it.

Despite this being the goal, if the BMI is your gospel of choice, Leigh would still be classed as overweight. Madness, I think many would agree, especially as this index fails to factor in how the individual feels about themselves, and how they look physically at varying weights.

When Leigh gets to thirteen stone, he might decide he needs to lose a little more, then again, he might wish to stay where he is. He may feel that he needs to gain a few pounds back. Who knows? Perhaps if I write a second book, I can catch up with Leigh and the many others who have shared their stories... I'd love to know, wouldn't you?

But for now, please forgive me, because I've jumped ahead and need to go back... thirty-four stone, five pounds... for those lucky never to have never experienced issues with their weight, this figure seems unbelievable. But for millions around the world, carrying an extra half a stone is often noticeable. Multiply what most would view an insignificant amount by ten and welcome a myriad of issues into your world. Push aside how you think you look in your new dress, or the oh-so-easy brushing off of the fact you've had to loosen your belt a notch or two, let alone, breathe in until you're almost blue, aesthetically speaking, gaining weight can shatter confidence like a claw hammer to glass. Once that confidence is stripped away, building it back to what it was can seem an impossible task.

Meeting Leigh, I instantly notice that he displays the same tricks I've employed on and off over the years—arms crossed tightly over the chest, which in his case could be simply down to comfort. I'd guess otherwise because overweight people, me included, often use it to hide their body shape, or as a non-verbal warning for others to keep away.

Jump to 2024, and Leigh currently weighs twenty-five stone, five pounds, which is a fantastic achievement in itself. Admittedly, he has regained some of the weight he had previously shed—from twenty-two stone, seven pounds—we've all been there, but Leigh works tirelessly to reach his personal target. His immediate aim is to be under twenty stone, and I have no doubt that he will get there.

At the start of his journey in 2017, he was wearing 9xl T-shirts and 68-inch waist trousers.

Now, well on his way to target, he slips into 3xl T-shirts and a 52-inch waist trousers.

This is something he should look upon proudly, which I hope in some way has gone to restoring any lost confidence. Gaining weight was the easy part, but shedding it takes strength, both mentally and physically. Thankfully, Leigh isn't alone on his journey.

Settled in a long-term relationship with the lovely Maria and leaning on his local *Slimming World* group for support, I ask what brought Leigh to this moment.

"I used to be a marathon runner in the 90's and played rugby for Wallasey. Then in 2001, disaster struck. I'd always wanted to do the London to Brighton ultra marathon... fifty miles in the day... I got to thirty-one miles and tripped on a brick and hurt my ankle and knee." I see sadness and regret in his eyes, that he was almost there. "If I hadn't hurt myself, I'd still be running to this day. I miss it." With conviction, he adds, "But I've jogged this year at the size I am now."

Sadly, more bad luck was to follow his injury. "In May 2010, I was made redundant from my job, and then I broke my ankle. That was the start of me overeating and I went downhill from then."

Gaining weight after an accident is a tale as old as time, then throw in worries about losing one's job, Leigh was forced to deal with what life had thrown at him the same way many of us have. "I was never really a big eater. Then, in 2015, quite suddenly, my mum passed away, and that started me on the path to overeating."

Grief is a leading factor when forming addictions—food, drink, drugs, sex... name any addiction and grief will have pushed a percentage of people into its destructive path. But once in the throes of it, seeing weight creep on means nothing until it gets to a point where a person, and the life once led seems unrecognisable. Leigh is no different. "From 2015 to 2017, I put on fifteen stone because I was constantly eating. You don't know you're doing it."

Leigh readily admits that his darkest moments were between 2015 and 2016 when he didn't want to do anything but pig out. There is strength in recognition. "Personal care became an issue. Showering—I struggled to stand so I had to sit on the floor inside the cubicle and shower that way. Not only that, but I found it difficult to clean myself after using the toilet, having to use a plastic stick with toilet paper on. Some might wonder why I have chosen to reveal that, but I want people to read this and realise they are not alone and that it happens to many of us. Obesity impacts what should be the simplest of tasks. Putting socks on was virtually impossible and because I couldn't get them on, I developed repeated issues with foot fungus. Walking even the shortest distances left me sweating profusely, and that was only from the front door to the car."

Once in the car, Leigh's size meant he could not fasten the seatbelt.

His health deteriorated to such a point that he required prescription glasses for failing eyesight, something that is no longer an issue since losing weight.

He was also reliant on a walker. "It was bad," he reflects, then recalling a trip to Cyprus with Maria. "I left for my holiday weighing twenty stone and returned a stone heavier."

He remembers his poor sleep patterns, saying that he found it difficult to keep his eyes open, and therefore slept most of the day away.

His moods were darker. "I hated people asking me for help." Not because he didn't want to, but physically, he was unable to do so. "Now, I'm the first to offer."

During this time, Maria's family became concerned about Leigh's increasing weight, and out of love for Maria, and concern for Leigh, numerous members broached the subject, only wishing to encourage him to re-engage in a healthier lifestyle. And while Maria was unaware of these hushed conversations, she later learned that her stepmum warned Leigh that he would lose Maria if he didn't lose weight and regain his fitness.

"That would never have happened." Maria is adamant on this, and thankfully, they are still together.

I query about Leigh's preferred foods—where does his weakness lie? "My main downfall is bread and cheese. I can eat a loaf of bread quite easily and if there is no bread, it's chocolate and crisps."

I ask him at what point is his strongest desire to eat, and like many of us stuck in that loop, his answer doesn't surprise, "Boredom. If I am doing something, maybe volunteering for AGE UK, I don't think of food, but sitting in front of the TV, I want to go and pick something up to eat."

How did the weight gain impact his social life?

"I had a best friend who I saw regularly, then I started putting weight on, and he stopped coming to see me. Not only that... the people that I used to socialise with, go on pub crawls with, I don't see them anymore either because I couldn't physically keep up with them. They turned their backs on me, not the other way around."

I wonder if any of these people are back in Leigh's life since successfully losing weight and regaining an element of physical fitness. "No, and if one of my old mates said hello to me now and asked me out for a drink, I'd tell them to get lost." Nobody would blame Leigh for how he feels towards his former school friends. But he explains his reasoning anyway. "Only remember the people that were there for you, and you didn't have to ask. Maria was always there for me, and they weren't. Now, I am past caring what people think." There is a touch of bitterness, but wouldn't we all feel the same way? I know I would.

And how does Leigh view himself now?

"I'm mentally proud of what I have achieved." And so he should be. "From being a recluse to being able to exercise... I look better because my clothes are going smaller. I do feel the difference. But with people who are overweight, it will never change. For instance, if I stay the same weight, I will never be able to go into certain shops and buy clothes. Bigger people can't go to Gucci 'cos they don't want to know you."

I do believe Leigh's assessment is valid, and correct, because designers don't hire overweight people as ambassadors for their brands, and if they do recognise plus size, it is for more calculated reasons, namely, to avoid shoutouts by a bandwagon-jumping press.

"These designers will never change. You'll never, ever, see somebody my size walk down the catwalk at London Fashion Week. Diversity, and all this trying to change is a load of rubbish. It will never happen for people who are overweight."

Although he has worked hard, found, and maintained well deserved success, what does he see when he looks in the mirror now? "You never ever look the same. You should never look in the mirror because you will always see a person who is overweight. But I am immensely proud of where I am, and what I've done. I'm a different person now. When I was thirty-four and a half stone, I wasn't physically capable of cooking, cleaning, or doing most things I did before, so everything fell to Maria—she had to cook, and take care of me, even though she was struggling with her own health issues. But that was then. Now I've lost weight I can do more."

Love between them is there in abundance, it's easy to see, but Leigh clarifies things for me with Maria's help. "I would rather do things for her because I love her so much and I don't want to see her in pain. It's all about caring for one another. Now, I do all the cooking and food preparation, and I do all of the dishes. I am there for Maria, and when I am not feeling my best, she is there for me."

Maria, who suffers from various health conditions and must have struggled during Leigh's less active period, agrees with his following statement. "We try and do as much as we can for each other."

Making one's vulnerabilities public is never easy, but Leigh credits *Slimming World* with giving him his life back.

Has being overweight caused any significant health issues? He points to his ankle and reveals a scar, explaining that "fluid built up in my ankle due to excess weight, resulting in an ulcer, caused by lack of movement and bad circulation." But since losing weight, the ulcer has gone, with only the scar remaining as the reminder of its existence. "I also found I was sleeping all day, but I don't have any conditions related to being overweight aside from hypertension, which made me a ticking time bomb—no diabetes either."

What is Leigh's life like now?

"I volunteer as a Tour Guide for AGE UK, and also support kids between the age of eight and eighteen at an organisation called HIVE, based on the Wirral."

Have his fitness levels improved as he has lost weight? "When I was at my heaviest, I met a guy called Hassan Ashley who taught me to box. He had all the patience in the world. He wrapped me up and looked after me. I trusted him and he was there for me. He would come to my house because I didn't want to go to a gym, and I would box in my basement. At the start, hitting the boxing bags, I was tired and struggling. Now, I can do two-minute rounds."

He must feel proud of his progress. "Hassan now works with Anthony Joshua, and I train with a lady called Angie Taylor who runs a boot camp to try and help people lose weight. But I feel so much better. Before I could just about walk and now, doing everyday tasks... to what it was then, now is easier."

Leigh enjoys mountain bike riding, but due to issues with his Achilles Tendon, he doesn't do it as much as he used to. But he is slowly getting back into it, and finds since losing weight, the aforementioned issues cause him less complications.

Aside from that, for the first time in ten years, he is seeking employment within the Mental Health sector, and believes his own struggles make him the ideal candidate to help others in need.

For him and Maria, marriage and children was something they had discussed, but with their combined health issues, they were also reluctant to bring a child into the world unless they could provide for them financially.

And while Leigh has recently hit fifty, and Maria, forty, children aren't an impossibility. It is obvious they would make wonderful parents. But they have their heads screwed on and acutely aware of their limited capabilities at the moment, have put their hearts aside, and ruled with their heads.

Once upon a time, they visited wedding venues, planning for their big day until the harsh realities of life took over. But they assure me that marriage in the not-too-distant future is on the cards.

With promises of I do, shimmering enticingly on the horizon, no couple are more deserving of that happy ever after.

With their backs against the wall, Leigh, and of course, Maria, continue to achieve so much together that it's only a matter of time until their dreams become reality.

MY JOURNEY - JUNE 2023

June 1

    A new month, and already we are halfway through 2023. Where has the time gone? Christmastime seems like only yesterday, and now we're on the verge of what I hope will become a blisteringly hot summer.
    The sun is shining and I'm not at all hungry. Regardless, there is no time to rest on my laurels, so it's back to the gym, which I am looking forward to, and a trip to the dentist afterwards, which I am definitely not in a rush to get to.
    I cycled 10.06 miles on level 13 in 43 minutes. Once again, it was unbearably hot in the gym, yet despite my eagerness to go, after three miles, I'd had enough and was tempted to go home. But I didn't want to leave until I'd hit the ten-mile mark at least. On my way out I passed the attendant at the desk and noticed she had a hoodie zipped right up to her neck—it was so warm because she had turned the air conditioning off. Calories burned is 403.
    Exiting the dentist, I'm not in the best of moods because my mouth is sore from her fiddling around so much. It seems I have a loud voice, but only a small mouth.
    "Open wider, if you can," Nicole said, as she almost jammed her fist in.
    I didn't bother to reply although my mind conjured a witty response.
    "I'm just going to use this to hold your tongue down." She waved a mini spatula-type instrument in front of me.
    But it's over and done with until my next appointment this coming Thursday, and hopefully a few more appointments after that means no more treatment, only check-ups.
    Then, I hoofed to the barbers, and by the time I arrived I was bright red in the face and sweating buckets—it wasn't just my jaw that was aching—my feet were throbbing too.

June 2
WEIGH-IN DAY

I'm peed off with myself today because I'd planned to go to weigh-in then had to miss it due to an impromptu visit from the in-laws. I wish I'd gone yesterday when I had the idea. Worse still, I am away next week so can't weigh-in then either.

June 5 & 6

Thank goodness the weekend is over, and I can regain some semblance of control. Have I fallen off plan? Oh, yes, quite spectacularly. But I am heading back to the gym to try and reverse some of the damage.

I managed to cycle 12.06 miles on level 11 in 53 minutes and have burned 501 calories.

I have not done my food shop, so the only thing in the house is snacky foods, so remaining on plan doesn't bode well.

Later that day, I knew my lack of preparation would lead me straight to the shop for goodies, and I was right.

Marco, you are self-sabotaging... stop it!

The following morning, I got up to go to the gym and quickly realised it wasn't going to happen as my stomach was cramping. I spent the morning on the loo, courtesy of my pig out last night. When will I ever learn?

Seems not anytime soon as I fell off plan again this evening.

I passed the mirror in my hallway and caught my reflection, and for the first time in years, I could see how different I look. With this fresh in my mind. It is more important than ever that my hard work doesn't go to waste, not now.

... "You've lost so much weight."
... "Surely you don't have much more, if any, to lose."
... "You look amazing."
... "Wow, you look so different."
... "You're not going to lose any more, are you?"

All comments I've heard from various people lately and as nice as it is to hear, none of it quiets my mind.

Far from perfect I keep telling myself the same thing over and over again... "I'm only human, I'm only human, I'm only human."

June 12

Back on plan, and to the gym. It took all of five minutes for me to regret going; as soon as I started to sweat, I'd had enough. But I persevered and cycled 12.11 on level 13 in 50 minutes, managing to burn off 488 calories. It won't be enough to undo the damage, but it is a start.

Dinner was meatballs (Yuk) with JD Seasoning, baby potatoes and mixed salad (Syn Free).

Fresh fruit and natural yoghurt with tropical granola filled in the gaps (5½ Syns).

June 13

After a terrible night sleep interrupted with tossing and turning, I gave up and slipped into a red-hot bath, which was the worst thing I could have done as I was already sweating by the time I walked to the gym.

Distance travelled was 7.01 miles, I really couldn't do any more than 7.01 today but managed to get up to level 10 and burn of 277 calories. My poor performance was nothing to do with my tiredness, more the sweltering heat in there.

Seated Leg Press – 95 presses, which isn't bad considering I haven't used this for a few weeks because I went overboard on it and hurt myself. But I am aware I need to vary my workout or there is a chance I will become bored. My aim is to start using other machines in there that will tone my upper body—bingo wings are about to start flapping, so I need to get started.

Total workout time was 41 Minutes. The gym manager really needs to do something about the air conditioning in there.

Not in the mood for anything substantial, so ate strawberries, black grapes & fat free natural yoghurt for lunch, while dinner was onions, peppers, mushrooms, baby potatoes and mixed salad. In-betweens was a repeat of lunch. (Syn Free)

It hasn't happened to me for a while, but I was as sick as a dog after dinner—I knew I didn't feel hungry.

June 14

Another scorcher of a day today, so I decided to give the gym a miss. I couldn't stand the thought of being boiled alive with inadequate air conditioning. So, I went for a forty-minute walk instead, popped into the barbers for a haircut and beard trim. *I look good but the scraggy neck is still there*. But I can do nothing about it right now. I walked home, soaked from excessive sweating. I cooked my lunch - fried eggs, Fry Light (Syn Free) & 2 x slices of Warburtons wholemeal bread (HEXB).

Dinner was Chilli with JD Seasoning, mushrooms, peppers, and canned tomatoes (Syn Free).

It's two days away but already I am getting nervous about Friday. Once more I was kicked out of the *Facebook* group for not weighing-in, so I went cap in hand and asked our supreme leader to add me back (Again!).

This is her reply: So, I'll be seeing you THIS WEEK?!?! X

It isn't a question, more of a command.

I did laugh because she really doesn't harass anyone about not coming to class. You either go or you don't. Not sure how helpful that is for members like me, but I am aware that she would have no time to herself if she chased her wayward members.

My reply: Yes, I am back on Fri. But I'm not leaving, ever! X

June 15

I'm aware I haven't put in as much time and effort at the gym. I really need to up my game because the more exercise I do, the less fibro symptoms I experience.

Seven miles cycled at level 13, burning 277 calories. Once again, it was unbearable hot in the gym, yet despite my eagerness to go, after three miles, I'd had enough and was tempted to leave. But I didn't want to, not until I'd hit ten miles at least. As soon as I hit the mark, I was out of there in a flash.

Seated Leg Press – 95 presses. (Feet Positioned High, Feet Positioned Together / Low & Feet Positioned Apart).

Total workout time was 41 minutes.

June 16
WEIGH-IN DAY

I almost tiptoed on to the scales, too scared to look. I needn't have been.

"4½ off."

"Really?"

"Yes! Well done."

"Thank you."

"You're smashing it, Marco." Shelly is always encouraging which means a lot to me. "And you've broken through to the next stone bracket."

"I'm the lightest I have been for years."

"You look amazing."

It also means I am 10½ pounds away from my chosen target. The end is in sight, but I am under no illusions—I could mess it up.

June 19

Yes, I've been off plan but if there is a positive, it is that I haven't over-indulged nearly as much as I usually would.

As true-life plot twists go, this is a biggie because I am starting to recognise my wins, albeit small ones, rather than focusing solely on those times I don't do as well as I know I can. *Is my mindset slowly changing?* I think so, and to be honest, it feels good not to constantly berate myself.

No gym today as I had pre-existing appointment I didn't want to cancel, and the rest of the week is going to be hit and miss because my diary is chocka-block.

I do aim for three sessions a week because I really need them, but not sure about tomorrow because I am going to the dentist. I will see how I feel afterward.

I'm within touching distance of target. I can't fail now.

June 23
WEIGH-IN DAY

Due to finishing the editing of my upcoming release, I missed the scales.

Once I'd finished work, I spent the next three hours walking around Liverpool, taking in the sights and sounds of the city. The hustle and bustle which I love... envious as I watch others eat and drink with abandon. I wonder if those I set my sights upon have ever been fat. Maybe yes, maybe no, but whatever the answer, it doesn't alter my journey.

During my walk-about, I never struggled at all, which is a far cry from my last mammoth trek. I felt stronger physically, especially in my legs.

June 26

My day started early, and by 8 am I was at another physiotherapy appointment. It was a good session.

"You have a lot more movement in your neck, Marco, and your body as a whole."

"I've noticed that too."

"It's a good thing."

"I think it's down to losing weight and forcing myself to turn my neck rather than my entire body when I have to."

"You're probably right."

"I don't feel as locked in, which instantly makes me feel better."

Though I had to take my top off again today, I didn't feel anywhere near as self-conscious as I did the first time.

While at Clatterbridge, I saw my aunty, who I haven't seen since my mum's funeral in 2012.

"Hello, Aunty Tricia."

She appeared genuinely confused, then realised who I was; well, I thought she did until five minutes later she asked, "Which one are you?".

"I'm Marco." I did understand the confusion because she is almost eighty and it has been a long time since we have seen one another.

"I would never have recognised you. You look completely different."

"I'm not as fat as I was."

"No, not at all, you're very slim, you look wonderful, and so like your mum."

So, I was pleased on many counts, mainly to see her after so many years, and for the compliment because my mum was considered beautiful.

It's strange how much pleasure I get from not being recognised anymore though. It proves how long I have travelled in my journey.

My whole week is mapped out and I already know I can't go to weigh-in this week again because I am away on Thursday and have pre-existing medical appointments on Friday morning. But I aim to stay on plan. On top of that, I have had to cancel another two medical appointments because I cannot fit them in, which means I will be waiting until August. They are important, but there is nothing I can do about it.

Straight after physiotherapy I went to the gym but did much less than I usually do.

I cycled 5.01 miles at level 14 and burned 204 calories. The heat inside the gym put me off stride once more. I'm certain Hell would have better air conditioning, so I abandoned the bike after twenty minutes and moved on. I felt bad but figured five was better than nothing.

Seated Leg Press – 120 presses. It's the first time I've used this since last week, but I really want to build my leg muscles and tone up my backside at the same time.

Total workout time was 45 minutes.

Straight afterwards I walked to the supermarket but didn't cook anything as I really couldn't be bothered, nor did I want food.

June 28

Starting the day at the gym, and though I aimed to do more than Monday, it wasn't to be. And while I really don't feel happy with myself until I have cycled at least ten miles, I have realised that it is the immense heat in the gym that zaps me of any energy I have as soon as I walk through the door. On colder days, I don't seem to struggle at all, but of late, I find working out a chore, but something I force myself to do.

I am also off plan and eating sweets like there is no tomorrow. Help!

Cycled 7.02 miles at level 14 with a burn of 279.8 calories. I really didn't want to be there today, but I pushed through, so all good. Seated Leg Press – 120 presses. I really enjoyed using this machine today but seemed to spend more time resting in between sets. I know I am fitter than this, but the heat robs me of vital energy. Workout time was 45 minutes.

I planned to start working on my upper body as my bingo wings are suddenly noticeable. I need to tone up as much as I can. But the gym was busy, and the machines were in use, so I didn't want to hang around as I had shopping to finish for Jon's 37th birthday in July.

Surgery is on my mind again, because I am terrified of losing a lot more weight and being faced with folds of excess skin.

June 29

Another day off plan, but at least I went to the gym and tried to burn off some of the calories I have consumed. Some might say my session was successful, but I would argue otherwise. I feel thoroughly defeated by it.

7.18 miles cycled at level 10 with 282.6 calories burned. Once again, the heat in the gym rendered me useless. I really couldn't wait to get out of there, and though I wanted to hit the ten-mile mark, I was physically unable to do so. Sweating so much makes me feel sick and uncomfortable. I am considering buying a neck fan from Amazon. But are they just a fad that don't really work?

Seated Leg Press – 105 presses. My legs felt like dead weights today, but I did what I could. While my legs are looking slim and toned, I am not happy with the top of my thighs—loose skin is unsightly. I imagine booking myself into BUPA for a whole-body tuck and telling the surgeon to knock me out and cut off the slack. It depresses me that I am putting in all this work... what am I going to be left with?

June 30

    The first appointment of the day is at the Pain Management Clinic to see the pharmacist about changing my medications—the tablets I am on now do not agree with me at all and make me feel sick, and worse, drowsy the following day. Hopefully the pharmacist will put me on the new medication which is being trialled for patients suffering from Fibromyalgia. Apparently, it only works for a small percentage of those taking it, but I am willing to try anything, if it means I don't feel like I can't move the following day.
    With those, and tablets for my allergies, plus creams for my burning skin, and folic acid replacements, multi-vitamins, and minerals to replace what I don't get from normal food, I should be rattling.
    Well, I had my appointment with the pharmacist, and she went through a whole list of medications, from Morphine to Tramadol to Ibuprofen, telling me why they will not work for my condition—I told her that I didn't think anything would work because not enough is known about the central nervous system, especially in the hope of stopping it from sending out pain signals. Anyway, she recommended one medication, but I wasn't thrilled.
    "This could work, but the side effect is weight gain."
    "Well, I don't want it."
    "Why not?"
    "I've spent years trying to lose weight, so putting me on medication that will reverse all of my hard work will have a detrimental effect not only on my physicality but also on my mental health."
    "Okay, I understand, so let's try you on something else."
    "As long as it doesn't make me balloon, I will try anything."
    So, I am to start next week on a dose of 30mg daily for two weeks, then after that, it is upped to 60mg daily, and then finally in six weeks, to the maximum of 90mg daily.
    While I dislike taking medication, I will try it.
    "It only works for 1 in 9 people, and if it hasn't done anything for you after six weeks, we can stop it and find something else."
    "Okay."
    "This particular medication can cause depression in some people leading to suicidal thoughts."
    "Oh, no." That is not me as a person.
    And here is the corker of a revelation she saved until last. "If you do notice a decline in your mental health, stop taking the tablets immediately and call your GP urgently."
    "What if I don't recognise that I am suicidal and I actually try something?"

"Don't worry too much though if it happens, it's only a chemical thing, and the effects should wear off quite quickly."

Hmm, right!

Immediately, I wasn't sold, but she's the expert and I'll try it, and hope I experience no negative side effects. But I know from experience that the gym helps reduce pain more than anything prescribed so far.

MY JOURNEY - JULY 2023

July 3

    Well, after another weekend, well two weeks of faffing about I am finally back on plan. What damage have I done? I am dreading weigh in this week, especially as I had worked so hard to get into my final stone bracket. Whatever I have gained, I know with hard work and determination, I can lose it again.
    No gym today as I have a dentist appointment to have my new crown fitted. I also have a cracked tooth at the back, but the dentist says this is due to me being sick so often, that the stomach acid is affecting my teeth.
    I'm trying not to think about it, but the back tooth has been mended. For how long, I have no idea.

July 4

    Still on plan, and zero appetite, although I want to gorge on chocolate and cakes. I'm going to the gym to take my mind off it.
    A disappointing 7.01 miles completed at level 10 with 202.8 calories burned. It is official. My strength and stamina have upped and left me, and while I am certain this is fibro related, I am annoyed because I felt I was doing amazingly well. Still, if seven miles is to be my new normal, it is better than nothing. I know I will try and do more when I feel that I can, but I know I can't push past my limitations.
    Seated Leg Press – 120 presses. Crikey, I think I was pressing too heavy weights today, and my legs were burning afterwards. I will pay for it later when my hips start to ache. Still, I do believe this exercise is strengthening my legs, so will keep at it.
    Workout time was 45 minutes.
    After the gym I popped in to my local bistro. I didn't eat but even if I had been hungry, I would have declined because I am so fussy with how they cook my food, I am sure I annoy them.

"No snotty bits in my eggs."

"Dry toast, please, and oh, can I please scan the barcode for the bread."

"Semi-skimmed milk, please."

"Can you please make sure my food is piping hot?" I can't eat warm food, and although this and the others might seem reasonable requests if one is running an establishment, I feel awkward asking all the time.

So, I had a cup of tea.

Back home, I had no idea what to do with myself. I didn't feel like writing. Jon and I are not talking and haven't been for days. Not that there is much conversation when we are on speaking terms lately—he is forever stuck in front of his PS5, and I am glued to my PC writing.

We seem to exist in different worlds while living under the same roof, and both of us need to make more of an effort. He is stubborn, and I am renowned for it, so a meeting in the middle is required. I love him wholeheartedly, and I know he loves me—sometimes we just drift, not that I like it, but I think it happens in many long-term relationships. Sometimes I don't feel supported by him, and I know he doesn't feel supported by me. We are very different personalities, and I know opposites attract. Still, I wish we could do more together both inside and out of the house.

Anyway, despite us not speaking, and the fact I didn't want any food, he cooked a roast dinner (6½ Syns), which was delicious, and strangely enough for me, the tastiest meal I have eaten in a long time.

I only ate one Yorkshire pudding, none of the meat, and left one roast potato. I ate most of the carrot, turnip, and peas. But two minutes later, I felt nauseous, and wrestled with myself, trying to keep the food down. I am sick of being sick if that makes sense. Jon is annoyed with me—perhaps he laced mine with *Ipecac.*

Anyway, five minutes later, the lot came back, which instantly made me question why I bother eating normal food when I have no appetite for it, desire to eat it, and it only ends up down the toilet anyway.

Instantly I was wrenched out of my mindset, and I could feel myself losing control, and that little voice urging me to get dressed and go to the shop. With no fruit in the house to pick at, I lay on the bed craving chocolate, cakes, and crisps because they never make sick.

But I resisted and as I write, it has just gone midnight. I won, but tomorrow is a new day that could bring failure, or success.

First thing in the morning I am going to the gym, then off to buy fruit and Greek yoghurt. If all else fails and I can't keep anything else down, that rarely makes me sick.

Right now, I am really fed up with SW because I am forced to deal with food, which is the least interesting thing in the world to me. Also, I am in a pickle with myself for being off plan for the last two weeks, my personal life is up the creek, and I don't have a paddle to navigate my way out of it, nor do I want to right now. Throw in daily vomiting, and my life is stuck on a loop and has become a chore. Something has got to give, but I will carry on because I know the alternative—put the weight back on and feel miserable every hour of every day or fight through this funk I am in.

Right now, I am sure it is a phase. I hope so anyway because I am not moody or grumpy by nature. But I feel like screaming my frustrations from the rooftops.

What I do need to do is book an appointment to see my GP—I feel like I am in the throes of an eating disorder, and while it is not anorexia or bulimia, my hatred of food is causing issues, and I feel that the constant vomiting is going to cause me more problems in the long run, not least dentally.

My friend believes that I am an unwilling bulimic and while I would never make light of any eating disorder, that is exactly how I feel although I have never been able to put it into words.

July 5

It is way past time for me to give my head a shake, in the hope it might knock some sense into me. I seem to replay everything in my mind, every bad decision, every time I have failed and fallen off plan. But what sticks is the fact I am approaching forty-nine with seemingly no more sense than I had as a teenager. I'm insecure about myself, and that pushes me into a circle that seems to spin me off my axis.

Grow up, Marco, and take accountability. Isn't that what it's all about; being accountable for my choices. *Yes, so deal with it.*

Lying in bed last night, in the throes of a bad mood, I realised I was shifting blame for my bad mood onto SW, but what I should stress right now is; I was wrong, and SW has been a lifeline. Yes, it forces me to deal with food, but in my desire to lose weight, I must eat healthily, or at least I strive to. So, I might throw up one big healthy meal, but if I can manage to keep an assortment of fruit or a tin of soup down—isn't that better than only eating sweets? It was all I was existing on before I rejoined SW anyway.

Now, I am back on plan, I am dreading mealtimes although I can't avoid them. What am I going to do?

I should confess, I was planning to stay for class for the first time ever, but realising whatever is going on with me and food has overtaken my life, I would feel like a fish out of water. Could anybody relate to my personal struggles even if I was to speak up in class?

A lot of the people who do stay for class, because they can't control their desire to overeat the food that I wish I didn't ever have to eat again, might think me bonkers.

This realisation has made me feel isolated and like giving up.

July 7
WEIGH-IN DAY

Due to the change in medication, I am absolutely exhausted having not slept for two nights, therefore no sessions at the gym. Plus I've got a banging headache and every part of my body hurts. So, it's understandable that I don't feel like speaking, let alone walking the five minutes to get weighed, but I will.

And I do.

Drumroll please... the results are in...

"4 on."

"On? Why do I bother to ask when I already know. It's not a surprise.

"It's a new week now, a fresh start."

I am upset and disappointed in myself, but it would have been so much worse had I not pushed myself back on plan.

I really wanted to stay for class, but I could barely keep my eyes open. I just want to go back home and crawl into my bed.

I'm such a pig... why can't I leave sweets, cakes, and crisps alone?

What really grates on me is the fact I am back in the nineteen stone bracket, again. I must work harder to get to target and beyond, or what is the point?

Not in the right frame of mind to be bothered with anything, and I know that is partly due to the medication making me feel rough.

This situation really is horrible, and I want to do better.

I keep telling myself I am only human, but right now, I feel anything but.

July 8

And the weekend comes around, and guess what, goodbye common sense.

Why do I do it?

When I set my mind to it, I can work the plan all week long and barely consume a Syn, but as soon as Friday arrives, I go crazy.

Can somebody please help me with this?

I can't be the only one that fails every weekend, can I?

July 9

Marco, you are an idiot!
This past week I have been eating a lot more Greek yoghurt than usual, believing it to be fat free.
Wrong!
I just cleaned out my fridge to find I have been eating the full fat variety. BLEEP, BLEEP, BLEEP, BLEEP, BLEEP... I'm usually more observant but because my usual brand was out of stock, I chose another and misread the label.

I'm furious with myself because I have been eating it for breakfast, lunch and using it as an in between, thinking I am within my Syn allowance... maybe my gain would not have been so great this week. Maybe it would, so there is no use crying over spilled milk.

But I move on...

July 10

Today would have been my parents' 52nd wedding anniversary, and for some reason I am more aware of the date than I usually am. Perhaps it is because my dad and I are once again estranged, and most of the rest of my family might as well not exist. I didn't realise, not until she had died, but my mum was the glue that held us all together. I only seem to see certain members of my family when they want something, and the others, not at all. Even my aunty, my dad's sister, who I was closer than close with from the day I was born doesn't bother anymore—that one stings a little because it seems that I cease to matter now—maybe I should just call her and tell her that I miss her.

Anyway, I plod on and did okay at the gym today, managing seven miles with 204.8 calories burned off on the bike. My levels varied from 7 to 15, but I averaged at 10.

July 12

I woke up this morning in agony and didn't have full movement of my shoulders or arms. I really cannot be bothered sticking to plan, or cooking, or shopping, or doing anything really.

Some good news... I did pass the Chronic Pain Management course I have been taking for the last three months. And while I am pleased to have achieved this, it taught me very little, aside from learning to listen to my body more, and that medical professionals really know very little about Fibromyalgia.

July 13

Woke up a little less sore that yesterday, which was a bonus because I had appointments, starting with the dentist. As I hadn't been to the gym, I need exercise so walked there and back and to my other appointments, trekking roughly three miles. Some exercise is better than none, right.

When I came home, I lay on my bed, and the revelation hit me immediately.

WRITING NOVELS x SELF EMPLOYMENT x RUNNING A HOUSEHOLD x CARING FOR PARTNER & PETS x WEIGHT LOSS JOURNEY x FIBROMYALGIA x EATING DISORDER.

One of the above would be enough to overwhelm a person functioning normally, but I am dealing with day-to-day life and too many other things on top, so why am I being hard on myself? Yeah, I've screwed up these last few weeks and had a little gain, but so what? I know I can lose that again, and more when the time is right. For now, I must prioritise my health and well-being, so if I am exhausted and have no energy to go anywhere, even to weigh in, I don't care, even if others feel let down.

Today is the first time I have seriously considered leaving SW to go it alone—well I do it alone anyway as I don't stay for class. But perhaps leaving SW would be one less pressure in my life. I have some decisions to make.

July 17

TODAY I STRUCK GOLD ON MY BODY MAGIC.

The last few days I have tried to get my mind back into some semblance of order, so I was thrilled to have hit my SW Body Magic target. Even though I have not been fit enough to go to the gym, I have been walking as much as possible to hit the required daily minutes, which paid off.

It seems no matter what I eat lately, I am sick. It makes mealtimes more stressful than ever.

July 18

HAPPY 37th BIRTHDAY, JON!

I stuffed my face in solidarity with him. *Any excuse.*

But what I did notice is; I hated every moment of eating, which makes me realise more than ever that I need to go back to see my GP and discuss moving onto a liquid / soup diet to give my body time to recover from the constant vomiting.

July 19

Back to the gym today. *Ah, feels like home!*
Exercise Bike Calories Burned: 365.3
Levels: 7 to 15, but averaged level 8.

I cycled 10.11 miles at level 8 and burned off 365.3 calories. I did this in three sets because it was the only way I could do it. After 3 miles, pain crept in, but I didn't want to give in. But I got to 10, and felt better for staggering the workout, and dropping the intensity level. Not sure I will ever get up to the lofty heights of 20 again, but stranger things have happened.

Seated Leg Press – 90 presses. I wanted to be very careful with this today, so didn't overdo it. Did it in six sets and was mindful of not lifting too heavy a weight.

Total workout time was 65 Minutes.

July 20

After a groggy start to my day, courtesy of my new medication, and the increased dose, I dragged myself out of bed and walked to the gym, determined to equal, or better yesterday's results.

Afterwards, hairdressers, then I grabbed a few bits of food, and headed home.

I am on and off plan and can't seem to make up my mind what I am doing.

July 21
WEIGH-IN DAY

I can't go because I have a pre-existing appointment at the Orthodontists, and the electrician is coming to do a yearly safety check.

Still, I don't know if I am going to go back, or if it is worth it? I don't seem to be getting far these days because too much in my life is standing in the way. But if I leave, I know I will pile on the pounds.

What the hell are you even considering it for?

As the day progressed, fibro kicked off worse than it ever has, leaving me in total agony. After three baths, trying to ease the pain, it is still there. Right now, I feel like I have been hit by something heavy and my body, from my chest down, is unbearably sore.July 22

Mind made up, and after a terrible sleep, I've decided it would be stupid and reckless to leave SW and that I am once again laying blame at the wrong door. Accountability is a word I need to remember. So, I will carry on as I am now, and just do my best. Nobody can ask for anything more of me, nor can I of myself.

I have come so far, and there is still a bit further to go to hit my target.

I WILL GET THERE, BELIEVE ME!!!

As for today, I am doing nothing but lying in bed. My body demands it, and although I hate it, I know when I am beaten.

July 23

Where has Summer gone? Rain is battering my windows, and I feel claustrophobic, eager to get out and explore, anywhere.

Instead, I lie in bed all day and watch the reboot of Quantum Leap. I love all things Sci-Fi, but this is a poor imitation of the series that I remembered from years ago. I want to abandon it, but I must see the series out so I can find out why Dr Song leapt into the past without telling anyone. I am such a geek!

Dinner was spiced parsnip & carrot soup... if I could do a green face emoji, I would, because it was disgusting and filled me with enough wind I could have inflated an air balloon.

Afterwards, I tuck into crisps, muffins, sweets, and sponge cake.

July 24

Back on plan today, just! I'm trying, although my mind is wandering to sweets.

I didn't go to the gym because I am trying to give my body a rest after last week, but I fully intend to go tomorrow. But I did walk for about an hour, so that's my Body Magic covered.

Already, I am dreading having to eat the food, but I am all stocked up with fruit, vegetables, and fat free natural yoghurt.

Dinner was roast potatoes (Syn Free) and gravy (1½Syns).

I ate what I could, and already I'm feeling sick. So, I came to my computer, hopeful that writing will keep my mind off what I've eaten.

July 25

I woke up feeling sick. These new tablets are knocking the stuffing out of me, and yes, they help with regulating sleep, but the following morning, it's like having the worst hangover. I agreed to keep trying with them for another six weeks and hope the side effects disappear. If not, it means moving onto something else.

But I told myself I was going to the gym come hell or high water, and I am!

I cycled 10.06 miles at level 8 with 350 calories burned. Within half a mile, my knee started to burn, but I pushed on for the full 35 minutes of the session to do 7.67. The next session only last for 5½ minutes, but I did manage to do 1.18. I took a breather to use the leg press, then went back for one final go. By this time, sweat was pouring off me and I felt uncomfortable but another 5½ minutes and I managed 1.21 miles.

Seated Leg Press – 120 presses. I was so busy watching other people exercise that this took my mind off my burning knee and aching legs. I managed a little more than yesterday, so all was well.

Total workout time was 61 minutes.

After the gym, I walked to the parcel shop to send a new pair of trousers back that fit me in the waist but are too baggy in the leg... one gust of wind up them and I'm joining Mary Poppins in the clouds. Anyway, afterwards, I took a stroll around the area I grew up in, passing my old family home, my best friends house and that of my friend Sara, who grew up with us and basically became another sibling to me. Memory Lane beckoned, and I found myself lost to the past—it wasn't sad, more reflective, but it made me miss my mum so much. I wish I could turn back the clock and go back.

On the way home, I called into the local Bistro for a cup of tea and had a lovely catch up with my old friend June. She is great fun and hasn't changed at all in nearly thirty years.

Lunch was bananas, strawberries, black Grapes, tropical granola & fat free natural yoghurt (5½ Syns). Tea with semi-skimmed milk (HEA) & sweetener.

Cooking dinner was abandoned as I really didn't feel like eating, but there was some food leftover from last night, so I had a small bowl of that.

July 26

Another session at the gym, but it was heaving.

I couldn't do everything that I wanted to do because the machines were all in use, but I managed to cycle 10.38 miles at level 8 while burning 370.2 calories. It took about twenty seconds for my knee to start throbbing. Typical!

But I carried on regardless. It looks like I'll have to pay another visit to my GP because the old complaint that I was referred to the physiotherapist about is getting worse. If it makes sense, there is a lump just under my kneecap that formed after I banged my knee, but now, it is getting bigger and it feels like the skin is struggling to stretch over it. The physiotherapist advised me to leave it alone until it became an issue because it means surgery with an eighteen-month recovery period, which will end my time at the gym. But it is causing problems now and has become another thing on a long list of maladies. Once more, the excess weight I am carrying does not help, so I battle on because I don't relish the idea of being overweight or unfit, and having to go under anaesthesia.

After the gym, I called in to the bistro, again. My old friend June was there so we had a good chat for about an hour and a half. She really does make me laugh, and like me, has zero filter. She says it as it is! At seventy, she isn't as agile as she once was, so I was trying to convince her to give Aquarobics a try—she has a disability scooter but isn't confident enough to use it. So, I said I would walk to her house, which is only ten minutes away from me at most and take her to leisure centre. I'd even go in the pool with her, and we could bob up and down together. Saying that, we would do more laughing than aerobics.

Lunch was poached eggs, beans, mushrooms, all cooked with Fry Light (Syn Free). Tea with semi-skimmed milk (HEXA) & sweetener. Dinner was pasta in a spicy tomato sauce (Syn Free). I found the recipe on the SW app, so as it was Jon's turn to cook, I left him to it. My thoughts... I wouldn't feed it to the dog... well actually I did, and she loved it. Jon hated his too and scraped it into the bin. Now, as much as I can take or leave food, I feel cheated and want chocolate. But I know that is my brain formulating an excuse for me to fall off plan. I won't do it! I finished the day with fresh fruit and fat free natural yoghurt and a handful of granola (5½ Syns). As much as I wanted to run to the shop and stock up on goodies, I was happy that I chose the healthier option instead.

July 27

Another washout of a day thanks to our non-existent summer, but I faced the gym, knowing there are 24 hours until I weigh in. I am dreading it, and while I want to get on the treadmill and run the pounds off, I am not physically capable, and at this weight, I'd probably break the machine.

July 28
WEIGH-IN DAY

After a horrible night's sleep, here I am, accompanied by my friend, who keeps telling me everything will be fine.

Donna is there, taking payments and after a brief chat, I was surprised she was unaware of my aversion to food, but as I don't stay for class, why would she know anything about me apart from what I look like and what I weigh.

I have been a nervous wreck all week because I am scared to stand on those scales, and as much as I wanted to hit target for ABBA next week, I've got more chance of Kylie Minogue knocking on my door and declaring her undying love.

Shelly is on the scales, patiently waiting.

I fidget with my hands a touch before her directive comes.

"Okay, get on and let's see."

I step on. *Here goes, fatty!* "I've been a pig this last two weeks."

"Have you?" She really is the best person to do this as she conveys kindness and understanding.

"Yeah, and I think I've put ten pounds on."

Why did I not stay on plan?

Why do I hate normal food so much?

Why?

Why?

Why?

Questions I can't answer.

My thoughts run wild as I turn my gaze downward hating every moment of this.

Why did I have to be the fatty of the family? My uncle and aunty would have been considered morbidly obese, so I obviously took after them.

Why are my brothers slim?

Why?

Genetically, I was thrown a curveball and could drive myself mad asking myself questions there are no answers to.

There is little point me droning on because it is my own doing.

DRUM ROLL... and the damage is...

"½ OFF."

"Off?" Had I misheard?

"Yes."

Well, I have never been as surprised with any result as I have with that. I'm sure I muttered an expletive under my breath. Yes, it is only ½ off, but in my mind, I felt heavier and thought I looked heavier. My friend kept reaffirming that I didn't look any different than I had the last few weeks. But I could have dropped on the spot as relief washed over me.

I had a lucky escape because I have not really stuck to plan and have pigged out. I won't be lucky next time, so I need to get my head back in the game.

Still, I am thrilled, and hot-footed it over to Liverpool to find new jeans, convinced I would have to find a branch of Big 'n' Bouncy. As it happens, my friend convinced me to buy them in a 36" waist. I dithered but I grabbed them anyway, and the bonus was they were on sale.

"You don't see yourself how I see you," she said. "They *will* fit."

I could have tried them on, but throughout the shopping trip, I had sweated worse than ever before which bothered me a lot, and I had no energy. But I had not slept the night before, and with Fibromyalgia, lack of sleep irritates the condition that always hovers in the background. I did it and must have walked around for four hours.

We went for dinner in Liverpool One and half an hour later, I vomited the lot back up. Vegan Cheesecake too... de-lic-ious! Regardless, it was a waste of money, but hey, not many calories absorbed. I remembered my friend's words... *unwilling bulimic.* I so wish I could keep food down. If I didn't laugh, I would cry.

When I got home, I was exhausted and climbed in to bed, then when I woke, I tried the jeans on—perfect fit! My friend was right. But I was thrilled I was in a smaller size.

"They fit," I texted with glee.

"Told you."

"I didn't think they would."

"You're too hard on yourself."

She is right. A lesson learned for us all... what we see when we look in the mirror is often skewed by how we see ourselves. The reality is, we never look as bad as we think we do.

I am extremely lucky that I have a friend who champions me, no matter what I weigh or look like!

July 29

Last night, I slept like a baby. It might have been excess tiredness that knocked me out, or the raspberry Mojito. Not sure which, but whatever, the uninterrupted sleep was appreciated.

The sun was shining for once, and rather than relax in my recliner in my beautiful garden listening to music, I did three loads of washing. THREE LOADS. It is one of life's greatest and unsolved mysteries how a household with two people, who work from home, can generate such huge quantities of laundry. And as Jon doesn't know how to work our washing machine, nor has he ever asked, it is left for me to do. Due to the lovely breeze, I hung everything on the line, which saved me paying through the nose for using my tumble dryer to BRITISH 'THIEVING BASTARDS' GAS, then the delivery from Iceland (the supermarket chain, not the country) arrived. I was up and down the stairs, and in and out of the garden like a blue-arsed fly.

I'm knackered.

"Do you fancy cheese pie for dinner?" I asked Jon. "With mashed potato and baked beans?" Mash is a trigger food for me and reminds of dinner times as a child—corned beef hash and beans, gross—I could balk at the thought of it.

"Not hungry yet," he replied.

Suits me, and with his chance to be catered for (again) lost, when he is hungry later, he will have to cook for himself.

Duties fulfilled, for the rest of the evening, I am going to lie on my bed, do nothing and watch Good Omens 2.

July 31

A visit to my GP's left me feeling fed up because he wouldn't agree to put me on a liquid / soup diet. Instead, he wants to get to the root of why I am regurgitating my food so frequently. He knows of my aversion to food in general but wants to see if the problem is physical or mental, considering I have no trouble keeping sweets, cakes, and crisps down.

I told him that I thought it a mixture of both, because I am physically sick so often that when I do eat, I am anxious knowing what is to come.

As I'm not a doctor, he advised the route he would prefer to take.

Some good news: he was massively impressed with my weight loss, congratulated me, and said he would not have recognised me had he not known who his next appointment was with.

That was nice to hear but doesn't help me with my food issues. So, I'll plod on the way I have been, knowing a few months down the line he will tell me what I already know.

I skipped the gym today but did walk to the doctors and back. I even took the long way round.

Came home and got stuck in a Tik Tok loop, watching a guy having his nostril hairs waxed. Tears were tripping me up, but I shouldn't laugh, especially as I am due to have mine done on Thursday, in readiness of my trip to London to see ABBA.

Saw my best friend, Sarah, who I love and adore. We've known one another since our first day at primary school so give or take, it's about 44 or 45 years of friendship. How lucky am I! No matter how the years pass, she always looks the same to me—gorgeous eyes with a mischievous twinkle, blonde hair and a dazzling smile—perfection! Sarah brought me some gifts and a birthday card. Insisting I open it in case it didn't fit, I was thrilled because she had bought me an *AllSaints* T-shirt I have seen but not had the courage to buy—it is totally me, and yes, it is a tiny bit too small, but I didn't want her to change it for the bigger size because in a few weeks it would become too big for me. As I am in between sizes, I don't think I look good in most things, but slimming down into my new T-shirt is a challenge and one I intend to win. As soon as I feel good in it, I will take a picture and send it to her.

MY JOURNEY – AUGUST 2023

August 1

Five days until I turn 49… my last year before the dreaded 5-0 comes to claim me. Saying that, no matter how much I grumble, I don't feel my age. I did think of having one of those body scans that tells me how old my body is, but I'm terrified it will come back at 84 or perhaps older.

I went for a walk today, rather than go to the gym.

My friend sent me a song to watch on YouTube—*I Ain't Been Licked*, by Diana Ross. She knew I would like it. And yes, the unfortunate title did amuse my juvenile mind and make me laugh. But the song's lyrics resonated as they talk about not being beaten. We could all learn a lot from them.

Keep holding me down,
But I rise,
Just to start again.
Keep holding me down,
But I rise,
Show 'em that I can.
Keep holding me down,
But I rise,
Found a brand-new dream.
Keep holding me down,
But I rise,
Just to prove one thing.

What an absolute banger of a tune.

While dancing about in my chair to that, I was trying to sort out life insurance. Crikey, what a palaver! The fact I have Fibromyalgia makes it ten times more difficult, and after listening to the dimwit insurance broker who called me three times from a withheld number before I answered, and repeat himself, desperate for the sale, I told him I wasn't interested and that I would go elsewhere.

"Well, let me assure you that there are only two or three companies that will touch a person who has Fibromyalgia, so if you tell me what other prices you were quoted and from where, I guarantee I will better them."

Instantly, I was ready to bite, especially after telling him multiple times I would not give him that information. Why do these people not listen? Did he really think he could fire questions and bamboozle me. Even in a coma, I could run rings around these shysters. So, I delivered my parting shot. "I can guarantee one thing too."

"May I ask what that is?"

"That you won't be getting my business." And then I hung up on the ambulance-chasing wanker. It's only once I'd ended the call that I realised he asked me what my waist size was... like I'm going to divulge such personal information to a stranger. I wouldn't even tell my own dad that.

Dinner was okay, but I actually kept my meal down and thoroughly enjoyed it. After sorting out the kitchen and dishwasher, I spent the rest of the day re-designing book covers which is something I really enjoy.

August 2

Not in the mood to eat but I am feeling good today. Nor can I be bothered to hoof to the gym and exercise, so I walk to the barbers to get my hair cut and beard trimmed in readiness for ABBA.

It was a bit of a struggle having my beard trimmed because the barber wanted to move my head and neck into position it did not want to go in. Yes, it is much better, and I have a lot more movement and rotation than previously, but I am far from back to the way I was, or anywhere close. Still, it was done, and then I requested to have my nose hairs waxed—he shoved two cotton buds with a mound of wax on up each nostril.

After a few minutes, he asked, "Are you ready?"

"Ye—" He didn't give me chance to finish before he pulled the first one out.

Did you hear me scream?

"Jesus Christ," I gasped as my feet shot out in front of me.

Then he yanked out the other, which mercifully wasn't as painful as the first.

Wiping the streams of tears running down my cheeks, he positioned the cotton buds into my eyeline, wanting to show me the clumps of hair clinging to them. I didn't need to see, especially after feeling them being ripped out.

I am positive it didn't hurt last time... I could be mistaken and may have blocked out the memory.

Now, I'm home, I need to sort out dinner.

Jon is poorly; his varicocele has flared up, so it looks like leftovers, which he loves, but this time, he wants mashed potato, so I will make a cottage pie. For me, nothing could convince me to eat that slop, but I do need to eat something, so will have the same as yesterday.

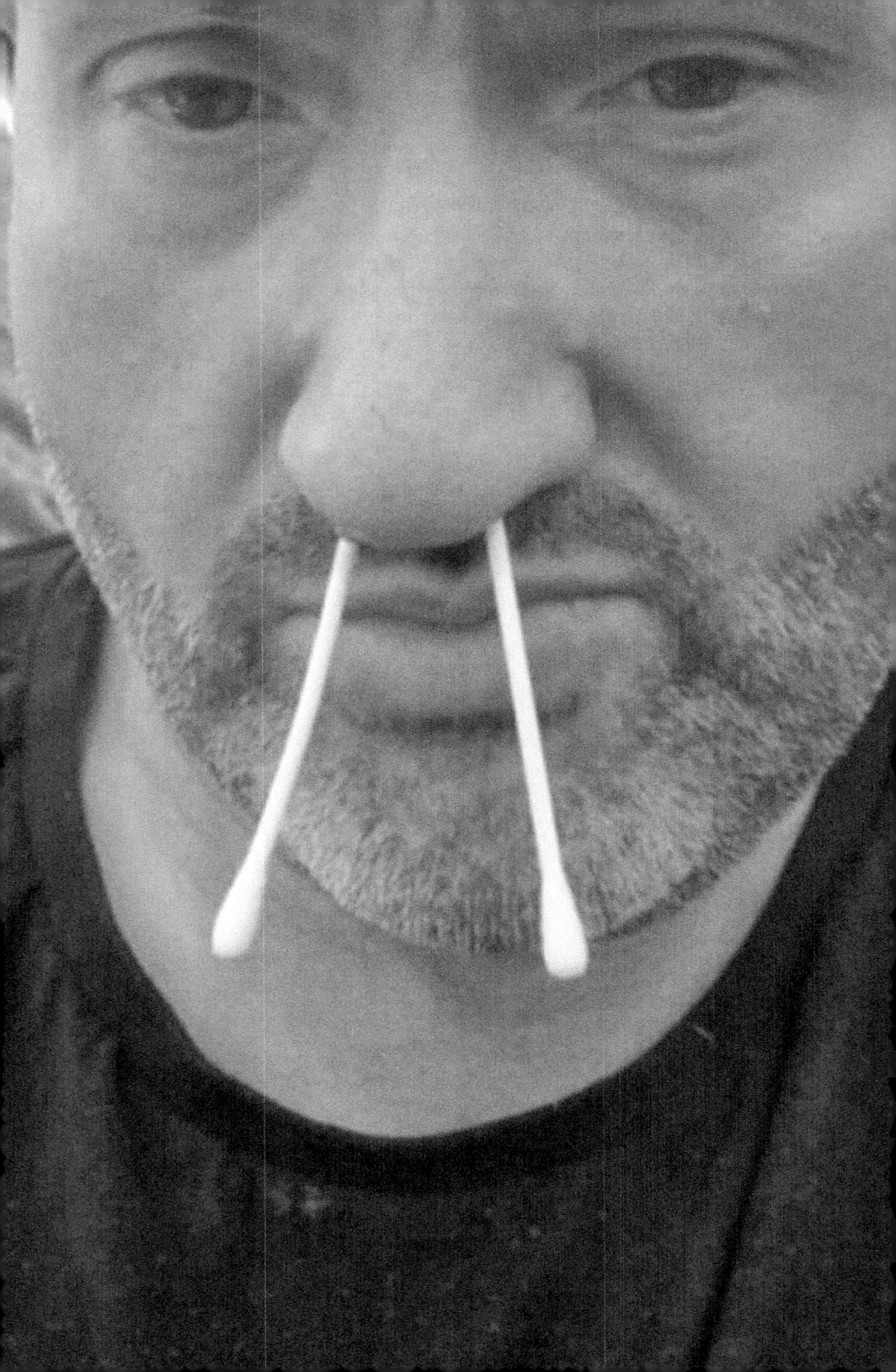

August 3

Lazy day today!

Aside from taking Sally to the vet as she is limping, I did nothing and felt guilty.

So, I walked up to the shops to get a few bits and bobs, wanting to make sure Jon had plenty of snacks while I am away.

And I've not been a pig food wise, so all said and done, not a bad day.

August 4

It is 6 am, and nobody should be awake at this unholy hour. But TODAY IS THE DAY!

ABBA, here I go... AGAIN!

I cannot wait, and though I did not hit target, tonight is all about fun, fun, fun.

While I am excited to be going with my friend, I will miss Jon and wish he was coming with us. He has volunteered to look after the dogs, and as he loves them as much as I do, there is nobody I trust more. Plus, he is feeling under the weather so the trip wouldn't have been ideal for him right now. When he is feeling better, and has shifted some more weight, we can plan special times together.

As my life often borders on farce, the trip wasn't without drama. So, rather than bore you with a monologue, I've listed everything for you...

1. Got off the train at Pudding Mill Lane Station at 12:08pm, which is just opposite the ABBA Arena. Tick.
2. Used Google Maps to locate our hotel which was about a mile away. Tick.
3. Got lost and ended up walking around in circles for an hour. Tick.
4. When we stopped people to ask for help, they looked at us as though we were Martians. Tick.
5. Finally arrived at our hotel at 14:14pm. Tick.
6. Sweating like a glass blowers' arse. Tick.
7. Feet on fire because I had to take my new trainers off and swap to flip flops. Tick.
8. Early Check-In sorted and paid the relevant fee. Tick.
9. Requested accessible twin room I had booked. Tick
10. Given a room on the seventh floor with floor to ceiling windows. Tick.

11. Found room and walked in to discover a double bed. Tick.
12. Back to reception to advise wrong room given. Tick.
13. Twatty Manager told me I had not booked a twin room. Tick.
14. Told Manager I had, and that I also called twice to confirm the booking. Tick.
15. Manager told me the staff had not done as requested. Tick.
16. Bit of a disagreement after Manager called me a liar. Tick.
17. Showed Manager the email with the twin room booking.
18. Rubbed his smug face in it. Tick.
19. No apology given. Tick.
20. Requested Early Check-In fee refund. Was only £10, but I was annoyed. Tick.
21. Manager instructs us to sit in the dining room and wait for the beds to be separated. Tick.
22. Manager returns forty minutes later and shouts across the room to advise room is ready. Tick.
23. Manager is a rude arsehole who needs to brush up on his customer service skills. Tick.
24. Back to room 704. Tick.
25. Is it a nice room? Very much so! Tick.
26. Am I too scared to look out of the windows because of sheer drop? Yes! Tick.
27. Close curtains to convince myself I am not vacationing in the clouds. Tick.
28. Moved bed and found Peanuts underneath. Tick.
29. Hinge that fastens beds together left hanging and I catch my foot on it. Tick.
30. Unpack and walk to Westfield Shopping Centre and find something to eat. Tick.
31. Nearly pass out at the sign advertising 4 small doughnuts for £10. Tick.
32. Find a small eatery, and my friend has heart failure when presented with the £35 bill for two tiny bowls of pasta. Tick.
33. I laughed and found it hysterically funny. Tick.
34. Ate a Nutella Muffin which glued my teeth together then stuck to the roof of my mouth. Tick.
35. My friend found it very funny, as did I when the same thing happened to her. Tick.

36. Back to the hotel for a nice relaxing bath. The tub was so small the water wouldn't have covered a tit mouse, let alone my belly. Tick.
37. Left towel, underwear, T-shirt, and mobile phone on the floor of the bathroom while I washed my bits. Tick.
38. Got out of the bath to find I was the star of a live action remake of The Poseidon Adventure. Tick.
39. Bathroom flooded. Water at least two inches deep. Tick.
40. Towel, underwear, T-shirt, and mobile phone soaked. Tick.
41. Friend in hysterics, laughing at my misfortune. Tick.
42. My friend used already sopping wet towels to mop up the water, wring them out and begin again. Tick.
43. My friend hurt her finger trying to dry the bathroom floor. Tick.
44. My friend eventually managed to dry the floor. Tick.
45. Copious amounts of vodka and diet Vimto drank before the concert. Tick.
46. Arrived at ABBA Arena, excited for the show.
47. WE HAD THE TIME OF OUR LIVES. TICK!
48. Woke up at 3 am with a gale force hangover. Tick!

I had the most amazing time, and the only thing that could have made it better would have been having Jon there too. We bicker like an old married couple, and it truly is six of one and half a dozen of the other, but for over a decade he has been my world. I wish we could spend more of these moments together, but with animals who suffer from separation anxiety, one of us always has to be there. I know people think we are crazy, but they are as priceless to us as children are to others, and it is the sacrifice to our relationship that won't always be an issue. Besides, Jon knows I want to do these things with him and that is all that matters.

Despite his absence, I truly enjoyed myself, but realised I didn't feel comfortable surrounded by people, and that is because I felt fat and ugly compared to them. Paranoia convinced me that they were staring at me. At the time though, it casts a shadow over what should be a joyous occasion. Why would anybody take any notice of me when they had ABBA to watch? Even with as much weight as I have lost, the fatty still lurks inside chipping away at my confidence. Plus, the damage fibro has done to my body these past few years really hit home. I won't let it get me down because I have a lot more weight to lose, and I want to get to the peak of my physical fitness—well, whatever my body can manage.

August 5

After an amazing night, I slept okay but was a little sore and thankfully the hangover had dissipated by the time I got out of bed. Wanted another bath but didn't fancy partaking in a remake of Titanic. So, I freshened my pits and went down for breakfast.

Went into London to the *Disney* Store then to the Harry Potter shop. Bought a few items then headed to Euston for the journey home.

Found the Pastie Shop. Jon had requested the extortionately priced chicken and mushroom pasties… 175 miles I travelled with them… if anybody reads this doubts my feelings for him, carrying baked goods from one end of the country to the other should scream true love!

One of the staff at the station escorted us to our carriage and as we were first on, secured the table seat. We were grateful of his assistance because I was sore from walking around London.

Was chucking it down when we walked out of the train station at Hamilton Square and I got soaked getting cash out of the machine, but I didn't care as I was excited to see Jon and my doggies. I had missed them all.

Spent the rest of the day relaxing in bed and watching TV with Jon and the babies.

Home Sweet Home!

August 6

Jon woke me at 11 am, which is very late for me. But he was excited for me to open my presents…

"Happy Birthday, babe."

"Thank you." 49 years old. Ugh. One step closer to 50. How fast the years have gone by, and I don't feel like I have achieved anything. "I feel old."

"You are," he joked. "Fifty soon."

He is not wrong, but I will deal with that catastrophe in twelve months.

As always, Jon thoroughly spoilt me. I'm thrilled with every gift and the thought that went into each one. The star of the show is a Samsung Galaxy Watch that I can track my fitness on.

My friends Sandie and Samantha arrived later than afternoon and spoiled me too. They had even baked cakes, which I had zero trouble scoffing.

I am a very lucky guy.

August 11

I've not really done anything since my birthday because Jon is poorly and can barely walk, and my little dog, Sally, who is sixteen and a half, has hurt her foot.

"Come to daddy." I talk to her as though she is human, and I can just imagine her thinking...

Not this plant pot again.

I smother her in kisses. "Daddy loves you." More kisses follow.

She tilts her head to the side and eyes me curiously. Nearly seventeen years on, she is used to me.

Both Jon and I guard our dogs, and cat, like prized treasures, but Jon is her human. I am fine with that because she knows she is loved.

I did take her to the vet last Thursday, but the tablets don't seem to be working. Still, she is happy enough, eating, drinking, chomping through treats and her beloved roast beef Monster Munch, and being her usual diva self. Perhaps it is just old age, and my time with her is running out. It doesn't bear thinking about, and when it does creep into my mind, I am so terrified of that moment and having to say goodbye, tears fill my eyes. But I tell myself to enjoy every moment with her that I have... she still wants to go out for a walk every night, but the vet has said no more. I did relent last night, and she ran like the wind. I don't understand how she can limp on one foot then run as fast as she does. That little girl is a mystery to me, but I love her with my whole heart.

So, with those two out of action, I am fetching and carrying, quite literally. I carry Sally outside to do her business, for a drink when she demands it, and am cooking and cleaning, amongst a host of other things.

I am missing the gym and craving exercise, but that must take a backseat because I can't leave either for two hours. I have noticed increasing pain, so my earlier thoughts about the more I do, the less pain I feel, seems to be the case.

Next week, I will be back for weigh-in, and Jon, all being well, is coming with me.

August 13

I am not in the mood to eat or do anything. I am exhausted and can barely stay awake for more than an hour. I must admit, I have never felt this weary. Is this a symptom of Fibromyalgia or am I coming down with something. After the ABBA concert, I hope it's not Covid.

Whatever it is, I'm going to bed and intend to stay there.

"Marco, dinner..." Jon cooked so I tried a few bites, but the meat tasted too meaty if that makes any sense. I gagged, but not hungry, that was probably more to do with it.

August 14

I desperately wanted to go back to the gym today, but I feel washed out. The weather is also grim, so I have not been shopping either, which means I don't have the necessary foods to stick to plan. Right now, I don't care. I just want my body to stop aching and itching.

"Have you eaten anything?" Jon queries.

"I don't want anything."

"You have to eat something."

"I might have some fruit later."

To stop Jon fussing, I tell him I have eaten a few things. A lie. It's nearly midnight, so I get into the bath for a long soak. My skin is burning and itching so I cover myself with sensitive Head & Shoulders shampoo in the hope it will stop the itch, and it does. Such a shame it doesn't tone up my wobbly bits at the same time because the manufacturers would strike gold.

Lying neck deep in water and listening to what I've called an 'Oldies' playlist, Transvision Vamp's 80's stomper *Baby I don't Care* blasts out. I want to sing along, but as I can't hold a tune and my throat is scratchy, I won't inflict my woeful voice on Jon, the dogs, or the neighbours.

August 15

I look and feel like crap. It seems that over-activity these last few months has finally caught up to me, and it doesn't feel good. I want to fall into a long, deep sleep. But Jon is still not 100%, so if I don't do the necessary household chores, they won't get done. I need food shopping and don't trust the home delivery people as they usually pick goods that is about to go out of date.

My cleaner is coming on Friday, so perhaps I can swerve the bigger stuff until she comes. Yes, I do like to clean before she comes, but this time, I might have to admit defeat.

So, in a bit of a funk, I dragged myself out of bed and made my way to ASDA. I was in a foul mood and with people walking in front of me without an apology, I was dangerously close to ramming them in the ankles with my trolley. I didn't, but I really wanted to.

August 16

Ever seen that movie, The Evil Dead? Yes, well, I look just like one of those creepy zombie things. My tan seems to have come off in the wash and I have the pallor of Casper the Friendly Ghost. It's not a good look, but that aside, I feel like poop, and don't do well when like this. I want to get up and go, but my get up and go has gone, leaving me stranded.

August 17
WEIGH-IN DAY

After waking at 5 am, I dragged myself out of bed determined to get my hair cut and beard trimmed. I did it, then went to weigh in.

"10½ on." Shelly says it like it means nothing but as ever this is no judgement from her, but plenty heaped on me, from me. Her support is invaluable, and I know she knows what it feels like. Still, I have to do it for myself. I'm too old to have my hand held.

"Oh, God, that's terrible."

"It's a new week, Marco."

I have not followed the plan for three weeks and this is what happens. Once more it seems I am far away from target. Will I ever get there?

August 22

Have felt so poorly since weigh-in that I barely care what I have and haven't eaten.

As it happens, I went back on plan yesterday and fell right off it.

Today has been a better day, although it started badly. I had every intention of going back to the gym, but felt so weary, I never made it. I'm not going to be too hard on myself and need to listen to my body. I will get back there, in time.

Lunch was fresh fruit, fat free natural yoghurt, and granola (5½ Syns).

I can't face anything else today.

August 25
WEIGH-IN DAY

These last few days have been awful, and I have felt so ill, yet managed to stick to plan. But life goes on and after a horrible sleep, where I must have got two hours at most, I slithered out of bed, still feeling like death warmed up and walked to weigh-in. By the time I got there, which is only ten minutes from my house on foot, at most, I was hot, and clammy, and in need of a sit down.

The room was empty aside from Donna, Helen, an old friend, who took payment, and the lady at the scales whose name I can never remember. Shelly—yes, that's her!

"I hate you!" Shelly joked.

"Oh, God, why?"

"Six and a half off."

I am so happy that after my mammoth 10½ on last week, I've lost 6½ of it... it's a great result, and despite illness, I have been more focused this week. Not perfect, but I noticed an improvement which ultimately paid off.

After weigh-in, I went to Liverpool shopping with my friend. What a nightmare! I couldn't catch my breath and had to keep sitting down to rest. I guess I still haven't recovered. But I did it, and checking my watch, I had burned off 2,227 calories and walked the equivalent of 9.9 miles throughout the day—no wonder I couldn't breathe!

August 26

Absolutely goosed, and had zero energy to do anything, so I spent most of the day in bed, aside from sorting out the dogs.

Spent the night in bed resting, watching *Are You Being Served?* and a few other programmes I've watched countless times over the years. I spent most of that time laughing hysterically at the same old jokes.

August 28

After wrestling with myself, I walked to the gym to find it was closed, totally forgetting again about Bank Holiday Monday.

I won't repeat the stream of expletives I muttered under my breath.

Back on plan but have been picking at food rather than planning and cooking.

Refusing to focus on the fact fibro-fog has pushed the simplest of things to the back of my cluttered brain, I'm reminded of the bank holidays when the gym was the last thing on my mind. Instead, I would usually jet off for city breaks around the world from Russia to Spain.

Many years ago, well before I met Jon, me and my friend decided to combine our third weekend away of the year with seeing 80's band Orchestral

Manoeuvres in the Dark live in Cologne, Germany, and as we'd been to the wonderful city many times before, we both felt safe wandering about.

We got talking to two German guys, who typically thought Mikey and me were a couple. Explaining that I was gay, and he was straight didn't seem to translate. People always assumed he was the gay one because he was effeminate and considered pretty for a man. Saying that, perhaps the fact Mikey had a pair of ladies' tights (stockings) pulled over his head confused them somewhat. Why was he wearing the tights? As I remember it and forgive me because I had sunk more than a few beers, we were told that German's have a custom for ladies on their hen nights—they carry a basket around and people purchase items from it for good luck—Mikey decided he didn't want anything from the basket and made an offer for the tights she was wearing, which was quickly accepted.

Anyway, sexuality aside, they invited us to a bar called Cox's—lovely, yes, great crowd and bouncing eighties music, but I was slightly unnerved by the wall-to-wall cabinets displaying sex toys of varying shapes and sizes.

What I didn't realise was; this bar catered to guys who liked bigger men… well that's putting it too politely… the-fatter-the-better, and as I was humungous at the time, I was seen as fresh meat. For the first time in my life, men seemed to come at me from all angles, offering to buy me drinks and suggesting things too lewd to mention in this book. This level of attention didn't sit well with me, and I felt out of my depth, especially being fancied for being a fatty, again. But there was one guy who recognised me from the OMD show, and he came over to speak to me, but did so in perfect German.

"Sorry, I don't speak German."

James, from London, soon switched to his native cockney tongue, and seemed quite enamoured with me, and if truth be told, the feeling was entirely mutual. Even though James wasn't my usual type and must have been twenty-five-years older than me, charm, and kindness emanated from every pore. The fact was, he could have had any man in the room, but he set his sights on me, singing my praises and declaring me quite loudly the hottest man in the room (I still cringe when I think of it).

We shared one hell of a snog, and he did invite me back to his hotel room. I declined because I was with Mikey and wouldn't have left him alone in a strange city, even though as a straight, skinny guy, he was perfectly safe in his surroundings.

Going through one of my many *I'm fugly* periods, the interest from James, and many others, bolstered my confidence. Still, despite me turning him down, we swapped numbers and kept in touch for years afterwards, only losing contact around the time I met Jon.

After we left Cox's, Mikey and I found ourselves in a club, recommended by a few guys from the previous bar. Paying to get in, the place bounced, and once I'd gotten over the pungent smell of poppers wafting in the air like cigarette smoke, I was in the mood to party hard.

We went to the bar, and I ordered two beers—I don't really drink beer, but it seemed the easiest thing to ask for when I don't speak the language.

Anyway, while standing at the bar, I suddenly felt a warm sensation on the back of my thigh.

"What the—" I knew something wasn't right, but this was the last thing I ever expected.

"Oh, shit, Marco..." Mikey exclaimed, trying to keep a straight face.

"What is it?"

"Look..." He nodded, casting his eyes downward, and when I turned around, a nearly naked muscle-bound guy, apart from a leather cap and boots straight out of Police Academy's Blue Oyster Bar, stood before me, willy out, wafting it about without a hint of shame. Then I looked down and realised what he'd done. The warm sensation I felt moments earlier defied belief; he'd peed on me, and as though it was the most normal thing in the world, he continued weeing, soaking the front of my jeans, cheekily wearing a big grin on his face.

"What the friggin' hell are you playing at?" I am no prude, but I have never been so shocked, disgusted, or angry. And while other people's kinks are theirs to enjoy, and I would never shame, ask me first. I would have told him to jog on, but manners matter as my good friend always tells me.

Typically, he didn't understand a word, but my angry expression is not easy to misunderstand so he simply turned the tap off and walked away.

Both the front and back of my jeans were stuck to me. With murder on my mind, and ready to rub his nose in it, Mikey was bent double, laughing hysterically at my misfortune.

"It could only happen to you, Marco."

"Dirty bastard," I yelled, but it seems I was the one in the wrong, judging by the horrified glares from other clubbers. In truth, I had no idea what I was walking into, and had I been pre-warned, there is no way I would have stepped foot in the place.

Though I should have left immediately, I didn't want to have to trek back across the Rhine to the hotel stinking of pee, so went to the toilet to try and clean myself up as best as I could beforehand. I had intended to take my jeans off, wash them as best I could and dry them under the hand dryers. But it only got worse from there—a man dressed from head to toe in rubber, including mask with open zipper where the mouth was, was drinking from the urinal.

He looked up, acknowledged me, said something with a thick German accent that sounded suspiciously like, I'm thirsty, and carried on.

Usually, I don't care what people do, or what floats their boat, but I'd just been peed on, without permission I might add, and as my palms hadn't been greased with a wad of Euros, I was raging and ready to explode. "Disgusting," I huffed as I turned, walking out, wanting to find another toilet.

I climbed the stairs to the next floor but should have followed my initial instincts to leave.

Without knowing, I'd dragged my shy, timid, straight friend to a sex club and each floor catered to a specific fetish. The ground floor, well you already know what that was about, but the second floor—plenty of swings but no roundabout in sight. Trust me when I say, I had not ventured into a park. While looking for another toilet, I walked past a few men enjoying the swings surrounded by eager volunteers... well, let's just say, they weren't reliving their youth... I am a man of the world, but I was quite embarrassed and rushed back downstairs to find Mikey.

We quickly exited and found a taxi. With Mikey's coat wrapped around my legs as best it could, we returned to the hotel so I could shower and change. Ready to rock, we ended up in another bar, even managing to laugh about our unexpected visit to a sex club, and the fact I had been an unwilling participant in the game of water sports.

After one too many beers, I thought I was hallucinating when I went to the loo to find Bertie Bassett standing at the urinal. Was I tripping? I hadn't taken anything, so apparently not. A group had entered the bar through another door and were dressed as confectionery characters. Weird I know. They were even carrying baskets full of liquorice—my idea of heaven, and I shoved my hand in each basket multiple times. As it happened, they all spoke easy-to-understand broken English and we had a laugh, dancing and singing until the early hours of the morning.

Sozzled, I intended to raise a toast, holding up the biggest glass of beer that I'd ever seen. In fact, I struggled to lift it. I was fascinated with the landlady, Irma, because she reminded me of Granny Clampett from The Beverly Hillbillies—I didn't tell her, not that she would have understood what I was saying anyway. Instead, I led the bar in a toast... "Up your bum and no babies," I chanted, juvenile to the last, and they all soon joined in.

I am positive that they didn't have a clue what they were saying, but Mikey and I found it childishly funny.

I seemed to be very popular in there and ended the night snogging a guy from Iraq. He couldn't speak a word of English, and I certainly didn't speak his language, but it was a good end to the long weekend.

That night, I was sick out of my hotel room window—I still blame the kebab.

A few days after arriving home, I received an email from Mikey. I hit play and gasped because he had recorded me on his mobile phone snogging the aforementioned Iraqi. I was too drunk and busy playing tonsil hockey to notice. What the heck was I thinking? Seeing the guy with horrified, but sober eyes, I didn't fancy him in the slightest and he was actually squeezing my moobs like he was milking a cow—touching me there is usually a no-no. I felt embarrassed seeing myself in such a state. Beer goggles ahoy! I could hear Mikey tittering in the background—it was a horrible reminder of my abysmal behaviour when drunk and all I saw was my big fat face squashed against his. I quickly deleted it and made him promise to do the same.

Still, it was a weekend to remember!

When going through my wallet, I found a receipt for the first bar we went into after we checked into our hotel—188 euros and that was just him and me drinking. How I didn't end up with alcoholic poisoning is a mystery. Such fun!

The next time Mikey and I met up was at an Erasure gig at Delamere Forest. I'd lost a lot of weight since our last trip to Cologne, and he didn't recognise me when I approached his car.

"Shit, mate, you look amazing."

"Do I?"

"Yeah, but you looked just as good before."

Lies, but I appreciated him more for saying it and it was testament to our friendship that he saw me for me.

Sadly, that period of weight loss didn't last long.

August 29

Sally woke me at 5 am barking, then again at 7 am, so when my alarm went off at 9, I rolled over and switched it off. I had planned to go to the gym, but I couldn't force myself out of bed. Will I ever get back there?

Jon is cooking today—there is a God.

Braised steak, onions, mushrooms, and potatoes for dinner (Syn Free), followed by fresh fruit and yoghurt with tropical granola (5½ Syns).

August 31

The last day of the month, and what a terrible summer it has been so far. Typical British weather, but at least we had those nice few months in May and June. What tan I had is gone, so time to get the fake stuff out.

I woke up late and dragged my too-tired-to-go-to-the-gym backside out of bed. While getting ready to go out to have my haircut and beard trimmed, I listened to a radio interview with Agnetha Fältskog, the blonde from ABBA. At the end of the interview, *The Winner Takes It All* played and as I preened myself in front of the mirror my life flashed before my eyes and for the first time, I felt terribly old, and looked it. I don't know what happened, perhaps it is Agnetha's voice or the childhood memories that song conjures, but as the song played my eyes filled with tears and immense sadness enveloped me. I realise I feel lost with no idea why. What does my future hold, and where do I go from here?

MY JOURNEY – SEPTEMBER 2023

September 1
WEIGH-IN DAY

How are we here already? Where has this year gone? Christmas is coming, and while it is exciting, the prospect of winter is terrifying. I hate the cold, but as luck would have it, the weather has turned, and the sun is shining. Better late than never.

I have been on plan, but I can't get weighed today as the plumber is coming. Then back-to-back appointments all day. Still, despite yesterday's mini-breakdown, and wondering about the direction in my life, I feel more positive and hopefully next week I will have a loss, obliterating the remainder of the ten and a half pounds I put on a few weeks ago.

September 2

Piggy day today, but I don't care.

My friend came for dinner, and we had a few drinks (Hello, Pina Colada Baileys—this might be the best tipple, EVER!), then we watched *My Big Fat Greek Wedding* 1 and 2 in readiness for seeing the third movie next Friday.

By the time the second movie finished it was 11:30 pm and I was knackered, more than ready to go to sleep. I blame the Bailey's.

I don't remember drifting off.

September 3

Glorious weather!

So, it's time to sunbathe and get a bit of colour on my cheeks. Armed with my *AirPods*, I relaxed on the recliner in my back garden for a few hours. The cat lay next to me and at one point I dozed off, only woken by him tapping my shoulder with his paw, wanting to be stroked.

I also used my weighted hula hoop today, and aside from the fact it takes some practice, I quite enjoyed it. An acquaintance of mine uses hers regularly and has lost inches from her waistline, and the reviews are glowing. The only problem is, there isn't enough space inside. I am terrified of the weighted ball flying off and breaking something.

September 5

Wow, another scorcher of a day, and way too hot to go to the gym. So, what else could I do but get the sun lounger out again.

Not quite on plan but not as off as I could have been. Trying to claw back a weekend of stuffing myself with twelve cupcakes, kindly supplied by my friend. I did give one to Jon but scoffed the rest.

September 6

It's gone 2 am and I cannot sleep. My house is like a pressure cooker, and the only downside to this amazing weather we are having.

Spent the afternoon sunbathing when I should be writing. I have been tentatively working on a new title called When They Met, It Was Murder, which will be book one in a cosey series called The Molly Mulgrew Mysteries. I am only thirty thousand words in so quite a way to go, then I plan on writing a book with Jon. Not sure how that will go because the last time he ensconced himself into my world was to do a read through of my debut novel, Promised Land Lane, and we nearly throttled one another.

It's been a while since I worked with Netta, and I doubt that we will again because sales aren't exactly blowing up, and we seem to have naturally drifted apart. Still, I choose to believe that exciting times are coming my way. I am even thinking of book signings, but that's a while down the road.

Still on plan but I'm snacking on sandwiches rather than planning. Suits me fine now.

September 7
WEIGH-IN DAY

I knew I wouldn't make it because I was not back until 2 pm, but I am definitely going next week.

This afternoon I had my first sports massage in ages. I was nervous because it was with a new therapist, but he seems like a decent guy.

"Your neck and shoulders are so stiff."

"I feel locked in."

"How long has it been like this, Marco?"

"I don't remember when it started."

We discussed what my previous therapist had done, and he devised a similar treatment plan and advised I also take up swimming. I wasn't nervous taking my top off, but he did say I could keep my shorts on. Phew! I wasn't wearing underwear.

After a quick warning not to touch my feet or the back of my legs, because doing so would mean me launching myself off the bed, I was ready. He laughed and said most of his patients loved their feet being massaged. I am NOT one of those people.

"Climb onto the bed," he said.

And then I noticed it. My last therapist had an automatic bed that looked sturdier than this contraption. This was more the typical massage apparatus that looked like a wallpapering table.

"Will this hold my weight?"

"Oh, yes, you'll be fine."

Gingerly, I climbed on, and positioned myself face down, terrified it would suddenly give way and I'd faceplant the tiled floor.

It didn't, but it took me a few minutes to relax.

I walked home in twenty-four minutes. I thoroughly enjoyed it but was rewarded with blisters on my heels thanks to new trainers not yet broken in. I won't make that mistake again but will definitely walk home on my next visit on the 21st.

I did get my second Gold Body Magic award, and while it prompted me to do it again, I won't bother because I am exercising anyway, and I gain nothing for the milestones.

September 8

It's a year to the day since Queen Elizabeth II died. Time is moving way too fast for my liking—I feel ancient.

After a gap of a few years, I met up with a lovely friend of mine, Pam, for a coffee. Following four hours of laughter, two hot chocolates and a large mug of tea (what was I thinking in this heat?) later, I met another friend as we had planned to see *My Big Fat Greek Wedding 3*. I absolutely loved it but felt a sweaty mess, cursing myself for not wearing shorts. I couldn't wait to get home and peel my jeans off.

September 9

Sleep came in fits and starts, but this old bladder of mine had me up and down like a whores' knickers, so when Jon woke me up at 9 am, I could barely open my eyes.

He was spending the day with friends at Chester Zoo. I refused to go because I am vehemently opposed to keeping animals' captive for entertainment purposes. Leave them where they are unless you are helping to save their species.

Anyway, while he was gone, I watched *Gilmore Girls* for what seems like the hundredth time and nodded off. As it was another scorcher of a day, and humid too, I basically slept in front of the fan with the dogs at the side of me. I love the heat, but I'm ready for autumn now. I'm typically British so give me a few weeks and I'll be moaning it's too cold.

I'm off-off-off-off plan and have polished off a huge tub of brownies from Costco, six bags of roast beef Hula Hoops, Pick & Mix, and it's not even dinner time.

September 10

So, it finally happened... last night I ate far too many sweets, cakes and crisps and felt FULL, and very sick. Will it put me off? We shall see.

Came downstairs this morning to see a puddle of water on the kitchen floor. No, the dogs hadn't left me a present. It had more to do with me not shutting the freezer door properly. Well, I wanted to defrost it, so it saved me getting the hairdryer out. The downside was a lot of food was spoiled so it had to go in the bin. There was no way I could cook it all and eat it. Steak, minced beef, burgers, pizzas... and way more than that. Such is life!

After cleaning up, I went food shopping so I can hop back on plan, starting with a full roast dinner planned for tomorrow.

I also stocked up on fresh fruit and fat free natural yoghurt.

Time is ticking. I must get to target.

Later that afternoon. I went to get my hair cut and beard trimmed and decided to walk. By the time I reached the salon, my T-shirt was stuck to me and sweat dripped down my forehead. So, I stood in front of the industrial sized fan in the salon and cooled off for five minutes, not that it made much difference because as soon as I moved, I melted again. The last thing I wanted then was to be fussed over by anyone. I think the barber wanted to slap me because I made him wash his hands before he touched me as he had just had a cigarette outside. He wasn't best pleased.

Sitting in front of the mirror, I thought, *God, I look old.* I'm supposed to be looking better as I lose weight, not haggard and saggy faced.

I called Jon during the walk home.

"I look so old."

"You're so superficial, Marco."

His own judgement riled me because he never once looked in the mirror in his slimmer days and wanted to change anything and he readily admitted to that. In fact, when we met, I told him that I was nowhere near his league. I believed he was too good for me. Now he is bigger, his size is all that he would change about himself. Lucky him! It's easy for people to deliver withering comments and think it acceptable. Not once during the conversation did he say that I looked good, offer any positivity, or relay that I was worrying over nothing. I could be bleeding from the eyes, and he wouldn't see past his own nose. Perhaps it's because he loves me as I am that he doesn't seem to see how I feel about myself.

Grumpy, I focused on the negatives which took me right back to the time I'd lost a lot of weight about twelve years ago. I'd gone out shopping for new clothes and took them to show my mum. She liked them, and was encouraging as usual, but my dad pulled a face when presented with my new jeans and scoffed.

"You're thirty-six, who do you think you are dressing like that?"

Of course, he revelled in putting me down and hit a nerve, and my mum gave him what for, so I shot right back, "You're the one driving a red sports car at 60. Who do you think you are?"

But that is typical of our tit-for-tat-I'm-going-to-win-and-you're-not-relationship. Jon's comments and remembering what my dad had said only reinforced that those closest to us can be the worst offenders when it comes to criticism, even if it doesn't come from a place of malice. They rarely think before opening their mouths—looking closer at themselves would work wonders.

Why do I bother?

Only this past Friday, I went out and bought Jon new shorts and T-Shirts for his trip to the zoo because he was worried what he had would leave him hot and sweaty. Easily sorted and I gladly did it. Shame he doesn't see me as kind and thoughtful because that's the person I like to think I am.

If I was talking to him through his headset from another country while pretending to fight an imaginary battle, he would offer all sorts of sage advice. I'm just the person that cooks his meals, runs around after him, and washes his clothes.

Anyway, screw everyone and their opinions. I'll keep my superficiality and judgements to myself. I know my strengths, and my weaknesses, and the former far outweigh the latter. Tough luck if certain people choose to ignore what is good about me.

September 11

Still seething over Jon's comments. But I let it go so it doesn't fester into something it shouldn't be. I am sure he didn't mean to annoy me... anyway...
Cooking a roast dinner today and trying to stick to plan. So, I don't want to look like Jabba the Hut until the end of my days. But sod other people and their opinions because I'm going to do this and if they don't like it, stuff them.

September 14

Feel better today than I have the last few days, so I'm off out to the shops. Retail therapy works wonders for me, but I already have far too many clothes and shoes. Ah, well, I'll find something to buy.
As soon as I step through the door, drop my bags and slump onto the sofa, my watch tells me I have walked four miles and 4387 steps. It's no wonder I'm knackered.

September 15
WEIGH-IN DAY

Back to face the scales and I am excited to see how much I have lost.
Drum roll... ONE stinking, rotten, solitary pound OFF.
I won't lie about how disappointed I am, but I should suck it up because it is a loss and there are many members who would be thrilled with that number.

September 16

The weekend is here, but so what?
I've done a hell of a lot of nothing today. In fact, I need to give myself a talking to. Get back to the gym, get writing, and get rid of more fat. Instead, of lying on my bed, stuffing my face with cakes, and wasting my days. Easier said than done when I am physically and mentally exhausted with no will or desire to cook or entertain anything healthy.

September 17

Jon and I were invited to our friend's house for a roast dinner. I didn't eat much of it at all which makes me feel guilty because she went to so much trouble.

Watched a concert live on the TV and shook the roof off the house because it was on so loud. I wished I could have been there because it looked like a great night.

September 23

Crappy week and I have achieved nothing. Fibromyalgia is beating me hard lately. I'm fed up having these same health issues, day in day out... fat and feeling like death warmed up is not a good combination.

But Strictly Come Dancing is back tonight so I will get off my bed and go downstairs to watch it. There is a chill in the air and winter is coming. I am dreading it because our summer has been awful. UK weather reports say we are going to have an Indian Summer in October, but that pig flying past my window says otherwise.

Jon and I watched Strictly together, which was nice because we rarely spend time together. I did suggest to my friend, Sandie, that we take ballroom classes... there goes another pig.

September 26

Feel like I am emerging from hibernation. I've felt so ill this past week but forced myself out yesterday to do an interview for this book. I even walked the three miles home, and while I felt like somebody had squeezed every drop of air from my lungs, I was glad I did it though. The blisters on my feet from new trainers tell another tale.

I've spent the day coughing so much I sound like a barking dog.

Typically, I feel like hell, so I don't want to cook, and as Jon is poorly too, picking up whatever I've got, neither does he.

September 27

Finally!

My second appointment with Dave at the Pain Management Clinic. I've had to cancel the last two due to illness. So, despite head-to-toe discomfort, I went with enthusiasm, and while I found the last session useful, this one, the opposite was true.

Why? I feel like I am being herded down a path that is not a comfortable fit for me.

I am not keen on group settings so Dave's idea to send me to a group that helps with sleep deprivation is my idea of hell. Yes, I really do need help finding a way to ensure a restful sleep, but I see no merit in sitting in a circle discussing it with others. I don't see how that will help me and will only cause anxiety.

"You need to turn all electrical devices off two hours before going to sleep to help calm your brain and maybe try some relaxation CD's..."

"I have tried them before."

"That's good, perhaps give them another go."

I remember the experience well... a friend gave me a CD with rainforest and waterfall sounds. While it was supposed to soothe me into a deep sleep, I was up and down all night long peeing, not to mention being irritated by parrots squawking in the background.

Usually, I would say, no that's not for me, but I couldn't be bothered and nodded, agreeing to book myself in. "I will do."

Hell will freeze over first.

That aside, what got me was this; we were talking about my symptoms and my aversion to bright lights, loud noises, and smells... I told him that I found it really hard to tolerate cigarette smoke, and that with my dad being a heavy smoker, it became more challenging to be around him because of the smell.

Anyway, he rudely interrupted me mid-sentence, exhaled (VERY LOUDLY), closed his eyes, rested his hands on his thighs, and said, "Breathe, Marco, just breathe it out...

"What?"

"Close your eyes and breathe... in... out... in... out... aaaaaaaah... in... out... in... aaaah... and out again..."

Knock yourself out mate, but I won't be joining in. I've made less noise and fuss while having an orgasm.

Instantly, I was irritated, not only by his rudeness, but also due to the fact I was expected to join in. Embarrassed, no way was I sitting there panting and deep breathing with a virtual stranger. It put me in mind of drama class when my teacher asked me to pretend that I was a dog with a bone in my mouth. Okay, fine, I had a bit more confidence at eight, so I dropped to my hands and knees, imagined I had a wagging tail and made barking sounds... "You have a bone in your mouth, Marco..." she remined me. Right then, it was apparent I would never be in contention for an Academy Award for Best Actor in a leading role. The shame and horror of that moment has never left me, so any public activity, or speaking leaves me cold.

Now, I've said my mind often wanders to the crazy, and this time was no different.

What's next? I thought. Will I be sitting cross-legged in a sage-infused wigwam, head to toe in a tie-dye kaftan, banging a drum while murdering a rendition of Kum Ba Ah My Lord?

Nope, not happening.

I couldn't wait to get out of there, so clammed up, hoping he would take the hint that I had nothing more to offer.

"Good talk," he added as he brought the session to a close. "Make an appointment at the desk for another eight weeks."

"Will do," I replied. But I WON'T!

I didn't. Instead, I went straight home and got back into bed.

Now, don't get me wrong, I am all for alternative therapies, medicines, and thinking, but group situations will only cause me unnecessary stress. And if he expected me to attend one of these workshop activities, the last thing I would be doing is practising deep breathing techniques—it was embarrassing enough with just him there doing it. I felt like I was intruding on a private moment—cringe!

So, I'm not impressed, but recognise this service does a lot of good even if it's not for me.

It is testament to the many embarrassing moments I've experienced over the years, and while this last one was health related, there was one time not related to my health that I have never forgotten...

I'd gone to the cinema with my friend to see a movie called *Wrong Turn*. That was my first mistake because those who know me personally are acutely aware that even though I often write in that genre, I have no stomach for horror. I can't bear to watch anything gory or sit through anything that will make me jump. Torture movies are also a no-no. I walked out of the cinema thirty minutes into a movie called *Hostel*, horrified somebody could have put such graphic scenes make believe or not, on film. Aside from that, every second I spent in an anxious mess, wondering what was coming next, so I bolted.

Anyway, my friend, Hilary, had not long lost her husband, Tim, in his early thirties, to leukaemia, and convinced me to go and see the movie with her. I adored her, and we'd both lost somebody special, so I'd suffer it, just to give her something else to think about for a few hours, even if it was her laughing at me jumping and screaming throughout the movie.

So, with trepidation we drove to Cheshire Oaks, ate gluttonously at Chiquito's first, then took our seats in the cinema, with me dreading what was coming. I nervously chewed handfuls of salted popcorn while waiting for the movie to start, and when it did, I wasn't prepared, not for teenagers being hunted in a remote American mountain region by inbred and grotesque cannibals.

Hating every moment, as the film progressed with continuing brutality, I could feel myself sliding down my seat.

The delicious popcorn was soon abandoned, and I shielded my eyes with salty fingers. So violent and scary was it, I reached the point where I couldn't stay any longer. Hiding my eyes was no problem, hearing it was slightly more difficult with no free hands or fingers—perhaps I should have stuffed my ears with the abandoned popcorn.

I leaned in and whispered into my friend's ear. "I can't watch anymore—I'll wait for you outside."

Alarmed, she grabbed my wrist. "You can't leave me here on my own."

"I can." Nothing could have forced me to stay until the end of the movie, so I stood up and made my way along the row, whispering apologies for disturbing others, and down the stairs from my seat on the back row.

When I was halfway down the staircase, the huge screen loomed large and right in my eye line, stupidly, I looked up as a cannibal grabbed the terrified girl which startled me so much, I screamed and jumped back, slipping on the step, and losing my footing.

Trying to stop myself while in freefall was useless because there was nothing for me to cling onto and seconds later, I landed on top of a poor unsuspecting guy who must have had heart failure at this nearly thirty stone colossi crashing on top him during a tense, frightening, part of the movie.

As I flailed about, I was almost deafened by a high-pitched scream.

I was certain it wasn't him that shrieked, so I assumed it was the girl sitting next to him.

"GET OFF ME, YA FAT CUNT," he bellowed, as the audience erupted into raucous laughter.

For a moment, I was disorientated by the darkness, and because my glasses sat askew (think Olive Rudge from *On the Buses*), I couldn't see very well. So, with only the screen providing very little light because this scene was typically set in the dark, as if it needed anything else to make it scarier, I fixed my glasses.

"I'm trying." I meant every word I hissed out through gritted teeth, but the problem was, when falling I'd wedged my foot under the chair in front of him and couldn't free myself.

As he wriggled underneath, trying to push me off him, I did manage to move but slipped further down, crushing his legs, which caused him to make more noise and fuss.

Shame held me tightly in its grip.

I could feel something sharp digging into my back, but there was no time to worry about that.

"YOU'RE FUCKING SQUASHING ME," he wailed, as an usher appeared, shining her torch directly at us, instantly enabling the packed auditorium to get a closer look at the commotion, rather than the poor girl getting shish-kebabbed on screen.

All I could hear aside from his continuing protests was riotous laughter.

Eventually, I managed to free myself with a gargantuan heave from the poor guy underneath me.

Mortified, and back on my feet, I dashed down the stairs as the audience continued to laugh.

I rushed into the main area as my lungs burned, desperately trying to catch my breath. It was humiliating. The hefty will understand when I say I hate being the focus of attention but falling on top of the guy brought the spotlight shining brightly upon me.

Humiliated and gasping for breath, I locked myself in the toilet cubicle and tried to calm myself down. Still, my heart was banging in my chest.

About twenty minutes later, I'd calmed down enough and slipped out of the toilet into a corner of the reception area as the audience finally made their way out.

When my friend eventually found me hiding in the corner, she burst out laughing.

"That was the funniest thing I've ever seen."

"I'm glad you found it so amusing." I must admit, I did laugh too because it was like a scene from a comedy sketch.

"Where did you go?" She was trying her best to keep a straight face, chewing on her lip, and failing miserably.

"What do you mean?"

"I came out to see if you were okay then went back in thinking you'd snuck back in through the other door."

"There was no way I was walking back in there, so I locked myself in the loo."

She linked her arm through mine, still chuckling. "Come on, let's go home."

As we were leaving, I wasn't prepared for confrontation, but it fast approached when a young athletic guy I didn't recognise marched over, with a girl in tow. "Oi, mate, can I have a word."

"Oh, God, that's *him*," my friend warned, sounding more than a little worried.

"Who do you mean?" Then I cottoned on and prepared myself, thinking he was going to kick off and berate me for falling on top of him. But I couldn't have been more wrong.

"I'm really sorry for saying those things to you, mate, but you frightened the shite out of me."

I was apologetic, and still embarrassed, yet thankful I hadn't injured him. "I hate scary movies–I'm really sorry, if I hurt you."

"You didn't hurt me," he tittered. "But you squashed my box of popcorn."

I wanted the ground to swallow me whole. "Oh, no, I'm sorry." That explained what had been digging into my back. My friend, and his girlfriend were now bent double laughing, and I saw the funny side of it too. "Please, let me buy you another box to take home with you."

"Nah, mate, it's fine, really." Then he laughed too. "I proper shit myself. It was like watching a film in 4D—one minute I'm all tensed up waiting for her to get killed then you landed on top of me."

We all burst out laughing because despite me being the butt of the joke, it was funny, and to be honest, if I'd have seen it happen to somebody else, I would have wet myself laughing. "I'm so embarrassed."

"I shouldn't have spoken to you like that, I'm not that guy, mate."

I wasn't offended, but pleased he saw the funny side. And I appreciated his apology, it meant a lot.

We shook hands and went our separate ways. I've never forgotten it, and I bet he never has either.

I still can't watch that awful movie.

MY JOURNEY - OCTOBER 2023

October 1

October is here already.
Where has this year gone?
It seems to have flown by, but not only that, I've felt so rough lately, I've slept time away.
What a day!
I invited my friend, Sandie, over for a roast dinner. I didn't count any of it. Yes, it was very nice, and I ate more than I usually would, but exhausted, it was a chore to cook it.
With dinner and dishes out of the way, I put the washing in the machine and programmed it. It's one of those new-fangled machines that talks (her name is Bianca—I didn't choose it, she told me what to call her) and has a touch screen display. My friend brushed past it which paused the cycle, then it wouldn't come back on, or respond to any command. So, after a lot of faffing we decided to open the hatch at the bottom of the machine in search of the switch that would release the door. As soon as she turned the valve water gushed out sending a small tidal wave rushing toward me. Thankfully, the back door was open, and I had the mop to hand so as the water continued to pour, I flicked it out of the back door.
Typically, Sandie was on her hands and knees laughing hysterically.
Talk about a comedy moment.
I nearly wet myself laughing at her laughing, and thankfully, the machine reset itself.

October 2

I feel relatively normal today, aside from a cough that doesn't want to go away, but I had to cancel my physiotherapist appointment this morning because I was too tired to get out of bed.

Eventually, I got up at 1 pm which is extremely late for me, and annoying because I hate sleeping the day away.

My body hurts, but I have an appointment with my GP on Friday so will discuss it with him then.

October 5
WEIGH-IN DAY

Feel like death and can't be any further off plan than I am but I am going to get weighed to see what damage I have done. I know I am sabotaging myself, but the constant battle to avoid sweets is a nightmare.

But I weighed in a day earlier than planned as I was right on the doorstep. Terrified, I stepped onto the scales but already knew I had gained.

"8½ on."

"Shit."

"That's in three weeks, and you'll turn it around."

I can't say I am not disappointed because target feels like it is slipping away from me.

HELP!

October 6

Jon is going away for the weekend with his family and won't be back until Monday. He is excited, and so am I because it will be nice for him to get out of the house and change up his routine.

Had an appointment to see my GP, who is amazing and isn't the type to wave my concerns away. He listens, which makes all the difference. Anyway, forty minutes later I emerged with a letter to take to my local X-ray department, which confirmed Pneumonia, which I was at the tail end of thankfully. Jon had been moaning at me for weeks to go and get my cough looked at.

Aside from that, he is referring me to the ENT (Ear. Nose & Throat) Department for a hearing test as I thought I had wax down my ears, which was causing the muffled sound.

"Nothing down there, Marco."

"They feel clogged."

"Your ear canals are the cleanest I've ever seen, which might mean hearing loss."

I'm not surprised as I had hearing aids from the age of ten until I was eighteen. My hearing was extremely poor, and I became an expert lip reader without realising, and because I never had vocal tone issues, nobody realised how deaf I was. I remember that first day at school wearing two hearing aids and crying, thinking I would be laughed at. Nobody said a word. Anyway, when I was offered a pioneering operation to restore my hearing at eighteen, and even though the risk was permanent deafness if it went wrong, I jumped at the chance. Now, age might just be the reason my hearing has worsened again. We shall see.

Sensibly, I booked a double appointment as there were other issues to discuss, namely the severe exhaustion I have been experiencing for months and the sweating. He gave me a prescription which should hopefully cool my body down and stop the sweats and has booked me in for numerous blood tests to rule out thyroid and other issues. If they come back clear, he thinks it will become apparent that I have chronic fatigue syndrome (CFS) as well as my old sparring partner, Fibromyalgia. It would explain a lot, but typical of my bad luck.

But, knowing is better than guessing.

There is no cure for CFS, but many have recovered from it, and are in remission. Regardless, I will have to take more care of myself than I do now, which also means I need to shift this excess weight, and fast. Not to mention, I need to get myself back to the gym.

October 10

I am shattered today but have made up my mind. I have to fight through this blip and get back to the gym, whether it be treadmill, or take the plunge and go swimming.

The good news is, I am back on plan, but for how long I don't know.

Dinner is chicken casserole, roast potatoes, carrot & turnip which is Syn Free.

October 12

So mad at myself because I didn't get up until 1 pm. I hate sleeping the day away, but I must have needed it.

I am still on plan, and today, I did something that I have never done before. I weighed myself on scales at home, curious to know if I had lost anything—I have, and that's good enough for me. So, I am looking forward to getting weighed.

For lunch I had two pieces of seeded bread with low fat cheese spread which cost me ten Syns, and every single one was worth it.

Leftover SW curry from last night but I didn't eat it all as Sally wanted it, so I picked all the chicken out. She devoured that, while I ate the sauce.

October 13
WEIGH-IN DAY

I never made it to weigh-in because Jon surprised me with S Club concert tickets. Plans were abandoned so I could get ready for the concert. How exciting! Their music takes me back to those amazing nights when I danced (not professionally, just badly) on the many podiums across Liverpool's nightclubs.

Annoyingly, due to an electrical fault in the arena, the concert was cancelled just as I was about to get dressed. It has been postponed until the 30th of October which gives me something to look forward to at least.

Bummed I missed weigh-in and went to all that effort for nothing.

October 15

This weekend I have stuffed my face, but not nearly as much as I usually do.

But for those interested... here goes... this is what I actually remember eating...

16 bags of roast beef Hula Hoops = 104 Syns
1 x bag of Haribo Star Mix = 8½ Syns.
16 x cupcakes = No idea on Syns.
6 x Cadbury's Fudge = 33 Syns.
3 x Snickers = 27 Syns.
Bottle of Pina Colada Bailey's = No idea how many Syns.

This means I have used nearly all of my week's Syn allowance. I should be horrified, but I'm not.

October 16

Sally woke me up early this morning barking to go out, so I dragged myself out of bed. Freezing cold, I picked her up and carried her downstairs, kissing her little nose. "It's a good job I love you Sally Ann..."

Went back to bed and woke up a few hours later.

Decided to get my hair cut and walked to the barbers. My hairdresser was off—damn it. Refusing the offer from the other guy to do it, I walked to get some food shopping, but most of the shelves were empty. What is going on? There is fighting in Israel and Gaza... are people stockpiling in case of war? I don't know, but I'll have to go back tomorrow.

October 17

I walked to get my hair cut and beard trimmed, and while in the chair, the barber mentioned hair transplants. Well, thank you very much! Fat, ugly, glasses, partially deaf, Fibromyalgia to name one of a few, and BALD! Just the reminder I needed.

When he had finished, he showed me some gruesome videos and photographs on his phone while he had the procedure done, plus the before and afters. It didn't sound too bad, but seeing it made me feel queasy. I watch Casualty through my fingers, so this was a step too far for me. Still, he continued with a rundown...

"Day one, nine hours," he said.

"That's a long time. Were you awake?"

"Sometimes I fell asleep."

"Well, I suppose nine hours and you have all your hair back isn't too bad."

"Day two was thirteen hours."

"Sod that."

"It didn't hurt." It looked like it did from what he showed me. "Where did you have it done?"

"Iraq, five hundred pounds."

IRAQ, as if, the inner me screamed, not that I said it to him. "Bargain," I replied, loaded with sarcasm.

"My hair will never fall out."

"Fab!"

Yes, he has an impressive head of hair, but there is no way I am stepping foot in Iraq, and that's not for any other reason than I can imagine how homosexuality is viewed there. Yes, the idea of a full head of (grey) hair is a wonderful thought but knowing my luck I'd be arrested.

What good am I in prison rocking a trendy haircut?

Dinner was chilli con carne with boiled potatoes (Syn Free), washed down with coconut ring biscuits, which once more pushed me over my allowance.

October 20
WEIGH-IN DAY

Slept through my alarm and missed weigh-in. So annoyed because I need to know where I am. Jon is toying with the idea of rejoining with me next week, so the aim is to go every week without fail. It is the only thing that will keep me on track.

October 21

Today was a lazy one, pigging out with Jon, while we watched our favourite programmes, and Strictly Come Dancing.
Roast beef Hula Hoops and Haribo were once again on the menu.

October 23

Last night was a horrible pain filled night. But I fought back with a four mile walk which left me a soggy mess. But I needed it. Back on plan but I'm in so much pain it hurts to eat.

October 24

Walked to the shopping centre and soon wished I hadn't. I forgot to take my tablet so looked like I'd had a bucket of water thrown over me by the time I arrived.
As a reward, I treated myself to six fresh cream doughnuts.
Before I get home, I slip off for a sunbed. Emerging from the tanning booth, my face shines brighter than ET's finger. Not only that, I feel like every part of my body has been flambéed.

October 27
WEIGH-IN DAY

I'm nervous, but it's got to be done.
"3 off. Well done."
"I hoped for more."
"A loss is a loss."
Shelly is right, and I should take every win.

MARCO LEWIS

October 30

S Club at the M&S Bank Arena in Liverpool tonight.

Excited, we made our way to Liverpool in the pouring rain, but the show was magical, and a total nostalgia trip. Towards the end of the show, the band were halfway through singing *Alive* when the stage lights cut out, plunging the arena into complete darkness.

A siren wailed, but I thought it was part of the show, until a voice over the Tannoy system warned, 'FIRE HAS BEEN DETECTED IN THE BUILDING, PLEASE EVACUATE.'

A chorus of boos rang out, but in darkness, if this was a genuine order, nobody could see anything, and as we were only eleven rows from the front, the evacuation points soon became clear—right at the back of the arena.

I wasn't worried or scared, more annoyed that the next song was my favourite, *Reach*.

Leading my friend out, I called Jon. "I'm not sure what is going on, but I wanted to hear your voice just in case... the arena is on fire, and we are being evacuated."

Then my phone signal went.

It was a good few minutes before we got outside, and I was able to call him.

"Sorry, my signal went."

"Frightened the life out of me, Marco." He was frantic by that point, but I was safe, and unbelievably miffed to have missed my favourite song.

If I am going to die, it's his voice I want to hear as I shuffle off this mortal coil.

Security told us to go home and that the band were not coming back on stage. You can imagine how angry I was to get to the train station to discover the band has gone back on stage and finished the show.

But it could have been worse, especially after what happened at the Ariana Grande concert in Manchester some years back.

RUTH'S STORY

Softly spoken, while conveying kindness and compassion, sixty-eight-year-old retiree, Ruth has been a member of her local *Slimming World* group for almost fifteen years, with the advantage of continuing her journey with the same consultant the entire time.

And while this past decade-and-a-half has been fulfilling and successful in many ways, it's not Ruth's first foray into the world of weight loss organisations. Having tried many others in her quest to lose weight, she has found the one that works for her after many false starts over the years.

"Every slimmer has a similar story, but with *Weight Watchers* and being diabetic I couldn't cope. If I'd had all my points, I was really stuck if my blood sugar dropped. Whereas with SW, I can have a few extra Syns or eat things like banana... or other fruits which are Syn free. It suits Type 1 Diabetes far better and I don't have to weigh anything. I couldn't keep WW up because it was unobtainable."

Happily married with two children, four grandchildren, and one great grandchild, Ruth still leads a busy life. "I qualified as a nurse in 1974 and kept my registration right up to when the pandemic hit—I love orthopaedics, so I did male orthopaedics, then I went into nurse training. I was matron for eight years."

I now see where her caring nature stems from.

Ruth is considered the mother hen of her local SW group, offering endless and valuable support to members who may be struggling, or for those who simply need somebody to talk to. "In group, I really enjoy seeing other members achieving and celebrating their awards, and also sharing some of my experiences of how I got to where I am... even recipes that may help them."

Regardless, she has no desire to become a consultant because of time constraints, namely caring for her 91-year-old mother. Despite this, she also volunteers at local charity shops two days a week.

Sitting across from her now, Ruth's doll-like figure shows no signs of ever being burdened by excess weight. But formerly 11 stone, 11lbs at her heaviest, Ruth has done exceedingly well to shrink to a healthier 8 stone, 5lbs.

At five foot tall, she sits within the normal range on the BMI scale but is determined to shed that one final pound which will take her back into her target range.

She readily admits to wanting to shed another four pounds but is happy with her current weight. "I'd like to be between 8 stone, 1lb to 8 stone, 4lbs because I know I can maintain that. If I do any different, I struggle with maintaining. I do go in and out of target, and I keep going to group because if I don't, I know I don't have the self-control to keep me where I need to be."

Ruth is an emotional eater, with stress triggering most of her binges. "I will use any emotion to indulge whether it is celebration, commiseration, or to simply alleviate boredom."

Health issues were and continue to factor into Ruth's desire to maintain her weight. With Type 1 diabetes, dealing with excess weight pushed her onto the path of a myriad of medical issues. "My blood sugars were out of control, and I was warned many times about the dangers of obesity and high blood sugars. Continuing issues would have resulted in, vision, kidneys, heart, nerve, and vascular problems. But I am now far less likely to suffer these problems, although I am still aware of the dangers of putting the weight back on."

How are Ruth's underlying issues now?

"My blood sugars are under control... if I behave myself! I wear a monitor now. Hopefully this time next year I will still be within my target range, and my blood tests, nerve and vascular tests results are within acceptable levels."

When did she first notice her weight gain?

"I've always had a weight issue and was always teased as a child for being fat. I wasn't horrendously overweight, but my whole family, my parents, and two brothers were on at me all of the time. They had nicknames for me."

I wonder if this family dynamic solidified Ruth's addiction to food.

Without prompting she answered this for me, "I comfort ate, and that was my way of keeping control. My parents never restricted my intake of food. I could eat what I wanted, but when I got a paper round at the newsagents... they had all the chocolate bars sat there. So, I'd go in to do my round and lo and behold, there was the caramel chocolate bars..."

Of course after she admitted her own diagnosis to addiction, I needed to know her biggest weakness.

"Peanut butter is my absolute downfall, but buffets also cause me problems as I cannot resist temptation. A little bit of this, everything is a little bit, then it becomes a huge amount. My saving grace is knowing my blood sugar will go up, and within about ninety minutes, I know I've had too much, and I don't feel so well."

With a family who cared but teased her, I asked, "was the weight gain from childhood to adult gradual?"

"When I got married, I was only a size 12, so I wasn't horrendously overweight, but then after I got married, I gained weight, probably due to comfort and shift work."

Ruth has come a long way, but you will agree that she has done amazingly well and has achieved what many of us can only dream of. Still, she admits to only looking at herself when having her hair done. "Other times, I avoid mirrors like the plague."

As busy as she seems to be, there must be some well-deserved down time, a favourite place where she can relax and forget about SW or maintaining her weight. "I've got some holidays booked. Me and my husband like train travel. We're doing Bavaria next year. We've done the Pyrenees, the Dolomites, Austria and Switzerland."

She later told me The Orient Express is on the bucket list and went on to explain, "It's one we'd like to do, and also travel around India on train. But with my mum needing so much care we tend to plan last minute. But we booked Bavaria and Transylvania because we haven't done that before. We journey down to London, through to France, Germany, where we stay over. We stop at every destination and stay in a hotel—it's all organised, and we go on different journeys every day. It's nine days. My husband is a train fanatic, and as I like knitting, I sit and knit beanie hats for the homeless during the journey. I love doing it, it's a hobby."

It's another example of Ruth's kind nature that even during vacation time, she is thinking of ways to help others. Ruth is also a fan of cruising, but how does that affect her weight?

"With cruising, most of it is healthy buffet meals, and you don't have to weigh anything, so there is never a problem."

Currently stable on her weight loss journey what does Ruth envision her future to be?

"My ultimate goal is to see my children and grandchildren happy and successful—our grandchildren don't keep us as busy, not now they're growing up because they have their own lives, but trying to get my mum sorted takes a lot of time up."

Putting aside family members, and her commitment to others, what about the lady herself... what is next for Ruth?

"For me, just to stay as healthy as I can for as long as I can. While I'm healthy, my husband and I can enjoy our lives which is great. My husband is seventy-five and still walks many miles—he's done the North Wales coastal walk, walked from Southport right the way down to Formby... he does that with his friend. Maintaining my health is so important because in the back of my mind is that voice... I want to see my family members grow into healthy, successful adults in whatever field they want to be in. Spending time with my children, grandchildren and great grandchild and being able to play with the little ones is important and makes me happy. For me, to stay as well as I can for as long as I can means I will be around to see that."

MY JOURNEY - NOVEMBER 2023

November 1 & 2

Where has this year gone? When I was a child, time never seemed to matter, and the four seasons seemed to trickle by. Now, they fly past me at breakneck speed. One foot feels like it is already in the grave.

I am still too far away from target, which bothers me incessantly, and while I am fully aware what actions will get me to target, the necessary will power to do it eludes me.

Aside from that, I really hate the autumn and winter seasons, and though only weeks into it, I am already craving the sunshine and can feel myself slipping into misery. Endless grey skies, reduced light and rain, rain, rain. Add on the constant want of things I shouldn't have, and this season sucks.

November 3
WEIGH-IN DAY

There is not a chance in hell of me stepping outside today, not to go shopping to Liverpool as planned or to weigh-in. I really loathe the cold and rain, not least because it has sent my fibro symptoms plummeting to an all-time low.

I WANT CAKE.

November 4

Although it is the last thing I want to do because of the rotten weather, Jon and I are heading to Prestatyn for his brothers 40th Birthday. It will be nice to see everyone on their turf for a change as I usually cannot go because of the dogs. But thanks to our wonderful friend Sandie, I know they will be safe.

Strange but true, I have only met Anthony, the birthday boy, once, four years ago when he returned with the rest of the family from New Zealand, the same time since we moved into this house, and even with fantastic neighbours who have been a blessing, it is time to move on.

Back to the party. The food aspect bothers me. I don't know from one day to the next how my body will react to food so throwing up in somebody else's bathroom is always a worry.

I needn't have worried because food wasn't an issue—my mother-in-law's skills for making poached eggs is legendary, and as somebody who is yet to master it (at nearly 50!) when offered, I simply couldn't say no. Two perfectly made eggs with English muffins went down a treat, and I was neither sick, nor eating past my Syns. Nope, I found myself craving more.

It was a lovely day, and I genuinely enjoyed being back in Prestatyn for a visit.

November 5

I have not stopped eating cakes, sweets, and crisps, and even washed them down with a vegetarian pizza from Domino's—I don't even like Dominos', so I don't know why I chose to eat that particular food. I never enjoy takeaway, but faced with the prospect of having to cook, I caved. Now, I am in agony and my shoulders feel like they have been yanked from their sockets.

Am I not supposed to be feeling better with weight loss? Yes, but I don't ever remember feeling as unwell as this at my heaviest. I am wondering how much the fat masked underlying issues.

November 6

Made a quick trip to the doctors this morning to drop a pee sample in for Jon. While there, I made an appointment to see my GP. I feel out of sorts and after stupidly googling my symptoms, I am more worried than ever about what this shoulder pain could be-chronic pancreatitis.

Writing this, I roll my eyes because it could be something completely different and easily treated. I usually tell Jon off for using the internet to diagnose problems, so I should know better.

Please don't think me a hypochondriac because I'm far from one. It just so happens that writing this book has seen the emergence of one health crisis after another. My weight loss journey has been marred by struggles with food addiction, food aversion, and chronic conditions such as Fibromyalgia thrust upon me. Right now, it seems like one more thing heaped on top of another.

On plan and have had a bowl of homemade spicy carrot and lentil soup which I enjoyed with wholemeal pitta bread, courtesy of Jon. It tasted delicious, and thankfully, there was no pain afterwards.

November 7

Managed to see my GP, and it was better news than *Google* led me to believe.

Due to Fibromyalgia, one of the drugs, Ibuprofen, proves essential, and while I have taken this on and off for years, it seems my body no longer likes it.

After relaying my symptoms and being asked to do certain movements with my arms, hands, and shoulders, plus having certain areas of my stomach and sides prodded, she told me that she thinks I have developed an intolerance to Ibuprofen which has caused inflammation in my stomach which in turn had caused pain in my left phrenic nerve connected to my shoulder. This is what is causing the pain. So, to stop this, I have to cease taking Ibuprofen which will probably cause a flare up. As the doctor agreed, I am in a catch 22 situation, so if I have to take Ibuprofen, I need tablets to protect my stomach. Whatever next? If I do take them, I am in pain and if I don't, I am still in pain. I can't win. But at least I know it isn't anything serious. As I was leaving her office, she told me that should my symptoms remain or worsen, I was to go back and see her for further tests. "I don't think it is anything to worry about though." Famous last words. Onwards I go.

Later on, I conducted an interview for the sequel to this book, and while trying to maintain a shred of professionalism, I found his story, and his never-ending sadness overwhelming me. I relate in so many ways, obviously for different reasons. But it hammers home how important it is for me to write this book.

November 9

Feel loads better today, but my stomach is still a little tender. Got up, looked in the mirror and didn't look well at all—in fact, I looked grey, and years older than my forty-nine years.

November 10

Jon has gone to visit relatives in Prestatyn for ten days and while I am fine with him being away, I will miss him, and so will the dogs. Sammy is already sitting on the stairs waiting for him to come home, and Sally is on alert, thinking he will walk through the door any moment.

This is a big part of their separation anxiety.

They were my mum's dogs, and after she died, we took them in because my dad was still working a lot. When she was alive, she never worked so spent all day with then. Now, they are rarely alone for more than two hours.

It is a big task, but after losing my mum, they don't understand that Jon is coming back, so I will spend the next ten days spoiling them even more than they already are.

It means sleepless nights because Sammy snores like a klaxon. But their happiness is all that matters to me. Still, it won't stop me digging out the ear plugs.

November 15

Went to view a new house today. Actually, it's a bungalow, which might be a blessing in disguise for my body while it's in revolt.

Finally cancelled my gym membership because my body isn't up to it, and there seems little point paying £34 per month when I can pause it and rejoin once I feel up to it.

November 17
WEIGH-IN DAY

I don't want to face it, but I have to. I have completely lost myself, but I know I can get back on plan.

"3½ on," Shelly whispered.

"It could have been worse."

November 18

I woke up this morning, soon realising that my backside was on fire. And no, it wasn't because I'd scoffed a Vindaloo the night before, more to do with the fact I'd fallen asleep and left my electric blanket on its highest setting. It's the closest I've ever come to being poached.

November 19

Another night of scoffing everything in sight because Jon isn't here. I have the worry of moving, packing and the thought of lifting all those boxes is not a welcome one.

November 20

Jon is finally home. It seemed like the longest ten days ever, and I really missed him.

Saw my dad for the first time today in months. Battling prostate cancer, which has spread, he looked remarkably well.

November 23

Spent the last three days packing and sorting the house out. Although we aren't moving until January, we want it all done by December, only keeping the essentials out.

While we will decorate the house for Christmas, we have decided no tree this year. It's too much hassle putting one up and then taking it down, and then moving, especially as Jon goes all out... he decorates it, then takes everything off, and begins again... he needs to set up his own business because the tree looked dazzling last year.

But I am so stressed that I can think of nothing else but moving. My house is a mess because boxes are everywhere, not to mention, emotionally, I have already vacated the place—the place could fall down, and I wouldn't care. Jon is in a filthy mood and spends his time shouting at me because he is stressed. I want to hit him with a shovel and bury him under the patio, but I don't. Right now, I want to run away. I'm not surprised moving house is high on the list of things that cause arguments.

MY JOURNEY – DECEMBER 2023

December 4

Seems like forever since I last checked in, but life has completely taken over and knocked me flat on my back. Packing for our move in January, my house is a mess which has left me with little desire to cook or to follow plan.

Today, I had a hearing test.

"You're hearing is getting worse." Jon has been saying it for a while, but I've not noticed anything because for the last thirty-two years, I've become accustomed to what I can and cannot hear. I don't think I need to go but I will.

Well, I am now the proud owner of two hearing aids.

Fat, deaf, blind, balding—all I need is a hump on my back and I can get a job at Notre Dame ringing the bells.

December 7
WEIGH-IN DAY

Determined to get to target, I had not bargained for bad news.

"Five on."

I really want to swear!

I am losing the fight, but I know I can turn it around. But this move and the mess in my house is consuming my life.

December 14
WEIGH-IN DAY

I haven't checked in because there has been nothing of worth happening, aside from the daily struggle that begins when I open my eyes. Tired doesn't cover it and even with nanna-naps, I am shattered, so I simply don't go. What's the point anyway? I've been so fed up this past week and considering quitting. I'm obviously meant to be fat.

CHEWING THE FAT

December 19

Busy, busy, so no time to do anything, let alone share my thoughts.

December 24

My little doggy, Sally, is not well at all. I am terrified this is it. But she surprised me when she tucked into pork, beef, and turkey, washed down with a butter cookie. Maybe I am worrying for nothing—who am I trying to convince?

I took her for a walk, and she seemed to enjoy it, although she was very tired. I carried her home nearly in tears, knowing in my heart that the end was coming. I pulled myself together and slapped on a smile before walking into the house. I know Jon's anxiety is through the roof, and as much as he worships Sally, she is also his support—he would be lost without her.

"She's going to be fine." I lied to Jon.

Miracles do happen, right?

December 25

I had everything pinned on a Christmas miracle, but it wasn't to be.

At 7 pm, Sally walked over the rainbow bridge and took a piece of us with her.

"We did the right thing," I kept saying.

"She might have come good," Jon sobbed out his misery.

"It was her time, babe." I could barely speak. "Even the vet said she would have done the same thing in our shoes."

"I miss her."

"So do I, but we love her enough to let her go."

To say mine, and Jon's, hearts are broken is an understatement but easing her pain and suffering was our last act of unwavering love for her. She went downhill fast, and after suffering a seizure this afternoon, I sobbed, knowing it was time to let her go. So, my dad drove us to the vet.

I felt horrible guilt telling the vet that we were ready, and I can still picture her looking at me, confused, wearing her little red bandage around her leg. I wonder if she knew. Still, I am mad at the world because I wasn't ready to say goodbye. But would I ever have been? Never!

Even though I've known Sally since she was a puppy, she loved Jon unquestionably; *he* was *her* person, so he held her as the vet administered the sedation. At every step she knew she wasn't alone and when the moment came, my gorgeous little girl buried her head in his armpit, closed her eyes, and drifted away peacefully.

We sobbed as the vet confirmed she was gone and stayed with her for twenty minutes stroking her and cuddling her. "We love you." I knelt and kissed her. God, even writing this, tears are falling down my cheeks. She was ours, as loved as a human child would be, and though she was a stubborn, badly behaved diva at times, she made me laugh, and smile, and brought Jon and me immeasurable joy that few humans ever have.

Coming home, nothing sits right because she is not here.

Jon rushed up stairs, and moments later, all I could hear were his wails of anguish. Nothing I can say will mean anything right now, so I don't utter empty words that won't help.

After nearly seventeen years, how are we meant to carry on without her?

When you've loved a dog to the end, you've known the deepest love. And the deepest pain.

December 26

Jon and I have spent the day in tears. Neither of us have any interest in anything or seeing anyone.

We just want Sally back.

I'm lost without her, but for Jon... Sally was his shadow, his baby, so he can't contemplate the fact that she is gone.

December 29

More tears fell when Sally finally came home today. Well not her, I wish, but her ashes, and while it is a comfort, it is also the final act, that this is really goodbye.

Every minute without her brings further distress and fresh grief. Losing a beloved pet leaves an emptiness that is impossible to fill.

Jon and I are absolutely broken, and while he can't hide his devastation, which is putting it mildly, that losing her has shattered him, I put a brave face on things, assuring him we did the right thing.

It doesn't mean I don't miss her every minute of the day, or that I don't fret for her. He just doesn't see me scroll through her pictures on my phone, kissing each one as I remember cuddling her and feeling her soft fur.

MY JOURNEY – JANUARY 2024

January 4
WEIGH-IN DAY

I can officially throw 2023 in the shit bin, but nothing that happened to me over this last year can compare to the sorrow and shock of losing Sally. I am still missing her like crazy, but told myself, new year, new start. So, why am I trying to convince myself of things I don't believe. We are allowed to grieve for her. My gorgeous little girl... it is a testament to how loved and adored she was, and still is.

I've screwed my diet up, so I begin again. This time, I need to lose the obsession with numbers so asked Donna to weigh me and not tell me anything until I hit target.

"How much do you think you've put on?" she asked.

"About a stone."

"Nowhere near."

So, we made a deal.

Donna will reveal my weight to me in four weeks. Hopefully, I will be close to where I was.

We are moving house tomorrow, and my stress levels are off the charts, so one less thing cluttering my already cluttered mind will be welcome.

January 5
MOVING DAY

The house move is done, and while I was pleased to be leaving, a part of me felt like I was leaving Sally behind. But we have her ashes, and her pawprints, so she is always with us.

Sammy is fretting terribly for her, but we will smother him with love, and his favourite treats.

Now, the hard part begins... unpacking.

January 6

I don't consider myself so unfit I cannot manage a house move, but I forgot to factor in fibro, which has reduced me to a shell of my former self. I am in agony. Every part of my body hurts, from the top of my head to my toenails.

Despite shopping for the healthy stuff, I still haven't managed to get back on plan because my new house is a mess, and all I want is for Sally to come back.

January 11

We're almost settled in our new home, and though there is a Sally-shaped hole in our lives, I can think back and chuckle at some of the things she got up to during her long and happy life. Her death has hit Jon terribly hard because she was his constant companion. He couldn't go to the bathroom, into another room, or move from the sofa without her wondering where he was or following him. Now, he doesn't quite know what to do with himself without her. She slept next to him every night... little things that drove him mad at the time, and now he would take endless sleepless nights just to have her back.

"Are you going to replace her?" Some have asked.

"Absolutely not."

"For two reasons, one she is IRREPLACABLE, and two, we have another dog, and a cat so know more heartbreak is looming. We can't sign ourselves up for any more than that."

Anyway, I am choosing to remember Sally with love and smiles, so today it is back to SW.

I can't give you an update because I haven't asked for one. My sister joined me today, signing up again, and I hope this time she manages to shift some weight and keep it off. Her health depends on it, and only a few days ago she was fitted with a blood pressure monitor. At 47, an overhaul of her lifestyle is long overdue. No judgement because we have all been there.

January 12
WEIGH-IN DAY

First things first. After an appointment with my GP, he is sending me for blood tests, again, to eliminate conditions that will hopefully lead them to confirm I have ME or chronic fatigue syndrome. I don't want it, but forewarned is forearmed.

I will worry about that when I have to.

For the first time in what seems like forever, I never missed a week, and actually weighed in. I don't know how much I gained but I assume I did.

A total first for me; I stayed for class with my sister, which was enlightening and spurred me on hearing other people talk about their struggle. I never spoke a word.

January 16

I woke up to find my garden resembling a winter wonderland. Ugh. I am not a fan of going out in the snow because I am terrified of falling.

I can't stress how good it is to have regained an element of control, and really do think staying for class last Friday was a great help. I don't want to know my weight right now.

January 18

Another day on plan, but it didn't start well.

For breakfast I had my usual fruit with natural yoghurt. Delicious... well I thought so until I realised the yoghurt was out of date and curdled. After hanging over the sink, I checked everything. I am usually fastidious when it comes to sell by dates.

Now we have moved house, I am already feeling isolated. Yes, I am in picturesque surroundings, but it's too quiet. I am used to hearing the flow of traffic and general footfall, but here the sound of silence is all encompassing.

Talking of moving house, I received a phone call from our old neighbour earlier to say that the tank in the loft exploded this afternoon and had destroyed the house, sending water cascading down the stairs. Apparently, every room in the house is ruined. The wooden floors are soaking wet. Dealing with that would have been a nightmare.

January 19
WEIGH-IN DAY

I went for early weigh-in but didn't stay for class as I had pre-existing appointments.

While I still don't want to know the numbers, Donna informed me that I had a LOSS, which is good enough for me. But why am I hiding from numbers? I'm big and ugly enough to take on the chin the damage I did before going back on plan.

January 20

I feel the pull of the gym so am looking into rejoining, but a different one closer to my new place.

Stuffed my face with junk food all day.

5 x Crème Eggs (45 Syns)

6 x Walker's bacon crisps (51 Syns)

That's nearly half of my weekly Syn allowance blown out of the water and I'm not even halfway through the week.

January 21

Went food shopping this morning and thank goodness I did because we have severe storm warnings. I'm not usually one to listen to weather reports, but I just opened the patio doors, and the blinds blew right back at me, and blasted me with freezing cold wind. I stepped into the garden and howling winds whipped around me. It was quite eerie, but as the table and barbecue covers had blown off, I had to fix them back on.

Stuffed my face again and have no idea how to Syn most of the food I ate.

Pizza and onion rings – no idea how many Syns.

5 x Crème Eggs (45 Syns)

January 22

Famous last words... back on plan.

Pasta, 5% mince, onions & mushrooms. (Syn Free). Sainsbury's lighter tomato & herb sauce for Bolognese (1½ Syns).

I actually enjoyed what I ate, but only managed a small amount.

1 x bag of Walker's ready salted crisps (6½ Syns).

January 23

As I am yet to rejoin the gym, I am going to take the opportunity to explore my new surroundings and go out for a walk. I'm not sure how far I will get before I am ready to drop, nor where I am going to, but some exercise is better than none.

My Samsung watch is fired up and ready to count my steps and distance, but driving wind and rain puts the blockers on exercise.

Stuck at home, trapped, and all I want to do is eat.

Although I like our new house, I feel like I did when we lived in Prestatyn—too far away from civilisation. Not sure if it is for me, or I need somewhere with more going on around me.

"I'm not moving again," Jon snaps. He would if I said I wanted to move to North Wales.

Lunch was bacon, egg, Fry Light. (Syn Free). 3 x slices of wholemeal bread (HEXB + 2½ Syns).

In-betweens, I tucked into 4 x individual Cadbury's Roses (10½ Syns) and Walkers ready salted crips. (6½ Syns).

Dinner was homemade potato and leek soup (Syn Free).

January 24

Freedom!

After being cooped up, it felt good to get out of the house.

I went to get my haircut, beard trimmed, plus a quick blast on the sun bed. I'm looking and feeling transparent at the moment, so a shade of colour is a necessity.

Hadn't banked on the sunbed being so cold when sliding on, but I soon warmed up.

Once home, I glanced at myself in the mirror—the double chin is still there, but I look a lot more refreshed than I did a couple of hours before.

Craving Cheerios so I treated myself to a serving, with skimmed milk of course. What I really want to get my hands on is a box of Crème Eggs, but I refrained.

Finally found the fabled SW Cauliflower Mac 'n' Cheese in Iceland and grabbed the last three from the freezer. Jon has been dying to try it and is struggling during times he would usually snack. Used my SW membership card and got 10% off the whole shop–bargain!

Busied myself with putting the shopping away and found a box of Crème Eggs in the fridge. I pushed them to the back of the shelf, and my mind. But now I have remembered that they are there, I hear them calling out to me, whispering for me to stick my tongue in the creamy centre. Yum!

Instead, I had a bowl of the homemade potato and leek soup again (Syn Free & HEXB).

For dinner tonight, although I don't want it, is braised steak with mushrooms & shallots, carrot & turnip, cabbage, Brussel sprouts (Syn Free) and gravy (1½ Syns).

MARCO LEWIS

January 26
WEIGH-IN DAY

Went for weigh-in with my sister. She did amazingly well with half a stone lost this week. That takes her total to ten pounds in two weeks.

I lost again but asked not to be told the figure. Still, a loss is a loss, and I am thrilled. But, good news, I was given a certificate awarding me Slimmer of the Week for last week.

Stayed for class and feel really positive.

Without shade, it is good to hear of other people's struggles first hand. I'm not the only one, but they seem a lovely bunch of people. Donna was in sparkling form, and I see why she is so popular.

Donna kindly stuck to our agreement and ignored me throughout class. I am shy until I get to know people, so being put on the spot would only embarrass me. Tammy won Slimmer of the Week and was given a well-deserved round of applause. Her cheeks glowed purple... she is so like me.

At the end of class, I won the raffle, so with good luck on my side, I went home and put money on the Euro Millions.

January 27

Didn't win the Euro Millions, but I did eat two slices of chocolate cake.

My dad and my brother, Ian, flew to Austria for two weeks of skiing. Lucky them!

I am intrigued by the idea of giving it another try, but I haven't been since January 1985—I was a shy, naïve, kid of eleven.

It was billed as a lad's holiday, so me, my dad, uncle Alan, and others jetted off for a week in Alpbach, western Austria. But two of the party ignored the memo and brought their girlfriends with them—annoying other members of the party in the process. I remember one of them—Tracey—a Page 3 model—blonde, stunning, but absolutely hopeless on anything aside from stilettos. Looking back, she must have been the most beautiful girl on the slopes—perfect hair, and makeup flawlessly applied despite the many times she went arse-over-tit in the snow, screaming for help.

She took a shine to my dad, and could often be heard yelling, "Oh, Dave, please help me..." in her best Penelope Pitstop damsel-in-distress-voice. Yuk!

My mum was furious when she found out two women had invaded what she had been assured was a lad's holiday. More so when she found out about the Page 3 model.

As holidays went, it definitely wasn't my favourite, especially after my dad greased my ski's without telling me. The abject terror I felt as I shot down the mountain like a bullet train has never been forgotten. I thought I had been doing brilliantly and had mastered the art of staying upright. But nobody taught me how to stop, so with the bottom of the mountain fast approaching thanks to the greased skis, and people edging closer, I threw myself over and rolled, and rolled, and rolled, to a stop, hurting my little finger. But I am jumping the gun.

Thinking back, it's no wonder my dad never took me again because the holiday was littered with catastrophes.

Timid as a child, and definitely not sporty or adventurous, I hadn't factored in the drag lifts.

Day One – the drag lift worked just fine, even if I was dragged up the slope by my booted ankle after losing my balance. I did manage to get it right the following day.

Day Two – I hadn't banked on how high the chair lifts were, so what seemed like dangling not far from The Kármán Line, the boundary between the Earth's atmosphere and outer space, my dad spoke…

"Are you ready?"

"What for?" I can vividly remember how scared I was dangling from this thin line of metal.

"Edge yourself off the seat and when the chair meets the snow, push yourself off and ski down the slope."

"Okay."

"Right, go!" And suddenly, he darted off the lift like an athlete, leaving me to miss my cue. What else could I do but go back down and around again. I didn't dare wave because he would have had a fit.

When I got back to the top, he was waiting, red-faced and furious. He never had any patience with me. But I had just as little with him. Nothing has changed.

I launched myself off the lift and managed to stay upright.

Wonderful. I enjoyed the day's skiing and found myself to be proficient when going at my own pace. Now, I was ready for the black run. Yeah, right!

The next day, confident on the chair lift, despite the height, and the knowledge I would soon have to launch myself off it, I swung my legs vigorously and looked down as one ski dropped and skied back down the mountain all by itself.

My dad's face said it all, but he bit his tongue this time.

At the top of the mountain, I somehow managed to manoeuvre myself off on one ski while he shot back down to retrieve my errant ski.

I was sitting in the snow enjoying the sun when he got back, but for some reason I couldn't get my ski boot to fasten into the clip on the ski.

"Use your pole, for Christ's sake," dad snapped, rapidly losing whatever patience he had left with me.

So, cack handed at the best of times, I used the pole. It slipped and jabbed him in the eye. He bent over, and for one moment, I thought his eyeball would be stuck to the spiky thing on the end of my pole. It wasn't... I am still alive, but God knows how. I wanted to laugh but didn't.

He abandoned me to my own devices after that, so I found my own groove, and other people to ski with. And for this eleven-year-old beginner, alone on the mountain, I was doing pretty well until I picked up speed. I think I gave a little yelp, and thankfully other skiers tried to help, roaring repeatedly the words, "SNOW PLOUGH, SNOW PLOUGH..." I finally managed to slow myself down as I skied right across the skis of those people trying to help me. Thankfully, they were good natured about it.

But then on my next run, the opposite happened as I kept slowing to a stop because my ski's kept clogging up.

"What's taking you so long getting from the top to the bottom?" Dad asked.

I told him the truth. Easily sorted. And that is where the ski wax made its appearance, and thinking about it, back then he would probably have been happy if I had skied off the edge of the mountain into a bottomless canyon... I dealt with it, but was glad to get home, happy never to have been dragged on a lads and dad's holiday again.

Jump to March, 1985, and my parents flew off for their own skiing holiday while I stayed behind with my wonderful nan.

When they got home, my mum only had one question for me. "Who waxed my skis?"

I had been using hers. "Dad did, why?"

She shot him daggers. "He knows damn well not to wax my skis."

"What happened?"

"I nearly broke my bloody neck, that's what." She was never a huge fan of skiing but went anyway. Her fear of heights and speed meant she was always nervous but standing at the top of the slope and edging herself over not expecting her skis to have been waxed... she must have been terrified when trees started whizzing past her.

Cue, hysterical laughter at the idea of my mum shooting down the slope at top speed.

I have never been skiing since, but maybe when I shift these last few tonnes of weight, I might take the chance. Not sure Jon would entertain the idea, but then again, my warped sense of humour means I would be in hysterics if he fell. Perhaps it's not the best idea...

January 30

Back on plan, but I am under no illusion as my head isn't in the game. Went to my dad's house to feed the fish and have a general tidy up, and when I got home is when I went hell for leather.

Multiple Cadbury's Roses (56 Syns)
6 x Pink & Whites (15 Syns)
Stew (Syn Free)
Leek & potato soup (Syn Free)
I used 71 Syns today, and I don't think I remembered everything I ate.

January 31

Back on plan.
I don't know why I'm not feeling it this week, but I am trying, and I will be going for weigh-in on Friday.
Spent £100 on new jeans—a small 36" waist, which look tiny... I am determined to feel good in them when I go to London in April.
Bacon, eggs, tomatoes (Syn Free)
Wholemeal bread (HEXB & 2 Syns)
SW Cauliflower Mac n Cheese (Syn Free & HEXA), I had really been looking forward to trying this, so cooked one for Jon and me.
"It's disgusting." I gagged at the bitter taste, reminding me of cottage cheese. "Do you want it?"
"Yeah, okay." So Jon finished it off, even though he wasn't overly keen either.
6 x Pink & Whites (15 Syns). DE-LIC-IOUS!
17½ Syns used today.

SOFIA'S STORY

I've conducted many interviews for this book, and although every person has their own story to tell, this one is no less fascinating because it taps into an ever-growing, evolving, and increasingly popular trend that many of us dip our toes in—style, hair, make-up and beauty. For some, image is oxygen—essential, all encompassing, and we pay increasing amounts in our quest to achieve perfection. But what about those who work in that world day in, day out—those who make the beautiful people evermore beautiful? What if that person bucks the trend to conform and doesn't maintain the perfect figure—how do their peers, and those who utilise that industry view those who tip the scales?

Sofia is quick to make her point. "People in the beauty industry aren't supposed to be fat, and if they are, they're scrutinised, almost alien."

Starting out twenty years ago as a hairdresser, then later re-training as a beautician, her opening statement isn't entirely unexpected.

Admittedly, I am extremely vain, but I don't walk in that world, so I ask her for clarity. "Just to clarify, what are people in the beauty industry supposed to be?"

She doesn't need to think about her answer because it's obvious that she's thought about this countless times over the years. "Slim, flawless, pretty, perfect figures, tits up here, not down there." She points to where she believes her breasts should sit, then at her stomach.

"Nothing about you seems out of place, and I'm no expert on women."

"It's how I see myself." She smoothed out the tiniest of wrinkles on her form-fitting trousers then brushes away something that only she can seemingly see.

She cares how she presents to the world, momentarily forgetting that this chat isn't about scrutinising her appearance. "Is that the image you've constructed of yourself, or is it that how you believe others see you?"

"I've had those stares and dirty looks from people on training courses."

"Why would people stare at you?" I'm probably asking the obvious, but this is Sofia's story, and I want to give her the opportunity to tell it how she sees it,

"Because I'm not considered slim, or pretty enough. I don't look like your typical hairdresser or beautician?"

"Is that the expected norm—society's opinion of what passes for slim and pretty?"

"It's accepted fact."

"Says who?"

Sofia glowers at me—she is deadly serious. "How can we sell something that we don't buy into ourselves?" She doesn't directly answer the question but offers her opinion as to why she considers herself out of favour with her peers. "How can I sell fat loss injections and still be fat, or walk about without a face full of slap and expect people to pay out good money to me for it?"

I could be wrong, but I fail to see the issue or fully accept that those seeking hair and beauty treatments truly care who delivers it, if they are qualified to do so. But that's something else entirely. Even so, if Sofia speaks the truth, she would still be considered attractive, stunning even, and while she might not be a size eight, her curves haven't diminished her beauty. They accentuate it. "I understand that mindset but is it really that important?"

"To you, maybe not, but for girls walking through my door, I'm trying to sell what is essentially a fantasy, but at my former size 24, and borderline 26 on a bad day, my reality wasn't something they wanted shoved in their faces—in fact, I've lost clients after their first appointment, and that wasn't because I'm not good at what I do—*I* put them off."

"You put them off?" That's quite a bold statement to make, and I need to get to the root of it.

"Yes, because of how I looked. I wasn't buying what I was selling, so they didn't believe I could deliver what they wanted. It really does make a difference."

There are flashes of hurt in her eyes, and briefly she turns away. She believes that she works in an industry that only accepts those it considers perfect, and as an outsider peering in, I don't know how much truth exists in her beliefs. However, this is Sofia's truth and it's obvious that what brings her joy also brings her pain. "That says more about the inadequacies of the beauty industry, and those shallow enough to be swallowed by it than you."

"You are very kind for saying that, Marco."

"I'm not blowing smoke up your arse, Sofia, but if those people who have judged you so harshly took a good look at themselves, they would see they are far from perfect because perfection doesn't exist."

"It's all a performance, but it's the industry I chose—the profession I love working in."

"Are you good at your chosen profession?"

"Damm good, yes," she claps back with confidence. "But it didn't stop the beautiful girls from looking down their noses at me, that they were walking into my shop a size 8, proud to show off their bodies, spray tan ready, and there I was squeezing into my tunic—well bulging out of it if you want the truth. I couldn't compete with that so made sure I worked hard and offered the best, and that my reputation preceded anything else that might put barriers up."

"Was it successful?"

"Yes, and I am brilliant at what I do, and I still love it. In fact, I can't ever see myself doing anything else. Didn't mean it wasn't hard at times, especially when I only ever got compliments when I lost a visible amount of weight. When I gained or when I looked flabbier, nobody said a word, when all it would have taken was, *Sofia, you look nice*, to make my day, and to stop me feeling like I had to retreat into myself or go home and eat a packet of biscuits to make me feel better, and I did that more often that you'd think."

"What was your top weight?"

"At my heaviest, I ballooned to almost twenty-three stone, and I'm only five-foot-three."

"Did you gain that weight purely through over-eating?"

"Eating junk food—chips, kebabs—drinking, recreational drugs—college and party culture. I learned early on that I fit in better as the loudmouth girl who could match the lad's beer for beer."

"So, you like to party, that's not a crime."

"I had more male friends than female, always have had, so I went hard, I still do."

"My best friend of forty-six years and counting is a girl."

"I respond better to men, Marco, and that's not because I was trying anything on, but I didn't feel like the girly-girl, even though I was fascinated by hair and makeup from a young age."

"If you don't mind me saying, you look very glamorous today."

"Thank you, I wanted to make the effort."

"For me, for this chat?"

"Well, yes, and no. I like to put my makeup on every day, and do my hair, dress nicely, because it keeps my mind occupied and away from what I can eat." She shifts uncomfortably in her seat, but she's the one who went above and beyond—for her, or for me, it doesn't matter. But I don't think she sees what I do—somebody who would turn many heads.

"You definitely make an impression, and it's not just waffle. I mean it—from my perspective, which might mean nothing, you are the epitome of a pretty girl, and I see how you slot into the beauty industry."

"I'm a walking advertisement now, because I have to be." Wearing a fitted trouser suit, and tight top that accentuates her on-show cleavage, whatever the past and how she was viewed then, right at this moment, she is what she sells.

"You don't have to explain yourself. I just wanted to draw the comparison of you not seeing yourself a girly-girl, to how you have presented yourself today."

"I know, but I work in the beauty industry, so I know how catty girls can be, and there are a lot of guys like that too. It's only getting worse thanks to shows like The Kardashians."

"Why that programme in particular?"

"It's their entire market, and how they sell themselves. They only have beauty and image to fall back on. Kim K paid to have a fat arse and is lauded for it. I have one naturally and I'm not good enough. Different standards for celebrities, and it filters down negatively to bigger girls like me."

I've never watched en episode of The Kardashians but from my understanding, most of them have a hand in the 'image' industry. "Are you judging them unfairly? Surely everyone is entitled to earn a living."

"Yes, I agree and maybe I am being a bitch, and I admit, I am a huge fan and have never missed an episode, but it's that corner of society that moulds young people's mindsets—beauty at all costs and the main criteria is to be slim and pretty. What about being a good person, or being kind?"

"I totally agree. And perhaps I am being harsh because I view the fashion industry exactly as you view the beauty and cosmetics industry."

"Yes, that's what I mean—if you see certain celebrities walk down the street without the glow up, you'd never recognise them—these girls who are Instagram famous, and make a fortune from their posts, without the make-up and the contouring, the extensions, and the filters, they look nothing like how they present themselves. It's all a mirage, fantasy—fake..."

"Again, I agree. But society seems to engage with that world on a terrifyingly increasing level."

"Yes, it does, and that world has enabled me to buy a house and pay my mortgage, so call me a hypocrite, and you'd be right. But some girls, like me, can't contour a size 20 out of existence, or hide who we really are." Emotion betters her, and she takes a moment.

My partner has an interest in makeup, so I've watched a few tutorial videos, and I do understand. "How did you try to hide your figure, or did you even bother to try?"

"God, yes, black clothes, baggy clothes, body shapers that felt like they were crushing me. I'd stand a certain way, breathing in, until I was sore. But who was I kidding?"

"Yourself, but we've all done it—I certainly have."

"So, you do get it."

"Absolutely. And just so there is absolute transparency between us, every word you have spoken, I do understand, and can certainly empathise."

"I'm not bitter, even though I know I come across like that, but I try to be decent and kind. I've been judged all my life for something I can't control, an addiction is what it is, although others laugh when I say it, and it hurts. I've lost friends because they've been too embarrassed to be seen with me."

"That's horrible. But once again, it says more about them than you."

"Still hurts to think my figure means more to some than who I am, and who they know me to be inside."

"In a perfect world, maybe, but tell me truthfully, why would you want friends like that?"

"I don't, not anymore. I won't lie though because I did want them in my life."

"Why were they embarrassed to be seen with you?

"Because I was too fat."

"Looking at you now, I don't see a fat person. Do you still see yourself that way?"

"Yes, and I always will." She thinks similarly to me because no matter how much weight I have lost, the mirror still shows me as I was.

"Why?"

"I'm never not going to struggle because I like a drink, and while I'm not an alcoholic, a good meal comes with a good bottle of wine."

"Do you drink every day?"

"Most days, yes."

"And what is your tipple of choice?"

"I try to stay on wine."

"Why only wine?"

"Because I can have it with soda, so it's not as fattening, and truthfully because Vodka goes down too easy."

"Do you think you have a problem with alcohol?"

"I'm not addicted to it, but my boyfriend, when he drinks, he smokes—it goes hand in hand."

"When you drink, do you tend to overeat?"

"I'm from a family that socialise a lot—my mum's side are Greek, so there is always food and drink on offer. She isn't happy unless we've all been fed, and if I don't eat what she serves, it's like a slap in the face. It doesn't help my addictive personality."

"I have a Greek Cypriot friend, and his Yia Yia always seemed to be cooking, and feeding him."

"That's my family, and no matter how many times I remind my mum that I'm on a diet, she shoves a plate of food under my nose anyway and tells me to eat, eat, eat—it's her favourite word, and no matter how much I eat, it's never enough."

"Forgive me but I am imagining that movie, *My Big Fat Greek Wedding*—good times with a tight-knit family. Some would give their hind teeth for that life."

She laughs, her face lighting up. "My world is exactly like that. Food is everything, and calories don't come into it. My family don't see fat, and I'm positive my mum thinks I'm going to starve to death."

"Because they love you for who you are."

"Yes, they do, but it's hard when I struggle to love myself."

"Have you ever?"

"Now and again, when I think I look good, or slimmer, I'm happy, but it's never love."

"On a scale of one to ten, how do you feel about yourself today?"

"Right now, a seven, maybe eight, but when the makeup comes off and the extensions are unclipped, a two at most."

"Is that acceptance—the seven or eight—remnants from your professional world?"

"I know how to paint myself pretty."

"And without the makeup and extensions, you don't rate yourself?"

"I don't look horrendous, but I prefer myself with the glow up."

"You aren't a fan of natural beauty?"

"Not on me, God, no. Fat, and natural isn't good, but fat with make-up works much better—just look at people like Gemma Collins, Oprah Winfrey and Melissa McCarthy—all big girls who look better with a glow up."

"In your eyes, yes, and I suppose they do it for similar reasons to you—image to the outside world is everything."

"All three have publicly struggled with their weight. But look at Oprah Winfrey now she has slimmed down and she has never looked better"

"Yes, she does look great, but she bought into *Weight Watchers*, plugged the hell out of it, then lost all her excess weight by taking Ozempic."

Sofia appears shocked, obviously not seeing it splashed all over the news. "Really?"

Oprah's hypocrisy isn't lost on me. "She went on record to admit it. And there is nothing wrong at all with using Ozempic or other such weight loss treatments if that is how you choose to lose weight, but it says a lot when a billionaire buys shares in a weight loss company, and promotes that diet, then uses drugs to achieve what she wants, rather than leaning on the company she part owns for support."

"At least she was honest about it."

"She admitted it when pressured to, and that is her right, to keep it to herself. But not everyone has Oprah's billions or promotes a diet only to use alternate means to achieve one's goal."

"It's naughty that she promoted *Weight Watchers* as the way to slim down then used Ozempic. I bet the members were pissed off—I know I would be, and truthfully, I would have left if I had been a member because I don't like being deceived."

"Have you ever taken Ozempic or something similar to help you lose weight?"

"I couldn't afford to even if I wanted to. I have bills to pay."

"I have considered Ozempic and discounted it just as quickly."

"For some, it's probably a miracle drug but then if I do start it, and my income shifts I'd have to come off it and end up right back where I was before and feeling resentful because of it." She has her head screwed on financially. "But there are some desperate enough not to care about the financial impact, I have to consider everything."

"You're doing it the right way, the sensible way—"

"The long way," she interrupts.

"Nothing worth doing is ever easy, I know that you know that, and so does every person struggling to lose or maintain weight."

"You did it, Marco."

"I'm still doing it, and I struggle daily, some more than others."

"How much have you lost because you look slim, and your legs look amazing in those jeans?"

Compliments never sit right but I appreciate her words. "That's very kind of you to say."

"I mean it, so how much?"

"Close to five stone, and I know people are impressed when I tell them, and so am I for getting there, but I have a long way to go."

"That's amazing, Marco."

"It's been a long road—surgery that left me in an intensive care unit for a week and an hour away from death, diets, bingeing—that circle you probably know all too well."

"It's hard to comprehend that this will be my life. But I must control what I eat because it's too easy to lose control."

"It doesn't have to consume your life though, Sofia."

"True. It usually does though."

"So, looking to the future—what are your plans?"

"To lose more weight, sensibly, stay healthy, get married, but not until I feel good in the perfect dress."

"When will that be?"

"I'll know when I get there. I'm trying so hard."

"That's all you can ask of yourself."

"I keep telling myself; that I'm in a better place than I was twelve months ago, and this time next year, I might look back on this and decide I'm where I want to be, and that's that—I can just be Mrs Jensen, and mum to my kids, rather than chasing something that I'm still not sure is attainable in the long term."

"Realistically, what is your target?"

"I'd say eleven stone—any less, I look ill, so yeah, I'm aiming for that." I see hope in her eyes, and with the smile creeping in, she has daydreamed this many times.

"And when you get there, what then?"

"I'll try to maintain it."

"What is the longest you've maintained your current weight, and what spurred you on?"

"I've been up and down so many times I've lost count, but my focus was to have a baby, and I couldn't do that at twenty-odd stone."

"Was it hard to keep that focus?"

"No, because the endgame meant I would have a baby of my own."

"And did you have children?"

"I have two."

"So, you can do anything you put your mind to?"

She grins, knowing where I am going. "Yeah, I know that I can. I just have to want something enough."

"Do you want to get to eleven stone enough?"

"Most days, yes."

"Then do it, and once you're there, game over, until the game of maintaining begins."

"That's a horrible thought."

"You've told me many times, and before this interview that you're always going to have issues with your weight, so accept where you are and what you have to do and live with it. Why fight what you know must happen?"

"I'm stubborn."

"But you're battling against something you actually want."

For the first time, she seems lost for words, and deep in thought. When she finally says something, it's not what I expected. "Why do I feel like I've been therapized?"

I chuckle because a few of those I have chatted to have said the same thing. "You haven't but remember that I am looking from the outside in; it's easier to see somebody else's problems than deal with my own."

"We're all like that, Marco."

"You mentioned your children—was it a struggle to conceive?

"I couldn't have kids—couldn't get pregnant no matter how hard I tried, it just never happened—all the doctors would say was, you're too fat, you smoke too much, stop drinking, your BMI is too high, unhealthy lifestyle, it was all put on my shoulders, and I was to blame."

"Playing Devil's Advocate, who do you think was to blame?"

"Me, but back then I wasn't ready to accept that my lifestyle interfered with my future, and when I couldn't get pregnant, my boyfriend, Paul, left me, but the worst thing about it was; my replacement was a skinnier version of me—loud, loved makeup, partied hard, but half the woman I was, and it hurt like hell, as though everything about me he wanted in somebody else, just not the fat girl."

"Did you ever talk to Paul about it?"

"My self-esteem was on the floor, so when he was drunk, I'd get the phone calls saying he missed me, and I'd fall for it every time and invite him round. We'd have sex then the next morning, I'd get the text telling me it meant nothing and that it wouldn't happen again. It did, too many times. So, my self-esteem was not only on the floor but trodden in too."

"I'm sorry."

"I did it to myself."

"Can you explain why?"

"I was the fat girl, so I took whatever I could get—cheating ex's—I was the 2 am girl."

"2 am girl... what does that mean?"

"It means I was the girl that was left on the dancefloor when the music stopped—nobody looked twice at me, then when the lights went up, any guy that hadn't pulled and was horny, there I was, the easy lay."

"I see." I don't quite know what to say.

"I knew it though."

"Doesn't make it palatable." It's hard to imagine Sofia at the end of the night, hoping that this is her only chance of intimacy, and with somebody she probably wouldn't have looked twice at.

"I wouldn't lower myself now though, not even if I was desperate."

"What's changed?"

"Me."

"How?"

"I found my self-respect, and that meant seeing the real me."

"What is the real you?"

"A woman who will always struggle with her weight, you're right, I know that. I've told you and anyone else that will listen the same thing. I'm never going to be perfect, it doesn't exist, so I need to stop crucifying myself for the unattainable."

"Was it really so bad?"

"You've been there—a fat person only sees the bad side of themselves, and then they project that side before somebody else can do it."

"I understand."

"It's not a poor me story, just fact. I was very overweight, I am still overweight, though I am ten stone lighter than I was."

"So, you're now around thirteen stone?" It's a remarkable achievement.

"Give or take, yes."

"That's amazing—that is something to be proud of."

"My doctor still tells me I'm obese." She brushes off what most of us would give almost anything for—that mammoth weight loss.

"Well, according to the BMI, you are, as am I. But put that aside, how do you feel about yourself now?"

"Better, fitter, more accepting although I still hate my body."

"Did you do that purposely?"

"What?"

"Three positives before the inevitable negative."

"Oh, yeah." She flashes me a curious stare—did she really think I wouldn't listen intently to what she has to say? "Two years ago, there would have been less positives."

"But there are positives, right?" Sometimes, we don't see the wood for the trees, and it takes another person, even a relative stranger, to point out the obvious.

"Yes, I think so."

"You are more accepting of yourself…"

"Of course, but there will never be a day I fully accept what I see in the mirror."

"Why not?"

"Saggy skin, stretch marks—reminders, and no matter how thin I get, I know what is there and no cream or beauty treatment will reverse that."

"Surgery... Is that an option? It's something I think about a lot."

"I do too."

"And...?"

"I want it, but I'm scared."

"So, what is the other option?" I really don't want to lead her to the answer that is glaringly obvious; I want her to see it for herself.

"I don't know."

"Maybe find a way to accept that you are a good, kind person and that you have somebody who loves you for you."

"But *I* don't love me for me."

"You have children..."

"Two girls."

"Do they love you?"

"Yes."

"Why?"

"Because I am their mum."

"That doesn't mean anything. Some children loathe their mothers, so why do your kids love you?"

"Because I love them, I care for them, I protect them, they feel safe because I make them feel safe."

"And...?"

"They know they are the most important people in my world."

"Do they care about your weight?"

"No. But one day, they might do."

"What about your partner?"

"Aiden adores me—he loves me fat or thin." Her face lights up at the mention of him. "I never thought I'd ever meet a man who loves me for me."

"It happens. Talk to me about him if you want to."

"He doesn't really want me to talk about him in detail, but he's in his late thirties, and works as an electrician—he just gets me and thinks I'm too hard on myself."

"Is he right in that assessment?"

"Yes," she admits, "but you know yourself; we are our worst critics."

"True. And does Aiden struggle with his weight?"

"No, and he never has. He goes to the gym every morning and works out. Yeah, he smokes when he's drunk, but that's it. He doesn't overeat, and he doesn't even have a sweet tooth—bastard—lucky him, and lucky me, because I found a good man, and he means everything to me."

"All three are your world."

"Absolutely, and without them, I'd be lost."

"So, if they are the most important people in your world, aside from your own, isn't their opinion the only ones that matter?"

"I've never thought of it like that."

"I have had the same doubts as you, Sofia, that I'm not good enough, that people look at me and hate what they see... why are we so bothered about the opinions of strangers?"

"I wish I wasn't."

"Then tell yourself what I try and tell myself."

"What's that?"

"Other people opinions of you are none of your business."

"It's not that easy, Marco."

"It's a good place to start because you're never going to win the approval of everybody you meet, so why bother trying?"

"I just want to feel that I fit in."

"Fit into what?" Societal expectations are a nightmare to navigate, and I have learned not to seek acceptance from anybody because it will never come or be what I want it to be.

"I want to be normal." There is sadness in her tone.

"What is normal, Sofia, does anybody even know what that is?"

"I don't have a clue."

"Then why are you chasing it?"

"I suppose society demands it of us."

"What for, the quest for what certain sections of society perceive as the perfect body?"

"I think so."

"Perfection doesn't exist, but somebody can get as close to that as they think they can."

"I'm way off."

I don't know why I have this particular thought, but I share it with Sofia. "Adam, my first ever boyfriend, people considered him the perfect specimen—bisexual, vain, and nobody was off limits when he wanted sex... he was extremely good looking to the point I hated going out in public with him because people made such a fuss of his appearance, and it made me feel bad about myself."

"Why?"

"Because I thought people would wonder why he was with me. And they did, and some even vocalised that, mainly girls who fancied him, which hurt."

"I feel like that sometimes, but I know my boyfriend loves me as I am."

"Well, Adam was narcissism personified and could never love anybody as much as he loved himself, and while I don't doubt there were feelings on his side, I think he chased me harder to win me over because it made him look better being next to me."

"That's not nice."

"No, but I think it's true, and I remember when I reached breaking point and dumped him, he was more upset that *I* had dumped *him*. He remarked that he couldn't believe that somebody who looked like me would walk away from somebody that looked like him."

"Sounds like you were well rid of him—wanker."

"I thought so too, and during our last conversation, I said to him, you might be gorgeous with an amazing body blah blah blah, but in twenty years' time when your looks fade and you can't be bothered going to the gym every day, you'll be left with nothing because you have no personality to fall back on."

"How did he take that?"

"He didn't like it and denied that would ever happen. But I've seen him since, and his looks did fade—he appears much older than his fifty years. He's balding, he's lost the muscular physique and gained a lot of weight—he looks nothing like he did at his prime. So, it comes to all of us, considered gorgeous or not. Nothing lasts forever, but I do know that I think more of myself than I used to, and so should you."

"I suppose because I am surrounded by good looking people who have better bodies than I ever will, I do feel inadequate."

"But they are coming to you to help them improve on something they want to change about themselves."

"Yes, they do."

"Everyone has a hang up, narcissistic, vain, arrogant—there is always something we don't like. I watch guys in the gym lifting weights, and some are well into their fifties and sixties—I don't believe every one of those men do it for the thrill—they want to maintain what they have, and even going into middle age and beyond, they are holding onto something that will one day be beyond them.

Her expression conveys disgust, and I wonder what is coming next. "I hate the gym, but I use make-up probably in the same way those guys use weights. Doesn't mean it works for me." Sofia's confidence flitters in and out, and I suspect like many of us, occasionally, she likes what she sees, but in the main, the negatives outweigh the positives.

"You look great—"

"You have to say that." Compliments don't sit right with her either, and I wonder how much damage has been done over the years, by her own thoughts and whatever negativity she has received from others.

"No, I don't have to say that, and I wouldn't lie to you. Remember, I am looking at you from a different perspective—I don't see women as sexual beings for start."

"Gay lads can be the worst though." I don't think it matters what gender or who a person is attracted to—human beings have the propensity to damage others, just from learning that behaviour from others. "I've worked with a few over the years who have been horrible to me."

"Oh, I know that from firsthand experience. But they still have that deep-rooted lack of confidence you and I do. They just deflect in the hope you won't see it."

"I wish we could all be kinder to one another, and I'm not blameless, I've done it."

"Done what?"

"Judged."

"So have I, and so have most others, even if they don't want to admit it. At the end of the day, we're human beings, and not one of us is perfect."

"I've been so miserable about it for so long, but now I'm sitting here talking openly for the first time with anybody, is it worth it, being unhappy because I'm a bit fat?"

"Do you think you are happy now?"

"Yeah, I am as happy as I can be because I have my kids, my partner and a family who adore me, but there's always that small part that is fighting against myself, which wears me out."

"Fighting what?"

"The urge to eat."

"How bad does it get?"

"Terrible sometimes, and mostly I give in and just eat then feel shitty afterwards."

"For bingeing?" I've been here too, as have most of those reading this book.

"Yes, but why am I so hard on myself? There are worse things I could do."

"Exactly."

"I work hard, and I'm a good mum and girlfriend, so what if I'm not a size 10?"

"Taking a good look at yourself right here and now, how do you feel about yourself, your appearance, or in general?"

"I look good right now, and it's not because I've spent two hours getting ready. I look good because I've kept the weight off, and I would like to lose more, but I've got to be realistic, and not think about my bloody BMI or my doctor throwing passive aggressive shade at me"

"What is your dream weight—be honest?"

"Realistically, eleven and a half stone, but I shouldn't think in those terms because it sets me up to fail from the start. I'd just like to be slimmer, not skinny, just normal—I can't see myself as a size 8 or a 10, it's not me, I just see myself running around with my kids without feeling like I'm gonna keel over, fighting to catch my breath."

"You will know when you get to that point."

"I'm doing better, and *Slimming World* helps, even though I hate going."

"Why do you hate it?"

"Because I should be able to do it by myself, Marco."

"I can't do it myself, and I've accepted that."

"Have you tried?"

"I've yo-yoed for thirty years, tried everything and like I said before, surgery that almost killed me, and I know going to my *Slimming World* class is the only place that has kept me in check. Ultimately, it's just me and my willpower when I close my eyes at night but being a member helps so much as does having a leader who knows what me and her members are going through."

"I dread weigh-ins."

"So do I but you keep going for a reason."

"Yeah, to keep me in check."

"See, we're not so dissimilar."

"Sometimes I think it's easier for men to be big."

"From a societal point of view, it probably is, but we do get judged and stared at as well. Plus, I'm gay, so I had that whole scene to navigate, and they aren't forgiving when it came to fatties."

"I bet, because I know, just like the industry I work in, gay world is superficial."

"Absolutely, it is. And I don't see any change, not really. Then again. I'm nearly fifty so haven't stepped foot in a gay bar since 2013."

"I remember when Adele became famous, people would always mention her."

"Why her specifically?"

"When I cried over being enormous, they'd say, look at Adele, like my life was anything like hers—I'm not a multi-millionaire living in L.A with access to chefs and personal trainers. But I knew what they meant, although an overweight singer is going to live through so much more scrutiny than the average person, so I felt for her. Then again, look at her now, rake thin, and you can't tell me it's because she stopped wanting kebabs and crisps."

I'm not a fan of Adele's music but can appreciate she has a fantastic voice, and no matter where she sits weight-wise, she was, and is a beautiful woman with a magnetic personality. I liked that she bucked the trend. Still, all the adulation and money in the world can't fight the implications of carrying excess weight for a long period of time. "It is probably a mix of things—getting older, her career, the fact she became a mother. But I agree, I don't think her weight loss erases those habits or behaviours when it comes to a poor diet. My habits are still there, and will always be just under the surface, as are yours."

"It takes me back full circle because it is image focused and that means everything in this day and age, and some of us just don't fit in."

"You don't think you do?"

"More than I did."

"Why?"

"Because I've lost weight and walk around dolled up most of the time. People look at me, yes, but it's not enough. A guy told me that I would be stunning if I lost weight, and that was only a few weeks ago." It highlights how cruel people can be. Sofia has heard the immortal words many of us have heard.

"I've had exactly the same thing said to me before today. It hurts, even if we do try to laugh it off."

"Yes, it does, and no matter how much I've lost, or how far I think I've come, it strips away every ounce of confidence I've managed to build up, even though Aiden tells me every day about how gorgeous I am."

"I wish I could tell you to ignore the negatives, but easier said than done."

"I don't want my kids to grow up ashamed of their bodies."

"Do your children struggle with their weight?"

"One does, yes, and I have to be really strict with her, and that's not me body shaming her, but gently re-enforcing the idea that eating healthier is a better choice."

"You don't want your daughter to face the same obstacles that you still face."

"Exactly, so when I want a burger and fries from *McDonalds*, or even if I want a night eating chocolate on the sofa, I can't because *I* am the example. I don't want Kira to grow up with the same issues that I have, but saying that, I am the parent and what I say goes, but I do it in a non-dictatorial way, almost, get her buy in, rather than her feeling forced to eat the fruit over the junk food."

"Clever parenting."

"She loves rabbit food, but has a sweet tooth, so rather than say no to sweets, I try moderation, and it seems to work—if she's anything like me, if I say no, she will only want it more and will start sneaking it, and stashing it, like I used to do."

"So, keeping your daughter on the right path has helped to keep you on yours?"

"I do everything for my kids, so if I can't pig out as often as I want to, it helps me, and her."

"That's a good thing."

"She wants me to go dancing with her."

"When are you going?"

"I'm not."

"Why not?" I know why, but I want her to speak her truth.

"Because I would feel too self-conscious."

"For five minutes, yes."

"Do you go to any classes?"

"Just to the gym, although I don't seem to go as much as I want to. But I do want to try *Clubbercise*. I'm trying to convince my sister to come with me."

"I hate the gym so much." It's the second time she has told me this.

"I like it, but it takes dedication."

"I don't like sweating, and I spend most of my time checking how I look in the mirror, and that my make-up hasn't melted."

"Beauty at all costs, huh?"

"It's in me, it's my life. And I use it to hide what I don't like about myself."

"You're only fooling yourself."

"Sometimes it's the only thing that gets me out the front door when I'm having a fat day."

"We all have those days."

"I don't think men have them like women do."

I press my hand against my heart. "This man does—and any given day I can wake up and feel fine then the next day, I feel like crap, even though nothing has changed from the day before."

"It's weird talking about this stuff to a man."

"Why?"

"I'd never discuss this with Aiden, and he is my partner."

"I get that but look at it like this; your words could inspire any given person reading this book, so isn't that a positive."

"I guess so."

"Aiden might read this book, and even though you don't talk to him in depth about this, reading your words might make him understand you a little better. You already said that he doesn't struggle with his weight, so he will never grasp how awful it feels to battle with food every single day."

"I hope so."

"Baring ones' soul isn't easy, I know that from writing this book, but you've done it."

"I didn't know if I would have anything to say."

"This book isn't about feeling sorry for myself or wanting sympathy, it's about the casual reader picking it up and realising we are struggling with an addiction, or for the reader who feels they are never going to get it under control; my words, your words, my leader's words... not feeling alone might mean so much, and even if only one person gets something from it, job done."

She reaches over and grabs my hand. "You're braver than me, Marco."

"Not really. You've done the same as me by sharing what you've shared."

"I do hope people who read it are kind and understanding."

"Some people will love it, some will criticise. Some people will write terrible reviews, some will message me to say they loved it while others will delight in telling me they hated it. What will be will be... once it is in the public domain, it doesn't belong to me anymore."

"I'd be shitting myself."

Her honesty is refreshing. "I've released so many books, some have had glowing reviews and others slated, it's the nature of the beast."

"I think it will do well, and I can't wait to read it too."

"Thank you. Now, before we close this chat, would you tell me what your ultimate goal is."

It takes her a while to answer but I wait and offer nothing. "Erm... I just want to be healthy, and to be an inspiration to my kids. I don't wanna be the fat mum at the school gates, for their sake as well as mine—I'm happier than I was this time last year, so I want to keep that, and to find a way to accept my body at whatever weight I am. I am determined to lose more weight but its going to be an uphill battle, I know that, so I guess my ultimate goal is to keep trying—if I do that, I know I'll get there."

MY JOURNEY – FEBRUARY 2024

February 1

February, already, and I have stuck to plan. It won't be enough to counteract the amount of junk food that I have shovelled in this week, but I'll face the music tomorrow.

Went shopping and took the long walk around the complex. In twenty-six minutes I managed 2,447 steps, which according to my go-go gadget watch, burned 164 calories. Better than a kick in the teeth I say.

I didn't want breakfast so waited for lunch and enjoyed eggs and tomatoes (Syn Free).

2 x slices of wholemeal bread (HEXB)

For my dinner I had, prawns, rocket, red onion, 40% less fat salad cheese (HEXA), and fat free vinaigrette dressing (2 Syns).

In-betweens, I scoffed 2 Skinny Whip bars (8 Syns, and well worth every single Syn—in fact, I wanted to eat both boxes but didn't.)

So, for today, I used a total of 10 Syns, and I know I should be using them all, but I was stuffed.

February 2
WEIGH-IN DAY

Even though I don't want to know the specifics, I am dreading stepping on those scales. But I am going, no matter what because time is ticking, and I have to get to target.

As I suspected, I gained.

"It's only a tiny gain, Marco."
"I can live with that."

Stayed for class, which I thoroughly enjoyed; it was a pleasure to be there as a member was awarded the title of SW's Greatest Loser, and no, that is not a slight, but a victory for the beautiful lady who received the well-deserved standing ovation, then motivated us all with a speech on how she lost weight, but added the importance of not making oneself feel guilty for falling off plan.

Another incentive to shift the weight; I have added another night onto my London trip in April to see the Frozen musical... ABBA Voyage, here I go, once again.

February 5

I had a restless sleep then woke up irritated, thinking I could hear bells ringing. But it turns out it was just a touch of tinnitus. Drove me nuts, so in the end I got up. Feel at a loss with myself today, and that I need to be exercising—the gym, anything. I have enquired about *Zumba* (again) and *Clubbercise* classes to up my fitness levels. I wish I could go to the gym but until my Rheumatologist gives me the go-ahead, there is little point signing back up to waste money.

Felt like stuffing my face today, but with 8 Crème Eggs in the fridge tempting me, I'm not surprised. But I don't give in.

I was shocked to see a news report this evening that King Charles has been diagnosed with cancer—sad news indeed. Cancer is a BITCH!

Dinner is baby potatoes, 5% mince with onions, mushrooms, and chilli peppers. (Syn Free), Sainsbury's lighter tomato & herb sauce for Bolognese (1½ Syns), but I only had a fraction of the jar. Strangely enough, I found this so tasty, which is unlike me. Tomorrow, I am planning on having it again. My taste buds might feel differently.

In-betweens are strawberries, bananas, black grapes & fat free Greek yoghurt (Syn Free), 6 x pink & whites (15 Syns), and 2 x peanut butter HiFi Bars (HEXB). I changed the brand of yoghurt... my eyes poured with water, and that sour aftertaste hit me at the sides of my jawbone.

Total Syns used today is 16½, but probably lower due to the over counting on the Bolognese sauce.

I still want chocolate!

February 6

Almost a week into February and I've done zero exercise, which is bothering me more and more as the days zoom by. What am I going to do? I woke up later than usual with sore shoulders, so dragged myself out of bed, intent on a long walk. Guess what... it's peeing down, and according to the weather report, snow is on the way.

Feel like stuffing my face but opt for something sensible.

As I woke up closer to lunch than breakfast, I combined the two and settled for bacon, eggs, mushroom, tomatoes & SW sausage patties (Syn Free). 3 x wholemeal toast. (HEXB & 2½ Syns). I cooked two of the patties but gave one to the dog. They tasted okay, but too meaty for my liking, if that makes sense.

With music blasting through my earphones, I carried on working on my new book. I am quite far into it but have so many other ideas for other books spinning around in my mind, I can't seem to focus my thoughts to get it done.

Dinner is going to be the same as last night, not that I'm the least bit hungry after eating so much.

I ended the day with fresh fruit and fat free Greek yoghurt (Syn Free).

February 7

Woke up at 2 am thinking about pie and pickled red cabbage. I am losing my mind. Turned over and went back to sleep, then woke up thinking about pink pancakes with lemon and lime juice on them. Yes, definitely losing it.

Dragged myself out of bed and decided to get my hair cut and beard trimmed.

Finally, the garden shed left by the previous owners has been knocked down and taken away. Now, we can start planning the layout of the garden, ready for Spring. I can't wait to plonk myself on the recliner, and to feel sunshine on my skin. Winter really does not suit me.

February 8

Off to dads to feed the fish. He's still abroad, but not sure how much skiing he is doing as the news reports show the slopes devoid of snow after an unusually warm January. I wonder if he's any good at grass skiing.

February 9
WEIGH-IN DAY

After a terrible night's sleep, where I was wide awake at 3 and 5 am. I dragged myself out of bed at 7.

I stood on the scales and spoke to Shelly. "I don't want numbers, but go on, tell me how much I've gained."

"You've stayed the same."

I can live with that. "Oh, good!"

"You need to stop being so hard on yourself."

"I'm not."

"You're always hard on yourself but you've done amazingly well, and I wish you'd see that."

She was right, and I should cut myself some slack because whatever I weigh right now, it is far less than when I started my journey.

My sister lost two-and-a-half pounds which took her loss to over a stone. I was thrilled for her!

My friend came round for dinner, but it wasn't exactly healthy eating.

5% minced beef, carrots, garden peas & onion with meat granules (1½ Syns)

Potatoes (Syn Free)

And yes, that all sounds fantastic, but I forgot to add that the mince was encased in delicious shortcrust pastry and the potatoes were cut into chips which were deep fried. How do I even begin to Syn that?

My friend and Jon managed two pies each, and thoroughly enjoyed them, but I only had one and took the other next door to my 89-year-old neighbour, Shelagh. She messaged me to say thank you, and to tell me I am a good cook.

February 10

I am absolutely shattered today, and although I got up at 9 am, and pottered about, doing dishes etc, I went back to bed to watch Star Trek and woke up at 3 pm, and that was only because Jon came into the bedroom to check on me. "You're still alive then…"

"What do you mean?"

"It's not like you to sleep this long."

He's right, it isn't, but I must have needed it.

Fast forward four hours and steam is coming out of my ears. Men, who bloody needs them? Well, right now, I am spitting blood. Twice today, Jon has annoyed me. First was the eye roll when I mentioned having a photo shoot done to promote this book. He knows I hate having my pictures taken and the thought of posing makes me feel nauseous.

"Why are you bothering? You hate having your picture taken."

"I know, but I need to do it."

Anyway, I asked a friend who is in the entertainment industry if she had a contact number for a decent, professional photographer that knew what they were doing and would consider how shy I am.

But there was no encouragement, only scathing comments because I hadn't asked him to come with me.

Bear in mind, nothing is booked and the main reason I didn't ask him was because I would feel self-conscious doing my best catalogue pose in front of him, and also because I want somebody there who knows the photographer, who can steer him or her around my insecurities enough to produce something I am happy to show in the book.

Add in the dog and cat, him coming would be a nightmare.

On second thoughts, I don't think I'll bother.

Right now, I am trying to stop the explosion but when it comes, and it will, the fall out won't be pretty.

February 11

Bored and needing some form of exercise, I decided to walk to the shop, which had both positives and negatives. I don't know the area, so went the wrong way, so a walk that should have taken me ten minutes, actually took thirty.

By the time I got to the shop, wearing a fluffy hoodie, sweat rolled off me.

I took a breather before I went into the shop, then grabbed what I wanted, and walked home, the right way, which only took the ten minutes it should have taken.

"Where have you been?" Jon asked.

"I got lost."

"Typical."

I could barely get a word out which proves how unfit I am again, which disappoints me because I worked so hard last year in the gym.

Still, I got good results, according to my watch: 3756 steps taken. 2.55 miles walked. 145.9 calories burned. If I could do that walk every day, it's better than nothing. Although I am considering buying myself an exercise bike. But I will hold off until I have seen the rheumatologist on Thursday.

February 12

Has Spring arrived early? Blue skies and moderately warm weather. It certainly feels like it. But I know rain and cold weather is due, but I'll take what I can get right now.

My mood is cheerier, until I called British Gas about my refund. They owe me £642.17, but according to their records, I owe them money. After two hours on the telephone and finally losing my patience with the man who could barely understand English and kept referring to me as *Mr Merseyside*—I kid you not—that I could not possibly owe them any money as I paid for my energy in advance, so I did not get quarterly bills. When he realised that I would not be fobbed off, he agreed to raise a complaint. In the meantime, I have requested a statement from my bank for every transaction to British Gas. Wankers!

Once I'd calmed down, I read the message from my dad that came through while I was on the phone.

He made it back from Austria in one piece but opened a letter this morning advising him of an appointment that had been made for today at 10 am. Obviously he has been away so had no idea. He just made it on time. The reason for the appointment; before he went on holiday, he sent a stool sample, as you do, over the age of fifty, and it came back with anomalies. He has to go to the Royal Liverpool Hospital on Friday for a colonoscopy. I can't bear any more bad news. Surely, he can't be unlucky enough for the cancer to have spread to his bowel. After explaining to the doctor he has recently completed chemotherapy and radiotherapy treatment, they said that could be the cause of the anomalies as the nerve endings in his backside could have died, releasing blood into his faeces. Fingers crossed. But it makes me wonder what is to come, and to be vigilant.

Lunch was two bananas, which I didn't really want, but after a home delivery from ASDA, Jon was on a rant about wasted food.

"You had to throw those other bananas away, so why order more?"

"Because I wanted to."

"It's a waste."

"So what?"

He is right, but to prove him wrong, I ate them and will eat the rest.

"You've bought radishes twice now and thrown both packs in the bin."

"I know."

And while I understand people are starving and wasting food is wrong, I don't need to be monitored.

Dinner tonight is homemade soup. I intend to have that all week because I am fed up with food in general and deciding what I do and don't want to eat.

February 13
PANCAKE DAY

I WANT PANCAKES!

But it's a slippery slope because I can't have one or two, and usually stop at ten. Anyway, I cheated and bought the ready-made mix—plain for me, and chocolate chip for Jon although he doesn't usually eat pancakes. He might prefer those. But I will hold off until I hit target, then treat myself.

Off to see my dad, and to have a cheeky sunbed. I am trying to get a bit of colour on my cheeks. I know I've said this before but I look much better with a tan, and in the absence of a holiday somewhere tropical, this is a good second best, I can't wait for the nicer weather so I can relax in the garden.

Dinner today is a repeat of yesterday. Chicken breast, carrots, celery, onion, potatoes, parsley, stock gels (Syn Free) & 2 x wholemeal toast. (HEXB).

Banana, strawberries, and black grapes (Syn Free).

2 x Skinny Whips bars (8 Syns)

Total Syns used today is 8.

February 14
VALENTINE'S DAY

I don't usually bother, and feel it's a tad commercialised, but I bought Jon a card and a huge bouquet of flowers.

"Aw, thanks, babe, they're gorgeous." He was thrilled—he loves flowers, so it was nice to see him smile. As I keep telling him I don't want or need anything, I got a lovely card, which I always appreciate more than gifts.

I'm still on plan. Come on, Marco, you can do this.

Jon's gran and grandad paid us a surprise visit today. It was lovely to see them both.

I had planned on eggs on toast but decided to have a cheese (HEXA) sandwich with 4 slices of brown Danish bread (HEXB & 5 Syns). I added a dollop of Branston Pickle (1 Syn).

Dinner was prawns, mixed leaf salad, onion, red pepper, balsamic vinegar (Syn Free) & Greek style salad cheese (HEXA).

Jelly (½ Syn) – I wanted to eat the other 4 pots in the fridge but didn't.

2 x Skinny Whips bars (8 Syns)

I only used 14 Syns today, but I am stuffed.

February 15

Got up and walked to a sports massage session—my first in about 2 months.

Took Sammy to the vet today because his whole right eye has turned blood red.

CHEWING THE FAT

February 16
WEIGH-IN DAY

"Half off, well done."

"Thank God." I am pleased about as I haven't been the best this past week.

Didn't stay for class as Jon and me were heading over to Liverpool for a pre-planned date. We weren't out long but still, I clocked in a good 7,342 steps.

My dad went into the Royal Liverpool Hospital for a colonoscopy—they were worried cancer had spread to his bowel, but thankfully, it's not the case. During his chemotherapy and radiotherapy, blood vessels were damaged which caused blood to accumulate in his stool. So, thankfully, there is nothing to worry about.

February 19

After four days off sheer gluttony, I am fed up. I talked myself back on plan, only to fall back off. I'm not going to berate myself because tomorrow is a new day. I bought an exercise bike for my office, so hopefully, Jon will build it for me. Despite my dad, and two brothers, having the ability to build a house and do everything needed within it, that particular gift bypassed me. I can cook a cracking roast dinner though, and oh, yes, write a book. We all have our strengths, right.

February 20

Why can't I control myself?

I started with the best of intentions and had roasted red pepper & tomato soup with crustless quiche (Syn Free), then had Domino's pizza, which I actually didn't enjoy, and never do. So, I buggered myself up for food I didn't like the taste of.

You're ridiculous, Marco. Grow up, you should know better.

February 23
WEIGH-IN DAY

I spent the whole week out of control, but I faced the scales, prepared for a mammoth gain.

"1½ on," Shelly whispered. "Just a little gain."

"It's way better than I expected."

My sister and me stayed for class, and while I don't think Donna meant for it to descend into something so personal for other members, who revealed a lot about themselves, it reinforced my idea that food addiction is often ignored.

But it also hammered home, that it is not simply food addiction that causes weight gain.

February 24
WEIGH-IN DAY

I spent hours on the toilet; the repercussions of eating junk food, and if that wasn't bad enough, I stubbed my toes on the corner of the wooden chest. I said a few silent swear words then tried to ignore the throbbing. I'm sure two of them are broken, judging by the bruising creeping up my foot.

KFC: 21 Syns.

Homemade coleslaw: 9 Syns.

5 x Crème Eggs: 45 Syns.

My daily allowance of 30 Syns has been obliterated and that is only a fraction of what I have eaten today.

Jon assembled my exercise bike, so I will be hammering that from tomorrow, broken toes and all.

February 26

Weekends are my Kryptonite—why can't I get past Friday without falling off plan? It seems impossible no matter how hard I try. But mostly, I have no problem during the week.

Back on plan. Our gardener is here, trying to get everything ship shape for spring.

Caught the back of my heel on a paving slab and took off a chunk. My heel was still bleeding three hours later. Between that and my sore toes, I can't get my trainers on. I'll be wearing flip flops to weigh-in this coming Friday.

Bacon, eggs, tomatoes (Syn Free). 2 x slices of wholemeal bread (HEXB).

Roast potatoes (Fry Light), minced beef, onions, carrots, mushrooms, cabbage, and courgettes (Syn Free). Gravy (1 Syn). Took a plate for my 89-year-old next door neighbour. I'd like to think somebody would look out for my nan if she were still alive.

25g Kellogg's Chocolate Cornflakes (4½ Syns) with semi-skimmed milk (HEXA)

7 x funsize Guiltless whip bars (14 Syns) – GIANT SIZE WOULD TASTE MUCH BETTER!

2 x Brooklea fat free vanilla Greek yoghurt (5 Syns) – DELICIOUS!

24½ Syns used today.

February 27

Had a lovely sleep and have noticed since I bought copper infused pillows, I suffered less tossing and turning and don't feel as exhausted as I used to.

Sammy's eye is much better and a lot less red. He has to go back for another check-up next week. He could be left with permanent damage to this eye, either through cataracts or irritation to his cornea. He's too old for surgery, but he has one good eye. I am hoping some vision is restored in the other.

Still on plan, but ready to fall off and stuff my face. *Don't do it!*

Jon has cooked a huge pan of homemade chicken and vegetable soup (Syn Free).

I've eaten so much today, and I'm still not satisfied because I want cake.

February 28

I slept fairly well last night, but I knew the engineer was coming at 9 am to fix the tumble dryer, so I couldn't settle, so as soon as the sun popped up, I jumped out of bed and hoovered the carpets and decided to wait until he had been to make myself something to eat.

I hate waiting around.

1:30 pm he finally arrived and fixed the dryer—the belt had snapped and got caught in the drum—and left a right mess in his wake. The kitchen floor tiles were filthy, so I cleaned the kitchen and cooked brunch for Jon and me.

Scrambled eggs, mushrooms & 3 x slices of wholemeal bread. (HEXB & 2½ Syns).

I left the cupboard door open, and forgot, then bashed my forehead off it—seeing stars, I uttered a few curse words, pressing the growing lump.

I caught up on my favourite programme of the moment, Vera, then troughed two bowls of homemade chicken and vegetable soup (Syn Free).

Forced myself to do some writing, and work on my author rebrand—all boring stuff but way past due.

4 x fun size Guiltless whip bars (8 Syns). Worth every single Syn.

February 29

    Is Jon supposed to propose to me today? I don't know what the rules are, but if he were to ask, hmm... I'm not wearing white.
    It's 9:47 pm and with no proposal forthcoming, I just got word that my Aunty Vera has died... you might remember that she was the one who uttered the words, "My God, you're obese," and I wanted to fling her into the open grave at my mum's funeral.
    Strangely, I feel sad at her passing, but I am now at that age where people pop off on a regular basis. It's strange that when young, mortality never comes into the equation—the older I get, the more I think about death. And thinking about death, I need to shift this weight as I refuse to be buried in a double wardrobe or be winched by emergency services out of the window.
    Sleep well, Aunty Vera.
Ps, Shockingly, her obituary is littered with spelling and grammar errors—I have warned my sister to make sure that if she does one for me when I snuff it, to make sure to use spell check. If not, I will come back as a ghost, sit on the end of her bed, and throw things at her.

MY JOURNEY - MARCH 2024

March 1
WEIGH-IN DAY

"Well done, you've stayed the same," Donna informed me with a smile.
"Great!"
Curiosity got the better of me so when I got home, I messaged Donna and asked for my weight.
20 STONE, the message read, sending me into a tailspin.
FAT, GREEDY BASTARD. I cursed myself repeatedly.
How much weight did I gain in December?
Devastation by the realisation that I am now two stone away from target lit a bloody big bonfire underneath my arse.
No more days off. I have to follow this plan seven days a week with no excuses.
To say I feel defeated is an understatement, but I will regain the upper hand.
I have six weeks left until I go to see *Frozen* in the West End, and I am determined to lose a stone, at least.
I'm not going next week, so I am hoping when I return on 15th March, I have lost something.

March 4

After stuffing my face all weekend, I woke up with determination that this is it. No more days off for me.
Today has been a strange one. I feel like I have eaten so much.
3 x veggie sausages, bacon, eggs, mushrooms & baked beans (Syn Free). 2 x slices of Neville's wholemeal bread (7 Syns).
Spaghetti Bolognese with 5% mince, onion, mushroom & fresh pasta (Syn Free). Tomato & herb Bolognese sauce (1 Syn).
6 x pink & whites (12 Syns).'
2 x Lindhal's Kvarg Quark pots (1 Syn).

Cheerios with semi skimmed milk (HEXA & HEXB).
25½ Syns used.

March 5

What a day! I did nothing, but I am shattered.

Looked at the clock. *8 am, what the hell am I doing awake?* Oh. yeah, I agreed to accompany my sister to the hairdressers because she is going to Bulgaria with my dad and brother tomorrow on a skiing trip. She fancied a bit of a makeover beforehand, especially after her stone and a half loss. The stylist did a great job, and Tammy was thrilled with it.

Afterwards, we went for a slimmer's breakfast in the local café, then back to my house before we had to leave again because she had booked herself in to have her nails done, eyebrows waxed and shaped, and her lashes tinted.

I am definitely the wrong person to accompany somebody for procedures that might be uncomfortable. As predicted, I was crying laughing as she made a strangulated noise when having her eyebrows waxed. But I laugh at everything so that's nothing new.

She looked great afterwards, but her T-Zone was red, and puffy. It put me in mind of the bumpy forehead of a Klingon from Star Trek. I did try not to laugh, honest.

March 6

Woke up to a picture from Tammy, sent from the plane. Her T-Zone is still red from the waxing which sent me into fits of laughter—*ever heard of cover up, dear sister?*

3 x Sainsbury's Be Good to Yourself sausages (3 Syns), bacon, eggs, mushrooms & tomato (Syn Free). 2 x slices of Neville's wholemeal bread (HEXB).

Dinner was mixed leaf salad, 40% less fat salad cheese, onions, and balsamic vinegar (Syn Free), which is my preferred food, but also enabled me to stuff my face with 2 x Lindhal's Kvarg Quark pots (1 Syn) and 4 x guiltless chocolate bar (8 Syns).

I closed today using 12 Syns. *Why didn't I eat the whole bag of chocolates?*

March 8
WEIGH-IN DAY

I couldn't attend weigh-in today, but I have gotten through my first Friday since re-joining SW without pigging out. I have been firmly on plan since Monday, and although I went shopping to Sainsbury's today and walked (slowly) past the Crème Eggs, I resisted temptation.

For the past five days, I have stuck rigorously to plan and feel like I haven't stopped eating, which isn't a good thing for me. But, uninterested in food most days, I have eaten free foods (as per usual), and used the Syns, which I am assured I must use, for things like crisps, yoghurts, and small bars of Guiltless chocolate. I don't feel like I have missed out. But I have developed an addiction to Lindhal's Kvarg Quark, especially the banoffee pie, and white chocolate pots. Heaven! I have eaten sixteen this week. But every ½ Syn per pot is counted.

22 Syns used today.

March 9

Haircut and beard trim today, followed by a tanning session. I do want to try a spray tan, but I don't fancy standing stark naked in front of a stranger cupping my meat and two veg… I can imagine the conversation.

"Marco, can you please lift your gunt. I need to spray under there."

"I beg your pardon…" And I storm out half-finished and tinted the same shade as a mahogany coffee table.

But I should look into it. Perhaps there is an automated type that I can use. Which takes me back to that episode of *Friends* when Ross tried one and it went spectacularly wrong—that would be me!

I am also thinking about colonic irrigation—I've even convinced my friend, Sandie, to go first in case it hurts. She *is* game, and so am I, but terrified in case undigested crème eggs get jammed in the pipe.

Syns used today is 25.

March 10

Today was a sad day because I am spending another Mother's Day without my beloved mum. I put a card up for her just in case she is floating about somewhere. She has never been, and will never be, forgotten.

Jon's parents and grandparents came for dinner. It is always nice to see them, and as his mum and gran are members of SW, the meal will be strictly on plan.

5% mince meatballs with JD Seasoning donner kebab mix, mixed salad leaves, tomatoes, onion, baby potatoes. (Syn Free). Wholemeal pitta bread (HEXB). Jon made falafel, which is 25½ Syns for the whole 150g packet. So, it depends how many Jon makes out of it. I didn't eat much at all—one meatball, a small bite of the pitta and one bite of the falafel—breakfast filled me up.

Later on I tucked into Cheerios with semi-skimmed milk (14 Syns & HEXA for the milk). I also tucked into guiltless chocolate bars plus 4 x Lindhal's Kvarg Quark and ended the day using 29 Syns.

March 11

SHATTERED on three hours sleep.

Miracles DO happen. For eight straight days I have remained on plan. I feel smaller and flatter in my stomach area, which is a good thing.

Went for a sunbed then to my dad's house to feed the fish and to turn the pond pump on—shattered, I struggled to keep my eyes open.

Came home and tucked into 3 x Lindhal's Kvarg Quark pots (1½ Syns), and for my dinner this evening, Jon has made a huge pan of chicken and vegetable soup—all Syn Free. But I will use my HEXB on a wholemeal pitta bread.

I am looking forward to weigh-in on Friday and am hoping for a loss—I have worked hard this week, but I know I have done some major damage, so if I stay the same until my body gets used to no days off, so be it.

March 12

Still on plan, and for those who have followed my journey, I hear you gasp. I didn't seem to miss that usual day off which always became three.

I have eaten sensibly today.

March 13

I am not struggling as I thought I would without eating junk food, although I seem to be going through Lindhal's Kvarg quark pots like they are going out of fashion. Jon went shopping today and bought me another twelve and that is after I've eaten about twenty since last Saturday. But at ½ per pot, they can't be too bad for me.

What I have noticed is my consumption of fruit has decreased so I need to make a conscious effort to up that once more.

March 14

Still on plan, which I am finding remarkably easy. But I am fed up... when are we due some sunshine? I'm sick of grey skies and rain, and the idea of living abroad is ever more appealing than ever.

But where?

Greece, or one of its islands currently sit at the top of the list.

I've always wanted to return to Corfu, having first ventured that way many years ago to work. I arrived during the 1998 FIFA World Cup and seemed to spend most of my time dancing—drunk—on top of bars.

I can't hear the song *Three Lions* without being transported back to that time, walking about with my face painted to resemble the UK flag. And I'm not even a football fan.

I remember vividly the moment I stepped off the plane and saw my friend Sue waiting for me with a stranger named Darren. The air was thick with the promise of adventure and the smell of jet fuel. My heart raced with excitement and a hint of unease as I embraced my friend, eager to see what this new chapter had in store for us.

Sue was beaming, her eyes twinkling in the throes of newfound love. I was determined to support her and make the most of our time together.

From the moment I met Darren, something didn't sit right with me. He had a way of looking at Sue, a possessive glint in his eye that made my skin crawl. And his hands, always lingering a little too long on her waist or shoulders. I could tell she was completely enamoured with him, but I couldn't shake the feeling that he was bad news.

As the days went by, I watched as Sue and Darren's relationship progressed at an alarming rate. Two weeks in and they were already madly in love, talking about a future together. I couldn't help but feel sceptical, knowing how quickly things can fizzle out. But I kept my opinions to myself, not wanting to rain on Sue's parade.

But my instincts proved to be true. The more time I spent with Darren, the more I saw the snake lurking inside. Worried, I tried to warn her, but she refused to listen.

Things quickly took a turn for the worse when I decided to cut my trip short and return home. Sue followed soon after, having broken things off with Darren. But that didn't stop him from trying to win her back. He would call and text constantly, even resorting to hiding in the bushes outside her house and jumping out at us late one night.

The terrible things Darren had supposedly done to Sue were unimaginable. And yet, despite it all, she couldn't resist his charm, and she eventually returned to Corfu with him.

During that time, I had met her next-door neighbour, Sandie, who I am still friends with now, and we bonded right from the off. We shared the same sense of humour, and I enjoyed spending time with her. But her husband, Gary, was a different story. He was always watching me with a wary eye, as if he could sense something brewing beneath the surface, that I was going to try and jump into bed with her—looking like a young Bryan Adams, he had more to worry about than her.

As the days passed, phone calls from our mutual friend Sue became more frantic and disturbing. She claimed to be held captive by Darren and begged for our help. But stranded 2,000 miles away, what could we do? Despite the distance, Sandie and I were determined to help somehow.

Late one night, after another harrowing call from Sue describing how Darren had purposely burned her, we made the decision to call the police. A PC arrived at Sandie's house, and we poured out our concerns and suspicions. As if on cue, Sue called again, screaming down the phone. It was as if she was being murdered right then. With a sense of urgency, we pleaded with the PC to listen to the screams and act.

Thankfully, he escalated the situation to higher authorities. It wasn't long before we received confirmation that Interpol would be getting involved.

I had returned to my old job after my trip to Corfu. Everything seemed to be slipping back to normality, until one day, while busy at work, the receptionist called to inform me that the police were waiting for me in the lobby. My heart raced as I made my way down, wondering what could have possibly happened. The officer asked for a statement and reassured me that once they heard back from Interpol, they would reach out to me and Sandie again.

Days turned into weeks, and still, we heard nothing. I tried to focus on my daily routine. Then, one day, while walking to my nan's house, a car screeched to a halt beside me. Two men in suits emerged, their expressions serious and unreadable. My stomach dropped as they approached.

"Mr. Lewis," one of them said in a low, menacing voice.

"Who's asking?" The two men standing in front of me flashed their identification, revealing themselves as detectives. I relaxed slightly but kept my guard up. "What do you want?"

"Your friend, Sue," one of them replied, his voice laced with suspicion.

"What about her?" My heart raced because I knew something was off.

"You and Mrs Sullivan filed a report that Sue had been abducted in Corfu," the other detective chimed in, his tone accusatory.

"Yes, we did," I confirmed.

"Well, we don't take too kindly to people that waste police time," the first detective snarled, coldly, his eyes boring into mine.

"We haven't wasted anyone's time," I retorted, my voice rising in defence.

At that moment, the first detective retrieved a file from the dashboard of his car and pulled out a stack of photos, handing them to me. My heart sank as I flipped through them. Each one showed Sue and Darren, her supposed abductor, strolling around Corfu, hand-in-hand, looking happy and in love.

"But she told us—" I began, my voice faltering as I realised that I didn't have a leg to stand on.

"I could arrest you and Mrs Sullivan for wasting police time," the second detective threatened, his eyes narrowing.

"But the police officer who called to Sandie's house heard her on the phone," I protested, my mind racing for a way out of this mess.

"Which officer would that be?" the first detective asked, his eyebrows raised in suspicion.

"I don't know his name but check with him and he will tell you what he heard. Sue called Sandie's house while he was there, and he heard her screaming. She was saying what Darren had done to her," I explained, panicking.

"If you're lying, I'll arrest you and your friend," the second detective warned, his voice stern.

"We haven't lied," I insisted, my heart pounding in my chest.

"We'll be in touch," the first detective said, as they both got back into their car and drove away.

I immediately called Sandie, my hands shaking as I relayed the terrifying encounter to her. We were lucky that the PC was able to corroborate our story, or we could have been facing serious charges.

Later, we found out that Darren was on licence from prison for gun running crimes. It was a shocking revelation that made me question everything I thought I knew about Sue and the people she associated with.

Sue's return to the country was like a tornado, stirring up old resentments and leaving a path of destruction in its wake.

She tried to make amends with Sandie and me, but we had already washed our hands of her.

But in a final act of malice, she reached out to my mum and revealed my deepest secret: that I was gay. She believed it would cause trouble, although it didn't. And to add insult to injury, she painted me as a heartless manipulator, using her as a prop in my charade.

My mum knew I was gay but didn't buy the added extras. Sue was twenty years my senior and often mistaken for Olive from *On the Buses*, a comedic character known for her dowdy, frumpy appearance, and oversexed personality. While we got along famously, she was nothing like the girls I had previously dated.

Sandie and I can laugh about it now, but back then, we were genuinely worried about being seen as complicit with her and Darren.

Not long ago, Sue found out Sandie's new telephone number and dared to call her. To say that Sandie gave her short thrift is an understatement.

March 15
WEIGH-IN DAY

DRUM ROLL, IF YOU PLEASE...
"7 off, well done," Shelly crowed.
"Wow, I'm pleased."
And Slimmer of the Week.

I am thrilled, and sticking to plan all week really does work. I am still 1½ stone from target, and I have been closer than this, but I am finally heading in the right direction again.

Couldn't stay for class as had to take Sammy to the vet for his follow-up appointment after he suffered hyphema in his eye from running into the patio door. Nearly had heart failure when I walked in and the first thing the vet said was, his lens has detached. After looking at his eye, she referred him to the eye vet in Runcorn and said they would call me. I had only been home an hour when they called and said I had to take him immediately. I don't mind admitting that I panicked. Arriving there, he was taken straight through by one of the nurses, and I was warned that he might require immediate surgery, but before then, they had to advise the cost would be £5845.00. I told them do whatever was needed. Thirty minutes later I was called in to be told that his lens had not detached, and surgery wasn't required. But, due to his injury, his tear ducts were damaged, and his eye had badly dried out. He required antibiotics, eye drops and eye gel. The vet, a lovely Scottish lady, told me that he did have a cataract and despite being in perfect health for a sixteen-year-old dog, surgery was not advisable for something that isn't an emergency. He still has one good eye which he will get used to relying on. I walked out £500 lighter, which is a small price to pay to make sure Sammy is on the mend. He's not going to be happy having the drops and gel in his eye for the next three weeks, at which point he has to go back for another check-up.

Still on plan, and never have I wanted chocolate more than I did after a stressful day. Instead, I ate three packets of Walker's French Fries and ate six guiltless chocolate bars—I am happy with that, but more so that I can stick to plan.

26 Syns used.

March 18

Another successful weekend on plan, which I found surprisingly easy. I don't know what the fixation with me was for Friday's and convincing myself that it should be a cheat day. I think it is embedded into most of us following any diet or healthy eating plan, that a day off is essential. The problem is that one day starts off well and good, until it slips to the whole weekend.

29½ Syns used on Saturday.

29 Syns used on Sunday.

Now I'm not saying I am cured of this cheat day nonsense, but I am trying my best and have told myself that I will strictly follow the plan until April 18th and 19th when I go to London to see Frozen and ABBA Voyage. I am going to try not to go mad, but that is my aim, and then I have told myself I must go back on plan until May 11th when I have a Eurovision Song Contest get together at my house. Even then, I will save my Syns to minimise damage.

Whatever happens, I now know the importance of sticking to plan.

Something I have realised these last few days; since abandoning cheat days, I have less tolerance to large volumes of food than I did before. Jon cooked a roast dinner yesterday and after three roast potatoes, a few carrots, parsnips, and a couple of spoonsful of mushy peas, I was done. I wanted to carry on, but I knew I would be sick. Still, I had 22 Syns left to use, so I indulged later that night on Lindahl Kvarg pots, French Fries crisps and guiltless bars.

Jet washed the flag stones in my back garden today—the couple who lived here before had obviously never heard of maintaining a garden but as I intend to have a few gatherings once the weather picks up, I want it to look good.

24½ Syns used today.

March 19

Still on plan.

Spent the morning jet washing my next-door neighbours back patio. The entire area was covered in moss, and slippery, so I thought I'd do it for her in case she lost her footing. I was absolutely filthy by the time I had finished, but she was thrilled, so it was worth it.

Came back in and cooked lunch for Jon and me, then sat down at my computer to help a friend design his new website and the ecommerce store attached to it. What a PITA that was, especially with AI trying to take over at every turn.

Had Syn Free homemade chicken and vegetable soup for dinner this evening. Struggling to eat my Syns today as my normal food intake amounts to only 2 Syns. So, I stuffed my face with guiltless bars. Strange really as I do feel guilty, but I keep getting told that the Syns are there to be used and as long as I count everything, I can eat anything I want.

Finally finished the day on 22 Syns. With 8 to spare, I couldn't fit anything else in.

March 20

Thankfully, the dog groomer had a cancellation, so she can fit Sammy in today, rather than 4th April. I had to postpone his last groom because of the damage to his eye. It seems a lot better, and less irritated, but it's a shame he can't see out of it. As long as he is happy and comfortable, that's all that matters to me.

Stuck to plan, and had mixed salad with feta cheese, and was sick as a dog—then I started to crave chocolate. But I didn't falter and chomped my way through more guiltless bars, while sticking to my Syn allowance.

28 Syns used.

March 21

Sick of the endless rain... I need some sun on this saggy old carcass of mine.

Still on plan—have I become boring following the rules? Probably, but the payoff will be worth it. Don't feel any lighter this week, so weigh-in tomorrow will be interesting.

28½ Syns used today. Thank goodness for Lindhal Kvarg pots and guiltless bars. It is difficult to eat my Syns because I prefer fruit and veg, which is always free. As I don't really drink, I can't use the Syns on that, and I am trying to avoid my normal go-to-goodies because once I start, I might find it hard to stop.

I did eat three bags of Walkers French Fries, but all sat comfortably within my allowance.

SW is a balancing act for me. But if I treat myself with yoghurts and guiltless bars, I don't feel like I am missing out.

28½ Syns used today.

March 22
WEIGH-IN DAY

Why do I feel more bunged up sticking to plan, than when rule breaking? I know a few people who have this problem, and it leaves me feeling bloated and nauseous.

Whatever, I got weighed and lost another 3 pounds so was thrilled. The lowest I got down to previously was 18, 10½, so I'm not too far off—I will get to target.

Stayed for class, and was awarded my certificates for bronze, silver, and gold Body Magic. All very nice, aside from Donna presenting me with them in front of the whole class—I really struggle with that level of attention, but it is an achievement in itself, and the rest of the group are so kind and encouraging.

Donna asked the group a question—if you could go back in time, what would you tell your younger self? Tammy nearly dropped on the spot at the prospect of public speaking. Regardless, I knew she would come to me, despite me asking her not to—I answered truthfully—to learn moderation and that if I didn't, I would enter my 40's obsessed with food, namely chocolate. I know why she tasked the group with this... it's not too long away until British summertime and she doesn't want us stepping into July and beyond regretting something we could have addressed now.

Came home and felt sick and exhausted so went to bed and slept for six hours. I got up, ate a few spoonful of chicken rice, then went back to bed.

March 25

Still on plan and have found it relatively easy. But I feel like I've slept the entire weekend away. I can't remember the last time I felt this wiped out. I think I am having a fibro flare-up. It will pass!

Dragged myself out to get my haircut, and to have my beard trimmed. Roasted myself alive on the sun shower and had to push the door open halfway through—the heat was unbearable.

26 Syns used today.

March 26

Surprise, surprise, I am still on plan and have just tucked into a large bowl of strawberries, bananas, and fat free quark—all Syn Free.

Watched an interesting debate on TV this afternoon. The question is, Should You Ever Tell Someone They Are Fat? Hmm, it depends on the person. It wouldn't bother me personally if somebody pointed out my excess weight as long as it was put in a constructive manner (Hello, Aunty Vera), and there was zero shaming. But it's not like fat people are unaware of their size—they are, I certainly am, and don't need anybody to point out the obvious to me. What business is it of anyone else's anyway?

What has happened to people accepting people for how they are?

Apparently, Britain is the fattest nation in Western Europe. Fifteen million adults are obese while thirty-four million adults are overweight. Men are five times more likely to get Type 2 diabetes while women are thirteen times more likely to develop Type 2 diabetes.

Yes, I do realise the UK has a problem, in fact, an obesity crisis, which is costing the NHS £11 billion per year, but smokers put a strain on the NHS too, as do people addicted to alcohol or drugs. The finger cannot be pointed solely on overweight people—it's grossly unfair, which is why debates like this stir up public feelings negatively towards those with food issues. The are worse things to be in this life than overweight. Does excess weight stop a person from being kind? Should it stop a doctor or a nurse from caring for obese patients unless they hit a healthy BMI? We all know carrying that excess weight can limit our capabilities from everyday tasks, to impacting our sex lives, but we're still human beings.

Fat shaming, or lifesaving, you decide.

29 Syns used today.

March 28
WEIGH-IN DAY

28½ Syns used yesterday.

For the first time in a long while, I feel genuinely annoyed.

½ ON. I know it is a tiny gain, but I've stuck to plan all week and used most of my Syns on a daily basis. So, I feel hacked off, but remain hopeful of a loss next week. Not going to lie though; my first thought was, sod it, I might as well take today off. But I won't. I am determined to get to target. So, forgetting my actual target for the moment, I want to get into the next stone bracket, which gives me 4½ to lose.

29½ Syns used today.

March 31
EASTER SUNDAY

Friday's Syns: 29.
Saturday's Syns: 28.

I have fourteen Easter Eggs in this house and ten Crème Eggs, and I have not touched a single one.

Still on plan and spent most of the morning preparing a roast dinner as I invited my dad and my sister for lunch—a full roast.

I did the full works, and even cooked rice pudding from scratch. They enjoyed it, which is the main thing. As per usual, I didn't eat a lot—two roast potatoes, a spoonful of mushy peas, Yorkshire pudding and gravy. After cooking it for hours, I didn't feel like it anyway, but it seems I am constantly stuffed up to the eyeballs with food, and as gross as this might be, since following the plan to the letter, I feel constipated and bloated, so have had to resort to medication to move myself along.

If I go to class on Friday and gain for the second week on the run, I will go nuts.

Today's Syns: 27.

MY JOURNEY – APRIL 2024

April 1

Two weeks until I go to see Frozen at Drury Lane Theatre, and the ABBA Voyage concert—how much can I lose in that time?

Still on plan. All easter eggs and Crème Eggs are present and accounted for. Surprisingly, it is easier to ignore them, but I will treat myself when I go to London, then hop right back onto plan before a planned pig out on 11th May for my Eurovision Party.

I don't feel like breakfast or lunch right now, but tonight, I am having homemade chicken and vegetable soup for dinner with wholemeal pitta.

"You're not eating enough," Jon reminds me often.

He is probably right, but he knows me well enough to know I am not a fan of food, so constantly having to shovel it in, and to meet my Syn quota, is bloody difficult, and trying.

"I know, but I'm fed up with it all."

I am sick of the sight of food—shopping, cooking, and eating. I've said it before but I wish somebody could invent a tablet so I would never have to eat again.

26½ Syns used today.

April 2

I had a terrible night's sleep, broken by constant visits to the toilet. Feeling more uncomfortable as the day progressed, I took something to help me along, and gosh did it ever—talk about a mad dash down the hallway.

Fancied a walk, so hoofed to the shop as Jon requested spaghetti with his Bolognese. I can't taste any difference between spaghetti and pasta, but he swears there is.

Anyway, on the way back, and weighted down with two litres of semi-skimmed milk for another batch of homemade rice pudding, tinned tomatoes, and four litres of diet Pepsi, I felt griping pains in my stomach, so took off along the road like Usain Bolt, desperate to get in doors before the worst happened—well, I only just made it in time and threw myself into the bathroom and let off a ruddy great big trump. False alarm, but I am still getting twinges. Still, it beats getting bunged up and should help towards a loss on Friday.

Prepared tonight's dinner—spaghetti Bolognese which clocks in at 1½ Syns for the Sainsburys tomato & herb light sauce. That's an over estimation for me though because I will only have a small amount.

Sat down this afternoon to do a bit of writing but got caught up in trying shoes on that used to be too tight for me. While not perfect, they seem a better fit than they were—Jon reckons people don't lose weight on their feet, so I did a bit of research.

This small snippet is from *Weight Watchers* US website.

Do feet get smaller when you lose weight?

In most cases, yes. While it may not be noticeable for everyone, weight loss does tend to result in smaller feet, says Lauren Wurster, DPM, a spokesperson for the American Podiatric Medical Association and a foot and ankle surgery specialist at Foot & Ankle Clinics of Arizona. Makes sense when you consider that weight loss reduces fat distribution all over the body, potentially affecting everything from breast size to skin appearance.

"The overall bony structure of the feet doesn't change, but the amount of soft tissue decreases," Dr Wurster says. Plus, as a person loses weight, pressure on feet comes down, too, which can reduce spreading and swelling, Dr Wurster continues. The result? Your shoes may feel looser than they used to.

Can weight loss change your shoe size?

Sometimes weight loss can shrink feet enough to change a person's shoe size. In one twelve-month study published in 2017, volunteers who lost fifty to one hundred pounds (through sleeve gastrectomy) saw their shoe sizes decrease by one full number on average.

And don't be surprised if you have to drop from, say, an EE width to a D width—your feet's side-to-side measurements may decrease with weight loss, as well. You can credit reduced pressure on your paws for that: The foot's tendons and ligaments stretch in response to weight from the rest of the body, says Rebecca Pruthi, DPM, a foot surgeon at Foot Care of Manhattan in New York City. Losing weight reduces some of that pressure, so the foot doesn't fan out as much, Dr Pruthi continues.

April 5
WEIGH IN DAY

I have spent the last three days in bed, sick—sore throat, runny nose, and watery eyes. Jon is convinced I have Covid, and as terrified as he is of catching it again, I am surprised he hasn't forced me into a hazmat suit and banished me to wallow in the garden shed.

But I have remained on plan (five weeks now without a slip, and I am so pleased with myself).

To be honest, I felt rough, and still do. Add chapped lips and a scabby nose from wiping it so often, and I don't want to go out of the house. But I have to as the scales call to me like siren song.

Braced myself and stepped on the scales. I turned to look at a glowing, slimmer-looking, Shelly, silently praying for good news. "If I've gained, I'm going to go mad." And after last week, I would have, but only with myself because I'd have been doing something wrong!

"How's seven and a half off for you?"

"What?"

"Seven and a half *off*. Well done, you're in the next stone bracket." I'm sure she wants to slap many of us who step on those scales because we are crushingly brutal to ourselves. But, to give her enormous credit, she bolsters us every week, and strangely enough, I am rarely afraid to face the scales because there is zero judgement from her, or any of the other ladies. They are on the same journey and know the score.

I was actually speechless at such a big loss, elated too but I felt bad because my sister had gained a pound. Still, she has had a loss eight out of ten weeks, and right now she is on medication and is struggling to go to the toilet. She will lose it next week I am sure because she is sticking to plan too, the longest she ever has.

Me and Tammy went to the butchers to get some Syn Free sausages, but the visit only made me feel nauseous as we were witness to a pig being sawn in half right in front of us. I know that is the point of a butcher, but I really didn't want to see, or hear it.

Back home and straight back to bed in hope that I feel human again tomorrow.

April 6

Woke up and still feel wretched, but marginally better than yesterday. Everything aches, and I blame Fibromyalgia for that because when I feel ill, that seems to flare up just to make me feel that little bit crappier. Frustrated, I did what I always do and tried to carry on. "Sod this." Defiantly, I got up, cooked myself poached eggs and tinned tomatoes with a wholemeal pitta bread, scoffed that down, even though I didn't really want it, then cracked on with the housework before jet washing the barbecue in readiness for the warmer weather—as if, it's England, remember—then felt rough again, so went back to bed.

Spent most of the day in bed but got up a few times to do bits of cleaning, washing dishes, mopping of floors, all the while sticking to plan when I really wanted to forget counting and tuck into the many Easter Eggs that are taunting me from about 20cm away.

Syns used today = 29½, and they were mainly on crisps and guiltless chocolate bars because I've eaten mostly free food today, aside from two tins of tomato soup.

April 7

Bloody dogs yapping again over the road—all five of appear to start at once, and their owners seem think the whole close wants to listen to it continuously. I am moody because I had a bad sleep and want to go and hammer on their door and tell them to S.T.F.U and learn to be more considerate to their neighbours. I know that all dogs bark, but their noise is incessant, and at times they sound genuinely distressed being left outside for so long. But Jon goes mad when I kick off, so I will bite my tongue and choose another moment before telling the owner what I think. Don't get me wrong, I love dogs, and prefer mine over 99% of human beings, but if mine barked when left unattended, I would bring them in, rather than allow them to cause a racket.

Rant over, what can I eat?

Thankfully, Jon is cooking meatballs, with salad and baby potatoes for dinner. All Syn Free—I really can't be bothered doing anything but moan as you can probably tell from the above diatribe.

April 8

Feel so much better today, so went out to do a little shopping—all good stuff that helps me remain on plan.

Came home and put a joint of beef in the oven, chopped and peeled the carrots and potatoes, then prepared the stock for the gravy.

My next-door neighbour messaged me to tell me that one of the fence panels had snapped in the wind. Typical. I went out to have a look, but not being the Bob the Builder type I have zero clue how to fix it, so I called my brother who said he will do it. I wouldn't have a clue how to change a fuse... still, as I once said to my dad, you can build a house, and I can write a book.

My expected parcel arrived. Two T-shirts from Peacocks—not wanting to spend a fortune on clothes that won't fit me for long I opted for cheap and cheerful that will match my new jeans and trousers purchased for London. I tried the first one on and my heart sank because I thought that I had ordered it a size too big, not wanting to spend the night tugging away at it. Then I tried the second one and felt that same panic thinking I'd gained weight. But then I realised both were a small fit. Don't get me wrong, both looked presentable, but to my critical eye, every lump and bump is visible.

28 Syns used today, and most of them were on crisps and guiltless bars.

April 9

Rain, rain, rain, rain, rain... when will it ever stop? It seems relentless lately, and rather than improving for Spring, well, I can see another cold and wet Summer.

I'm bored and have cabin fever, but the furthest I went was to the back gate to bring the bins in. Then, as I was dragging the second one in, I bashed the side of my foot against the wheel—rather than turn the air blue, which is what I wanted to do, I gritted my teeth and tried to pretend it didn't hurt. Five minutes later, I have the monster of all bruises on the side of my foot.

Once that was sorted, I peeled the veg for dinner—basically a rehash of yesterday's dinner but with roast potatoes rather than new potatoes.

Jon put his order in. "I fancy curry."

"Okay." So I put a whole chicken in the oven, but I'm not good at handling raw meat, or anything that still resembles an animal, so I gagged a few times, especially after taking the cellophane from around the chicken and its legs parted indecently wide.

So, not only was I having to deal with the hole where its head was, but its bottom half was gaping too.

Revolting! Once it was cooked, it was still too hot to take out of the baking dish by hand, so I rammed a carving knife down its neck and out through its hoop—disgusting.

I bet he decides against curry tonight and wants a roast dinner too.

28 Syns used again today.

CHEWING THE FAT

April 10

I woke up at 6:15 am, got up, then slipped back into bed for an hour before waking at 12:10 pm. Annoyed I had slept the morning away, I jumped out of bed and cleaned the kitchen. Sitting down to watch *Neighbours*, I opened my yoghurt, had a spoonful, and gagged—it was out of date and tasted worse than cottage cheese—disgusting.

Still on plan though and had homemade chicken and vegetable soup for dinner with a wholemeal pitta.

Getting excited for my trip to London next week, but I wish Jon was coming too.

April 12
WEIGH-IN DAY

Still on plan, so am looking forward to weigh-in. Getting closer to target, which is exciting.

Came home from class, fuming, disappointed, disheartened and livid.

"3½ on."

"How?" I really don't understand how I have gained when I have stuck to plan religiously, and forgotten nothing I have eaten, nor have I failed to write it into my daily planner. People have said it is something that I have done, and it's not the plan failing me... I have wracked my brain trying to think how I might have screwed up, but I am certain I haven't. I know I have been struggling to go to the toilet, but it can't be that—so I have to take it on the chin and hope for a loss in two weeks. I am further away from my target again and have jumped back up into the higher stone bracket. F@*K! Getting there means everything, so this setback I didn't need, or want.

But I won't let it knock me off plan—I am taking Jon to COSMO in Liverpool and then I have my trip to London next Thursday and Friday and know I won't follow it strictly, but I will be right back on it on Saturday—perhaps I shouldn't aim for a loss at my next weigh-in.

April 14

Sunday, and still on plan, and still reeling from Friday's gain. But I said I wasn't going to let it derail me, and I intend to stick to that, even though this weekend has dragged worse than usual.

April 15

My planned trip to London on Thursday and Friday has had to be postponed to July due to my friend's dad falling ill following a stroke last year. She wanted me to go without her, but it was not an option for me as she had been looking forward to it. So, trying to avoid disaster, I called the Drury Lane Theatre this morning, and emailed the ABBA Arena, and the tickets were swapped easily, and without question. The train journey was cancelled and rescheduled and the hotel was the same, albeit £60 dearer due to the time of year.

Even though I am disappointed, it gives me something to look forward to, and the added bonus is I will have lost more weight, plus the weather should be warmer.

After sorting out London, I went to get my haircut and beard trimmed, and despite the gale force winds, I walked home and got in 5000 steps. I was dithering, but I am looking fresh for the concert tomorrow night.

As I am taking Jon out to COSMO beforehand, I have eaten free foods all day, and will do the same tomorrow, so I don't have to be so strict while in the restaurant. I had been worried about it, but I have got to live. Still, I will be back on plan Wednesday morning... some might think I won't fall off plan, but odds on I will.

April 16

Date night with Jon.
COSMO first, which is a worry because it is an all-you-can-eat style restaurant, and where cake is concerned, I am a bottomless pit.
Afterwards we are off to see his favourite band, Blue, at the Philharmonic.

April 17

We had a great night at the Blue concert, but I was mortified to see they were filming the event for an ITV programme. I was terrified of being captured wobbling on screen, so it dulled my enjoyment somewhat, and at one point I noticed the TV camera focused on me, so I deliberately shoved my finger up my nose, knowing they wouldn't use that shot—well, I hope they don't because I am going to look like a right tit if they do.

Anyway, before the gig, we ate at COSMO. I told myself to be sensible, so ate three pieces of chicken in sweet and sour sauce, a spoonful of pilau rice—all good, but then things went downhill fast. Cake, my ultimate downfall doesn't come in slices, but 2cm x 2cm squares—I had eight, and okay, you might say, that still doesn't equate to a huge amount. But then, I went back for another eight squares, followed by salted popcorn and Haribo eggs. Oh, the guilt was horrible! Yes, I know it could have been much worse, but at that point I was stuffed and quickly realised that the goodies I had avoided while staying strictly on plan did not satisfy me. I knew I had not missed eating them, but the thought was more powerful than the deed. Quite the revelation, and I understood I have the power over food and not the other way around. Saying that, five minutes after I ate all of the above, I rushed off to the bathroom and threw the lot back up... I should remember that I am not a fan of food, and some foods rather than others do make me violently sick. The earlier feelings of guilt dissipated slightly, but I am not naïve enough to believe that vomiting entirely erased the calories I ate. I was taken back to the fact that I do not enjoy food, nor do I enjoy spending £25 on food simply to yak it back up.

Still, Jon and I had a good night, and when I woke up this morning, I had let go of the guilt because I am human and far from perfect. I take it for what it was—a nice night out with my partner.

I didn't bother trying to count Syns yesterday because I knew I would fall off plan—what is done is done, and I have moved on.

But that was then, and today is today—and to my credit, I went straight back on plan without any problems or feeling like I was missing out—splurge over, until my Eurovision party on 11th May.

Syns used today = 25½.

April 18

I should be in London today, instead I am cooking breakfast. I'm not bothered at all really about the trip being postponed as I still have something to look forward to. As a consolation prize, Jon has informed me that he is cooking us dinner this evening and we are going to watch Frozen 1 and 2... it's very nice of him as he hates the movies, or so he says.

April 19
WEIGH-IN DAY

I had booked a holiday from fat club, and could have gone due to my cancelled trip, but I am having my hallway floor laminated instead. Still on plan, so I am looking forward to what I hope will be a decent loss next week.

Jon cooked me a lovely meal last night and we sat down to Frozen 1—he analysed every part of the script and complained all the way through about Elsa, so I didn't make him watch the second movie.

April 20

Still on plan, but I wanted to eat, eat, eat today, although I didn't.

Instead, I used the twenty remaining Syns, and ate forty mini flump marshmallows. Did I feel guilty? Yes, because I felt like I was cheating, but at ½ per flump, I had the Syns, and there are no rules for them. I enjoyed every single one which took away the craving to eat one of the seventeen easter eggs in eyeshot.

April 21

A brand-new week, but most days roll into one for me now. Today is a different matter entirely as it is Jon's yearly cancer check. A couple of years ago, he had bladder cancer, which they caught early thankfully. This is his second annual checkup, so three more years and if it doesn't recur, he should be fine.

Still on plan and because today is what it is, I prepared a meal yesterday from the SW magazine—beef & paprika stew—it smelled like a pair of Jon's old socks. But I am hoping as it finishes cooking today while we are at the hospital, that aroma is replaced by something that will make me want to eat it.

I didn't enjoy it, but what's new? Jon and my friend enjoyed it, and said it was delicious.

April 23

Jon got the all-clear. Thank God because he is my world.

Still on plan but bunged up—I never had any problems going to the toilet and feel like I am carrying a dead weight inside me.

I've eaten so many flumps this past week trying to top up my Syns, it wouldn't surprise me if I'm clogged up with them. Saying that, I don't regret a single one I've scoffed.

Fingers crossed I have some form of movement, or it doesn't bode well for weigh-in on Friday.

If this carries on, I will have to go and see my GP.

April 24

A visit from the in-laws today, so Jon has cooked a pan of Syn Free soup... they are also members of SW, so it makes things so much easier when trying to decide what to eat.

Those who are trying to lose weight will know how it feels constantly having to decide what to cook. I hate it, and factor in shopping for it, making the decisions, then preparing it—I'd rather not bother and settle for a tin of tomato soup.

April 25
WEIGH-IN DAY

I'm nervous, but I don't know why. Well, I do know—I have stuck to plan, for two weeks, except for that one day. But I still haven't been to the loo, and I know if I step onto those scales and see another gain, I will not be impressed. It definitely won't put me off plan, but it will bother me.

Wish me luck!

Just got back from class and I am thrilled to report that I lost a whopping seven pounds, which moves me 1½ pounds away from a total loss of 4 stone, and only 7½lbs from target.

How wonderful—I can finally see the finishing line for this part of my journey. Now, time to really focus and get to where I need to.

Chicken rogan josh with JD Seasoning, and salt & pepper chips for dinner tonight. All Syn Free but I didn't enjoy it at all—I really do give up even contemplating the notion of liking what I eat as it rarely happens.

Syns used today = 29½.

April 28

Remained on plan all weekend, and still on plan today, but sick as a pig.

Thinking about food and having to eat so much is really driving me mad. Cooked a healthy meal and spent two hours throwing up afterwards.

Syns used Saturday = 30.

Syns used today = 30.

April 29

A good day overall but I thought a lot about my Uncle Alan, who was killed in an accident twenty-seven years ago today. We were extremely close, and I wonder what he would be like had he not been in the wrong place at the wrong time. I inherited my love of music from him, and wish he was still here.

Rejoined the gym, and my sister is joining too. She is doing so well, and I am happy she has taken this step to aid her own weight loss.

Strange as it might seem to some people, that as soon as I walked in, I realised how much I had missed it, and settled right back into my old routine. Although I didn't push it, and stayed for only forty minutes, I am proud of what I achieved.

I cycled 6.97 Miles at level 5 and burned 214 calories. I was surprised I got back into the swing of things so easily, and I would have done more, but my sister only joined today and accompanied me on the bike, so she didn't overdo it. I'm already looking forward to tomorrow.

Seated Leg Press – 40 presses. I had forgotten how hard this is, but it will do wonders for the strength in my legs.

I had planned to do some gardening with Jon, but the weather wasn't up to much, and with the wind, I stayed inside and caught up on a Netflix.

Cooked again, all Syn Free, and surprise, surprise, I was sick again. Tomorrow, and for the next few days, I am sticking with homemade soup. Fed up with eating only to spend hours with my head down the toilet.

Syns used = 29.

April 30

Up at 8 am, and back to the gym.

I managed 10.04 miles at level 5 and burned 317.1 calories in 51 minutes. I found this fairly easy, but as soon as I stepped off the bike, I felt the dull ache in my legs. Getting out of the car half an hour later, I felt bow-legged, and like I'd just got off a horse.

Still on plan.

Came home and cooked homemade vegetable soup—Jon usually does it, but this tasted surprisingly good. Better still, I wasn't sick afterwards.
Syns used = 28.

ALISON'S STORY

It must have been about nineteen years ago when I wandered nervously into Alison's *Weight Watchers* class. After defecting from another leader's class where I had largely been ignored and unsupported, I wasn't sure if I was breaking an unwritten rule.

From the moment we met, Alison's support buoyed me, and quickly, we became good friends. But as my failures racked up, I left, re-joined, left again, re-joined, then finally, I walked away, and got stuck on that cycle. Today is the first time since 2017 that we have seen one another face to face.

Unsurprisingly, time has been her best friend, and after a quick hello and a hug, I ask if she has a painting of herself in the attic, a la, Dorian Grey. It would make a lot of sense. Still blonde, still glamorous, sparkling, and effervescent, forever uber-stylish, with that same girlish grin and twinkle in her eye, it seems not much has changed at all. Same lady, different surroundings.

We find a quiet corner for our chat, and I ask my first question—one a lady should never be asked, with the option for her to decline to reveal her age if she so wishes.

Without hesitation Alison tells me, but as I have no concept of age in others, I am genuinely shocked when she reveals the truth. "Would you believe that I am now 64?"

I had no idea and told her so—in my mind, I am the only person that ages.

Working as a Travel Advisor for Jet2, and part-time, as a *Slimming World* consultant since 2023, I wonder if she could she be on the cusp of retirement? "I'm carrying on as long as I enjoy it. That's what I did with *Weight Watchers*... I'll carry on at *Slimming World* as long as I have something to give."

Married to Peter, and devoted to her precious son, Harrison, in all the years I have known Alison, she has epitomised the Duracell bunny—never stopping and seeing her in action while leading her class before our chat, there is no change in that respect either. Like all consultants, she gives a lot to her members, and probably doesn't fit the corporate mould, or what *Weight Watchers* or *Slimming World* would expect—there is a lot of heart, and encouragement, and heavy emphasis on the individual, rather than the group as a collective.

Alison explains her decision to leave *Weight Watchers* in 2020 after a quarter of a century. "I became disillusioned by *Weight Watchers*, and the change of plan which my members weren't keen on. We had red, green and purple plans and while I knew the company innovated every two years, I was initially fine with it. But the last change, members were talking to one another; some were losing more than others on the different coloured plans. Some lost five pounds on green while others lost two on purple, so inevitably, they wanted to switch. Eventually, they became frustrated. Then, three of my classes were changed to multi-venue, and my members hated it. My stock levels were also impacted, I couldn't offer what they needed, and to be honest, I think the whole thing was fizzling out. Then Oprah Winfrey bought into the company and there was a change of CEO... it went in the wrong direction, and neither me nor my members liked it."

It must have been hard walking away after being so dedicated as a leader for twenty-two years.

"Yes, it was, but then we had Covid and while I had good attendance on my Zoom classes and we had fun, there was a cull on leaders. As a five-time diamond leader, and a Jean Nidetch (founder of *Weight Watchers*) winner, my job was safe. Then, just as classes resumed, redundancy was being offered company wide, so after a chat with my husband, I decided that I had seen the best years at *Weight Watchers*. The targets became unrealistic, and to be honest, I was never driven by targets, more my members and their journey, so, it was time to go."

In 2022, two years after leaving her position at *Weight Watchers*, she joined *Slimming World* as a member, knowing all too well how easy it would be to regain the weight she had managed to keep off.

Then, in 2023, she became a consultant with the tools at her disposal to transfer decades worth of knowledge into her new role—while still remaining at her target weight.

Currently nine stone, twelve pounds, she sits within the BMI recommendation of eight stone ten pounds and ten stone, six pounds.

At her lightest, she states, "I was probably eight stone, ten, which was too light for me. Everybody said that I looked washed out." After a brief discussion, she agrees that a person struggles to win favour in the weight game—too fat—lose weight, too thin—put a bit on.

But at her heaviest, the start of her weight loss journey, Alison was fourteen stone, twelve pounds.

"My journey began when I took a good, hard look at myself in the mirror. I knew it couldn't carry on, and that I was the only one who could do anything about my situation. I didn't know where to start because I'd never been to a weight loss class before. As it turned out, there was a *Weight Watchers* class down the bottom of my road. I joined, and my leader, Kathy, was amazing. She was my inspiration."

How did she adapt to following a healthier-eating plan? Did she stick to it?

"More or less. I still had weekends off, and holidays, but I've always been conscious of what I've eaten calorie wise so if I ate something that was high in calories, it was my choice to do it."

Did those days off impact her weight loss progress, and if so, how?

"Admittedly, I was a slow loser and plodded because all I was thinking of each week was a loss. That was my focus. Everyone wants a big loss week in, week out, and all I was looking for was a steady loss. As long as I lost each week, I was fine."

From start to finish, how long was the journey?

"It took about three and a half years for me to hit target, but I had a break in that time after falling pregnant with Harrison. He was born prematurely, so I didn't put much weight on. I lost the last two stone when I went back."

I ask Alison to talk me through her transition from member to leader, and then finally, to diamond leader?

"My *Weight Watchers* leader, Kathy, told me that she thought I would make a great leader, and I didn't really believe her because it wasn't something I had ever thought about. Then she put my name down, so I went for an interview which I thought was just a preliminary interview, and to my surprise, I was offered the job—seventeen and a half years I worked as a *Weight Watchers* leader."

"Bidding farewell to something that had meant so much to you for so many years must have been hard to come to terms with."

She is pragmatic about her decision. "It was time to go."

Saying goodbye to that part of her life didn't mean Alison had reached the end of her journey. But I am eager to know at what weight she is at her happiest with herself.

I'd say between nine and a half stone, and nine stone, ten pounds."

Is control and accountability still an important part of Alison's daily life?

"I'm more confident when my weight is under control. But, then again, I've always been a glass half full person, so I try and turn situations from not so great to better. Of course I'm still critical of myself."

In what ways is she critical of herself?

"When I put a dress on, I always ask Peter what I look like from behind... he doesn't get it and jokingly asks if I'm going to enter a room walking backwards... I'm conscious about it. I have a smaller waist, and I'm curvy. But I always worry. I like to take care of myself. I'm a feminine, girly-girl. I like to sparkle. I like to be different."

Is weight loss, and maintaining her figure, the only things that bring confidence? "No, because I've always had confidence if I believed in something. I was good at my job. Losing weight just makes me feel better about me. I've never struggled with things like public speaking... I've always been able to do that. But with losing weight and keeping it off, I felt better inside, healthier, buzzing with the fact that I felt good about myself."

How does Alison maintain her current weight, and if there are gains, how does she manage to get back on track?

"I just basically try and be as active as possible. I can't promise I'll go to the gym or run a mile on the treadmill. I do what I do when I can. I watch my diet, I walk the dogs, do fitness classes at home. I don't have time for the gym, and even if I did, it would be a waste of money... I wouldn't go because I hate the gym. I'd only have to walk through the doors and wonder how long it would be before I could leave. I will always do a class if I can get to one. But realistically, I do what I can within the limits I have."

With her in-depth knowledge of both *Weight Watchers* and *Slimming World*, which plan does she follow?

"I only follow the *Slimming World* plan, but I do have an overall gauge of what calories are in what foods. I know that anything high in fat is high in Syns, or if something is high in sugar, there are Syns. I follow the basis of *Slimming World*, that free foods are the healthy stuff. Then I do what I do... I know what is going to be high Syns, but I still check, and it's my decision if I eat it or not."

What is her trigger to overeat or indulge in foods that might not be the healthiest option?

"Tiredness. Not boredom because I'm never bored. My go to—the quick fix. And while it's not necessarily overeating, I'm consuming higher calories. I've always eaten healthy even when I was bigger. I was a snacker—high calories like sandwiches. We didn't have the choices back then that we have now, with half fat cheese and low-calorie stuff... toast was quick, grab and go, and that helped pile my weight on."

What is her relationship with food now?

"I eat to live because if I don't eat to live, I won't have good health, and that has always been my mantra, even before *Weight Watchers*. I don't constantly think about food. I get up in the morning and have two cups of tea, then I don't feel hungry. I can go until about 3 pm before I think about eating. I try my best to be at my best. I don't always succeed but I try to be the best of me that I can."

What tempts her—sweets, cakes, crisps...?

"Marshmallows... microwaved... they go really gooey, and Pink & Whites... only when I'm desperate, or tired... in the microwave, they expand... or Colin the Caterpillar squidgy sweets, only those. I'm not a chocolate or a cake girl, and I love baking but don't eat it. Chocolate can live in my fridge for ages, and I won't eat that either.

And what are her downfalls... that one thing she simply cannot leave alone.

"Turkish Delight is my downfall. Once I start, I can't stop... the sugary stuff with the powder... I love it, and every Christmas, my husband buys me a box of it. Not the huge box, but the one with about eight pieces in..."

Does she eat it all in one sitting?

"When Peter and Harrison go out to walk the dog, I sit down and watch a movie, and I eat the lot. It's not a great amount, but if there was twelve pieces, I'd feel sick but still eat the lot. I can't have it in the house—I'd struggle to resist it—rose-flavoured things, I could sit and eat the lot and would begrudge sharing it."

I wonder if either Peter or Harrison struggle with food, and does her role as a consultant play any part in what the family eat collectively?

"Harrison only struggled in university because of the lifestyle... easy, cheap, junk food and now he's back home, I don't have to watch what he eats because he has always been a sensible eater anyway. He loves vegetables, just not fresh tomatoes. Don't get me wrong, he does like pizza, and junk food, but he's always eaten cauliflower, peas, carrots, asparagus, whereas with Peter, he's retired but isn't as active as he was. He is still active but there has been a lifestyle change."

Has retirement had an adverse effect on his weight, and do you crack the whip if his weight increases?

"He works really hard to keep his weight down, but I know what he wants and how he feels because he tells me. So, I go hard and ask why he is eating it if he knows it will make him gain weight. He tells me he eats it because he likes it."

Before this chat, I had the pleasure of sitting in on Alison's class, of which Peter is a paying member. While he spoke honestly about his weight gain, and despite being married to the consultant, she still held him accountable because he is probably the one member she knows inside out.

"Peter is an amazing cook and does cook the healthiest meals. It's snacking with him, which is why I'm hard on him."

I discuss her class, and how she interacted with her members. It's obvious she cares deeply, and that has never changed.

"My passion is to get members where they want to be."

From my perspective, every person who wished to contribute was given their moment to shine, and whether they had lost, gained or remained the same, there was no judgement, just encouragement.

"Accountability is everything. We make choices and tonight's class was about choices."

I fully agree with her summation, and it does come down to that one word—accountability—without it, the path to weight loss is a much harder journey to navigate.

"Sometimes we don't get the loss we want... I had one member who lost seventeen pounds the first week, but it can't be sustained and that's hard for some people to grasp. But I always ask, would you rather lose consistently every week than have a big loss every now and again?"

I know this from my own experience of losing eighteen pounds in one week. It isn't sustainable and only leads to disappointment.

Aside from her tireless work as a consultant, when is she at most content?

"With my family and friends, they make me happy."

What about food—where does that factor in?

"Food doesn't make me happy because it is a by-product. Whether I eat it or don't, it doesn't make me happy. I have to eat to stay alive."

What does she honestly think about the struggle many of us have experienced, and continue to do so with food?

"Food is an addiction... and people are judged for it. I understand why even if I disagree with it. People judge the book by the cover, and what really matters is what's inside, and that's why I love doing what I do because I get to know the members personally. I see their ups and downs, and everything in between. I'm a sparkly person and it's followed me throughout my life, so I like to sprinkle some of that to my members."

As our chat draws to a close, I ask Alison what her ultimate goal is? As a former diamond leader with *Weight Watchers*, would she like to progress within *Slimming World* and climb the corporate ladder?

"I don't want to be a big boss anywhere. My ultimate goal, if anything, is just to stay as happy as I am today. It might be cliché, but I'd love to see Harrison continue to be the person that he is. I'd like to see him mature, maybe get married... kids or no kids, just seeing him happy. I don't have any big ambitions anymore. I just want to continue to be as happy as I am now."

With that in mind, where does she see herself in the short term? "Hopefully, still where I am, helping my members as much as I can and keeping check on my weight and health. I don't have grand ambitions. I just want to go and enjoy my life."

MY JOURNEY – MAY 2024

May 2

Only four days back in and already I hate the alarm going off at 8 am. Still, I dragged myself out of bed, and even though I have been dreading it over the last twenty-four hours, I did it.

Killer Whale on the starboard bow...

Yes folks, that's right, I finally took the plunge and went swimming.

How on Earth did I pluck up the courage to do it?

Well, if it wasn't for my sister wanting to go, I would have procrastinated until Hell froze over.

Walking out from the changing rooms was the worst part and despite the embarrassment of showing my upper body, which almost made me turn around and get changed, I walked into the pool. I enjoyed my swim and did fourteen lengths backstroke. I wanted to swim properly but I hadn't bought any goggles and had my contact lenses in. I was worried they would slip out and leave me struggling to see. But contacts or not, and even with distinct lanes, I found myself moving diagonally instead of going straight. At one point I swam to the bottom of the pool and come up for air as a woman swam past. "JESUS CHRIST," she yelled, obviously shocked as she hadn't seen me. My sister and niece laughed, as I would have done, and then when finishing another length, I almost swam into the wall until my niece put her hand out to stop me. God help me without contacts.

Anyway, challenge over, and without that fear holding me back, I will aim to go for a swim a few times per week.

Came home and cooked a Syn Free breakfast but wish I hadn't bothered as I feel sick.

Weigh-in tomorrow, and I am dreading it, and not because I haven't stuck to plan, and exercised, but because I feel heavier.

Syns used 28.

May 3
WEIGH-IN DAY

Here I go again.

½ OFF. How do I feel about it? While I am happy it is a loss, and a loss is always reason to celebrate, I was hoping for 1½ as it would have taken me to four stone. But I am sure I will get there next week.

Stayed for class—it was lovely to see one of the ladies reach target, especially knowing I am not too far off. Right now, I am half a stone away from target.

Syns used: 20½.

May 4

Still on plan, but woke up ravenous for sweets, crisps, and chocolate—this is a first for me since following plan, and while I have had mild cravings, this morning, I wanted everything. But I refrained, wondering why the desire to go off plan is coming at me thick and fast—FLUMPS. I blame flumps. I think eating so many of them, even though they are counted in my Syns, I am craving everything else I used to shovel down. I won't give in! In the meantime, I will put a stop to them for a few days and see if I settle down again.

Cooked spaghetti Bolognese for dinner, and while I usually add a few extra spices—Jon likes his food spicy—me definitely not—I decided to add a chilli pepper. All fine and dandy, until I dished up and tasted it. Then I realised what I had done. Rather than my usual green chilli pepper I chopped up a scotch bonnet (and pips) and threw it in the slow cooker. It definitely had a kick to it, but I only ate a tiny bit. Jon enjoyed it, but his nose was running throughout. I took a plate in for my elderly next-door neighbour and warned her it was spicy. But she said it would be fine and that she would be careful.

Twenty minutes later, I got a message from her on *WhatsApp*: *OMG, That WAS spicy, and delicious!*

Syns used: 28.

May 5

Finally received the revised cover for CHEWING THE FAT—I wasn't keen on the previous version but this new design I like very much. Re-designing it makes the release so much more real, knowing that the close of this book will be written on the day I hit target. Then everything is ready to go to my editor before release. I am nervous at how the book will be received.

While lying in bed last night a news report popped up on my phone with the headline Britain's 'heaviest man' dies from organ failure week before 34th birthday. Reading the article, apparently at his heaviest, he weighed a colossal forty-seven stone, and there will be more readers than not who question how he could ever get close to that figure. Well, for those of us in the know, weight creeps on, and although a person could be two stone, ten stone, or twenty stone overweight, realisation often comes too late and usually at that point where losing it seems impossible.

Once I'd finished reading, I felt sad for him, that he couldn't find a way back to life, but also horrified knowing that in 2020 he had collapsed and had to be airlifted by crane from a third-floor apartment by a team of more than thirty firefighters.

"That was the most devastating time of my life," he said.

"The terrifying part of it all was the amount of people outside. I did watch [the film] The Whale and it did feel like a horror movie to me. I said to my mum, don't watch it. I turned it off and I started crying.

"I cried myself to sleep at that film. It was very upsetting for me because now I thought I'm Britain's fattest man, that's what people are going to think of me," he added.

His words hammer home society's distaste for people who are overweight—the fact he had to be airlifted out of his home due to an emergency with crowds gawping says it all.

Rest In Peace, Jason Holton.

Syns used: 22.

May 7

Back to the gym this morning. It was closed yesterday for Bank Holiday.

Distance cycled today was 10.04 miles at level 6, burning 334 calories. I did this with ease and would have done much more but we had planned to go swimming.

Swimming – 8 lengths. Not sure how many calories I would have burned because I swam really slowly.

Total exercise time was 125 minutes.

Left the gym and went to Liverpool with my sister and my dad. Came home and ate a bowl of homemade soup, then varnished the garden table.

Got the fright of my life; Jon was trying to make an appointment with his GP and noticed an addition to his medical file. It basically said there was cancer in his bladder. He instantly went into panic mode, while I hid mine and tried to calm him down. He couldn't get any sense from the receptionist at the GP surgery, so I rang the hospital and spoke to his urologist's secretary, who confirmed it was an old note from the initial diagnosis a few years back. She confirmed that his latest round of tests and scans showed no cancer, and only a healthy bladder. Thank goodness. Apparently, when reports are sent from the hospital to the GP, they list the conditions in reverse, so it appeared the cancer had returned. Bloody stupid if you ask me and could upset a lot of people.

Went to bed with a thumping headache at 2 pm and woke up at 7 pm.

Had dinner at 9 pm in readiness for a catch up with my friend in California. I ate more than I wanted, which was nothing, and had a belly ache.

Syns used: 26.

May 8

Back to the gym.

I cycled 10.02 miles at level 6, managing to burn 338.9 calories in 53 minutes. Sweat was rolling off me, but I continued, wanting to hit the ten-mile mark. I aim to increase the miles to twenty per day in time.

Syns used: 26½.

May 9

Not going to the gym because I have a huge blister on my heel from my mammoth trek around Cheshire Oaks last week, and it doesn't seem to want to heal. I'm getting home from the gym with blood in my shoe, so taking a few days off should see it right. As it is a warm day, I finished painting the planters and arranged the patio with Jon.

Not feeling like solid food at the moment, so put on a pan of homemade vegetable soup.

May 10
WEIGH-IN DAY

I stood on the scales, desperately wanting to lose one pound, which will take me to a four stone loss and closer to target.

"6½ OFF," Shelly told me with a smile. "And you've got your four stone award."

To say I was thrilled is an understatement, and while it is an amazing result, that pesky ½ pound keeps me from target. But in total, I have now lost 4 Stone, 5½ pounds.

I was also awarded Slimmer of the Week, and though proud of myself, I do get embarrassed when the group cheers me on. But it is amazing to have that support, especially from Donna and my fellow classmates. The plan really does work, and I am on my way to target, and then the next phase of my journey begins.

Stuck to plan, especially knowing that tomorrow I am having a little party for the Eurovision Song Contest.

Jon has made chocolate and vanilla cupcakes and even though he asked me if I wanted one, I declined, but even looking at them, I can see the Syns practically oozing out of them.

May 11

Tonight is the annual Eurovision Song Contest, so it is an excuse to throw a little soiree—me, Jon, my sister, and friend. I have already told myself I am not sticking to plan, and seeing the mound of goodies on offer, I don't stand a chance.

But I am not going to be hard on myself—I have stuck to plan almost religiously since March 5th, and as Donna keeps reminding us, we are human.

I will hop back on plan first thing Monday with a trip to the gym (hard work will be urgently required), but thankfully, I am not at weigh-in next week as I have pre-existing appointments. So, I have a little extra time to undo any damage I might do.

I will check in on Monday and be truthful about how far off plan I fell.

May 13

After a gluttonous weekend, I am back on plan this morning. I don't feel guilty. Why should I? I did it, now I move on knowing there are many more days this coming year where I will do what I need to do. I won't ace them all.

Breakfast was 3 x Shredded Wheat with skimmed milk: 3½ Syns plus HEXA & HEXB.

Saturday was the biggest blow out I have had in a long time, and I did say I would be honest about what I ate, so here goes...

1 x McDonald's Hamburger with onion and tomato sauce: 13 Syns.

5 x McDonald's Cheese & Herb Bites: 12 Syns.

Walkes Sensations Mature Cheddar & Chill Chutney Crisps: 72 Syns.

2 x Crusty rolls: 18 Syns.

2 x Mature Cheddar Cheese slices: 5 Syns.

M&S Deli-Style Coleslaw: 8½ Syns.

Chocolate Cake: I have no idea how to Syn it as my friend made it from scratch. Heaven on a plate though!

Trifle: 5 Syns.

BUBS (Sweets): I have no idea how to Syn these either.

Liquorice laces: 10 Syns.

1 x Baileys Colada: 4 Syns.

Total Syns used for Saturday = 147½, and that doesn't include what I can't find the Syn value for. I would triple the total, which is substantially more than my allotted 210 Syns per week.

On Sunday morning. I woke up feeling sluggish, exhausted, and sick, but I carried on stuffing my face anyway. Whilst I never ate as much as I did on Saturday, I still went crazier than normal.

3 x Crusty Cobs: 27 Syns.

Ham: Syn Free.

Salad: Syn Free.

2 x Mature Cheddar Cheese Slices: 5 Syns

M&S Deli-Style Coleslaw: 8½ Syns

Chocolate Cake: No idea!

BUBS (Sweets): I have no idea how to Syn these either.

Total Syns used for Saturday = 40½, which is a lot lower than yesterday. Still, there are items I cannot count. Without seeming dramatic, I wouldn't be surprised if I have swallowed 1000 Syns this past weekend. It is what it is, and I can't change it, nor will I fixate on it, but I am paying the price because this morning, I jumped out of bed, rushed to the toilet, and any concerns I had about being constipated soon shot down the pan as I sat for an hour squirming, remembering that awful feeling, that junk food makes me feel awful inside and out.

Looking back, did I enjoy being off plan and what I ate? No, I can't say that I did and while eating it I realised I hadn't missed it. But what I had missed was the idea of eating unchecked.

Anyway, new day, new week, and back to the gym.

I cycled 10.35 miles at level 7, burning 340.9 calories. I found this fairly easy and need to start upping miles cycled again.

Seated Leg Press – 60 presses.

Swimming – Baked alive in the gym, I was glad to jump into the pool, even if I did only manage a paltry two lengths before the mums with tums group forced us out.

Back from the gym, got changed then headed for my first sports massage in months. My neck has been very sore and stiff these last few weeks, so I need to book in more regularly. I was pleased my therapist's comments on how much weight I had lost. He was genuinely surprised by the results and congratulated me.

Dinner was Syn Free Chilli courtesy of Jon, followed by Lindahl Kvarg desserts (1 Syn). Neither tasted good when I threw the lot back up. Note to self; STOP eating rice.

I felt a bit peckish later on so had 3 x Shredded Wheat with Skimmed Milk: 10½ Syns plus HEXA.

Total Syns used today = 15.

May 14

A terrible night's sleep, which was to be expected after my sports massage. Every turn in the night was agony, so I skipped the gym. It wasn't helped by strange dreams of seeing myself lying in a hospital bed, comatose— but that's not the strangest part—this all took place in the middle of a Blockbuster store as customers were picking their DVD's and choosing what Ben & Jerry's Ice Cream to have as I lay there, aware but unable to talk to ask somebody to get me out of there. I have no clue what dreams mean, if anything, but my take on it is this; it was less Sleeping Beauty and more the fact I hate to be the centre of attention.

Got up, and although I didn't want food, I had breakfast anyway; 3 x Shredded Wheat with skimmed milk: 3½ Syns plus HEXA & HEXB. Then I put the ingredients for SW Rice Pudding in the slow cooker. I will eat this over the next few days. I have crafted my own recipe using semi-skimmed milk and have switched the sweetener granules for the tablets. If I want it any sweeter once cooked, I will sprinkle the granules on and count it that way.

Dinner is leftover chilli, but I will have fry light roast potatoes instead of rice. I don't fancy another night with my head hanging over toilet.

May 15

Still on plan, well not exactly, as I haven't used all of my Syns. But I am still feeling bloated from the weekend. I need to get back to it 100% because when I next get weighed on 24th May, I want to be closer to a five stone loss, and more importantly, at target.

Back to the gym.

12.01 miles cycled at level 6 with a burn of 397.9 calories. I could have continued, but Tammy had finished on the treadmill and hung over my shoulder.

Seated Leg Press – 40 presses. I wanted to do more, but the gym was suddenly heaving, and people were milling about, anxious to use the machines.

Total workout time was 40 Minutes.

Came home and had 3 x Shredded Wheat with skimmed milk for breakfast. I followed that with 2 x Lindahl Kvarg yoghurts.

I skipped lunch because I had not long eaten, and thoroughly enjoyed homemade chicken and vegetable soup for dinner.

Flumps made a reappearance, as did fresh fruit with fat free quark to round out the day.

May 16

Still on plan, and back to the gym but it wasn't my best effort today.

A paltry 7.36 miles managed at level 6 with 242 calories burned. I simply couldn't do any more and struggled to get this far. Disappointed, but I have to listen to my body.

Seated Leg Press – 40 presses. I really struggled with this but persevered for as long as I could.

I was in agony when I got home, and my neck had locked so I couldn't turn my head. I took a strong painkiller and went to bed, exhausted and miserable.

Hash browns, homemade chicken and vegetable soup today with Lindahl Kvarg yoghurts. I scoffed down two bags of crisps because it was easy, but I didn't fall off plan. I would have preferred something healthier, but needs must when I can't be bothered eating, or cooking. Jon offered to make me dinner, but I declined.

Syns used: 20, and now I am going back to bed.

May 17
WEIGH-IN DAY

No weigh-in today because I have two hospital appointments. But I am eager to know how much damage I did last weekend, or whether I got away with it. Whatever happens, I will be at class next week in the hope of losing that ½ pound, which will take me to target.

Hospital was a waste of time; just to be told they can do nothing to help my fibro and that the recommended medication they could give me only works for one in twenty-five people—I will try it, but I don't hold out any hope. So, I plod on...

Still on plan. I cooked beef goulash with fry light roast potatoes, cauliflower, and green beans, which was all Syn Free. Filled myself up with flumps, yoghurts and shredded wheat with semi-skimmed milk.

May 18

The sun is shining, so I got stuck into some maintenance in the back garden. Boring. How my dad and brothers do this sort of stuff day in, and day out baffles me. Bad luck, or perhaps good luck, I ran out of wood filler so that brought an end to that. Tomorrow I will go and buy more and finish the job.

Cooked breakfast and ate it on the garden table with Jon.

May 20

Still on plan. Back to the gym this morning.

A more respectable 10.37 miles cycled today at level 7 with 355.6 calories burned. Sweat rolled off me and I seemed to spend the duration of the session dabbing at my face with my towel.

Seated Leg Press – 120 presses. I found this quite easy today, even though I did get off walking like I'd just got off a horse.

Syns used today = 29½, which is quite a lot, but I did top them up with crisps and marshmallows.

May 21

Shattered when I woke up but dragged myself out of bed to go to the gym.

10.72 miles today at level 7 and another 372.8 calories shed. Once again, I sweated profusely.

Seated Leg Press – 60 presses. I could definitely feel the burn when I got off this.

Came home to change my T-shirt, then went to the garden centre with Jon, Tammy and my dog, Sammy. He had never been there before, so he was fascinated with new surroundings and wanted to wander. It's one of the most boring places for me, and Jon turns into a dragon, annoyed by the fact I choose anything with colour—I'm not a fan of a green garden if you get what I mean, whereas he knows the names of all plants and when they flower. I don't care as long as there are pops of colour everywhere.

Took the plants home then went to get my haircut and beard trimmed. As soon as I got out of the car, I felt like I'd been hit by a bus. Instantly, I felt nauseous and devoid of energy. Sitting in the chair, I could easily have fallen asleep, but waited until I got home, when I went to bed for five hours.

Homemade vegetable soup came courtesy of Jon, and I felt a lot better.

Syns used today = 23½. It's been a struggle, and I topped those up with crisps and marshmallows again. Still, nothing to feel guilty for because I have had my five vegetables today, fruit, and eaten my healthy extras.

May 22

Up and out for the gym.

Mother, and Gran in-law due to visit today. They are bringing Jon's brother, Adam, because he is moving back to New Zealand, the place he considers home, next week, so it's kind of a goodbye as we don't know when we will see him again.

We had a nice afternoon. All but Adam is following SW, so lunch was Syn Free. But it was bittersweet for Jon, who was very upset saying farewell to his little brother. I wish him all the luck in the world.

Syns used = 23½.

May 23

Not going to the gym today as Jon has a medical appointment, but the weather is so awful, for once I was glad not to have to go out.

The downside is, without my mind occupied and focused, I want to eat everything, and by everything, I mean the seventeen easter eggs still on my shelf and the fifty crème eggs in my freezer.

But I don't. Instead I tell myself not to undo all the hard work I have put in, and that tomorrow could mean I reach my goal. With that mindset, I am nervous. What if I've gained? I know I had a pre-booked couple of days off two weeks ago, but I've been on plan before then, and since. If I have there is always next week, but I don't mind admitting, I am nervous.

May 24
WEIGH-IN DAY

Could today be the day?
As a non-believer, I don't pray but I wouldn't mind whatever help is out there right now. If somebody is listening, please move those scales in the right direction.
Pooping myself because this could be a day to celebrate or anti-climactic.
With just ½ pound to get to target, that small amount would mean so much.
I just got back, and drum roll...
Weighing in at 17 stone, 12 pounds, and with a loss of 2½ pounds...

I DID IT!

After a rollercoaster journey, I finally hit my personal target weight.

MIRACLES DO HAPPEN!

CONGRATULATIONS TO ME!

Yes, I could have gotten here a lot sooner, but I did it my way, which isn't exactly the right way. But it worked for me, and when I did finally realise that I had to follow the plan wholeheartedly, I know that valuable lessons had been learned.
Even though there were times I thought I would give in, I knew I had to hold on. I put my faith in the plan, hoping that if I summoned strength from deep within myself, more than I ever dreamed possible, victory would be mine.
I won't lie and say it wasn't a quiet, reflective, emotional, deeply satisfying, and gratifying moment because it was, and now I'm here, as well as pride, I take a deep breath, in readiness because my journey is not over, nor will it ever be.
For those who may be confused, when I joined *Slimming World*, I specified the weight I would be happy with in the short term, but as good as I think that I look and feel right now, I have more work to do. And, yes, I could maintain

this weight, but according to the pesky BMI, I am still obese, and I completely agree, but won't drop to their suggested number. I have another leg of the journey to navigate before I slip into the healthy category.

So, closing this book, opens another, which I have cheekily titled, 'YOU'RE FAT, STOP EATING'. Due for release at the close of 2025, it will journal the final leg of this journey, which is to lose another four stone.

Why don't you join me... https://geni.us/ck173

While some might gasp, I am setting vanity aside, knowing that I must do everything I can to look after myself, especially now I am dealing with chronic illness.

Maybe I'm crazy, I probably am, but I've come so far that I really think the endgame can be achieved.

So, right here is where I sign off, for now.

But before I go...

I wrote this book about *my* experiences, about how hard losing weight, and keeping it off, is, but also to try and shine a positive light on those people battling alongside me. And to the reader, struggling or not, I hope that you can see that our individual and collective journeys are always going to be fraught and fantastic, filled with ups, downs and all that comes in between.

As human beings, we have the capacity to bury our heads in the sand, but there's no escaping what needs to be done if something is worth achieving. It won't be easy—and that's okay because that's life and who said it's meant to be a walk in the park?

You have seen a snapshot of my life over an almost three-year period, and snippets from so many other wonderful people, and for joining the joyride, I thank you.

I can't put my pen down without conveying my eternal gratitude to those wonderful people who shared their story within these pages—Sofia, Sarah-Jane, Ruth, Danny, Alison, Leigh, Dave, & Maggie Jane—I know how hard it was for them to give so much of themselves.

Digging deep into oneself, facing the truth, then allowing strangers a ringside seat is harder than you might think, but they did so with humility, grace, style, and aplomb... you are all superstars in my eyes.

I remain positive that our readers have taken inspiration from you all sharing that part of yourself.

The lovely ladies on the scales, and in no particular order—Shelly, Dawn, Helen, Debbie, Julie, Marie, Neeta, Rachel, Lin, Alana, Ruth, Ursulla, Vicki, Margie & Wendy... thank you for your kindness and encouragement, and more importantly, your ability to see our ups and down without judgement, while only showering us with compassion and understanding.

A special mention must go to the lady that has kept me on track even when she probably wanted to shake some sense into me. Take a bow, Donna Wade, leader of our tribe. Thank you for sharing your story because there will be many who are inspired by you, just as I am. For your support, guidance and patience, you have my eternal gratitude. I'm not the only one who feels this way, and rightly so.

It is my sincere hope that whoever picks this book up is inspired, buoyed, and comforted by the knowledge that we all know the fight and feel lifted to that place where they feel able to start, continue, or re-start their journey— we are not alone because we will always be a part of this community.

And even though we might be at opposite ends of the country, on far flung continents, or at different stages in this lifelong journey, we stand united, and from me personally, I wish you all love, light, health, and happiness.

See you on life's highway, my friends.

Yours in solidarity...

Marco Lewis

Acknowledgements

To Jon – we're almost thirteen years in and that doesn't happen for nothing. Ours is a true and real love, and I wouldn't want to be without you… forever and a day, I love you, Marco xxx

To Maggie Jane Schuler – your guidance has been worth its weight in gold. Thank you for helping me shape this book into something I am proud of, and for sharing your story. I look forward to meeting you for cocktails in the near future xxx

To Tammy – my sister, and diet comrade. I remember mum laughing and saying she had two fatties and two skinnies (LOL – cheek, we know what side she placed us on), so if anyone in my life understands where I am coming from, it is definitely you. You're my only sister, and I count myself lucky you joined me on this journey. Love you very much xxx

To Sofia Athanasiou – Your story highlighted your struggles working in the industry that you love. Your beauty and grace shines through and I am not the only person to see that. Thank you for sharing your world with us.

To Sarah-Jane Dalton – You were terrified to share your story, but I am so happy that you gave me a chance because your life has been quite remarkable and will inspire those who read this book. Thank you.

To Ruth Gort – A classy lady who embodies kindness. From your endless support on the *Slimming World* group page to sharing your own journey, the world needs more people like you. Thank you.

To Danny Mainwaring – I am rarely shocked, but your story stumped me. I struggle to imagine how you are still standing, but you are. Please know there is so much for you to look forward to, and that the past should remain there. I thank you for sharing part of yourself and know you will emerge victorious.

To Alison Moreton. How long has it been? We met when you were a leader for *Weight Watchers*, and your support was invaluable. We even spent an unforgettable night crossing a Cliff Richard concert off our bucket lists, and a night surrounded by screaming women waving their bloomers has got to bond two people (LOL). I am so happy you get to pass on your knowledge to members of *Slimming World* now.

To Leigh Sheldon – Thank you for sharing your story with us. I know life has been difficult these last few years, but you will get there, I know it.

To Dave Sellman – It took a while, but we finally got there. Your story is invaluable and offers another perspective about the struggle with weight. Thank you for sharing it with us.

To Donna Wade – I feel like I've known you forever and getting to know you that little bit better whilst doing this book, I see that we are spookily similar. I thought you didn't like me, but I see it now—you only have so much to give of yourself because there are so many people in your life who need a piece of you. You do a fantastic job for so many, thank you.

To my team of beta readers, Gloria, Michelle, Sue, Shirley, Janet & Paula – Your help was invaluable. Thank you.

To all the others I've met along the way, the good, the bad and the different. You're all part of my journey and it wouldn't have been the same without you.

Help is available when you want it.

If you are struggling with your weight, in the first instance visit your General Practitioner for help and advice:
Or find a weight loss organisation that works for you.
I am not advocating for any of the below organisations but have added their links because they are featured in the book and have been a part of my journey.

Slimming World https://www.slimmingworld.co.uk/
Weight Watchers: https://www.weightwatchers.com
LighterLife: https://www.lighterlife.com
Overeaters Anonymous: https://www.oa.org
Overeaters Anonymous (Find a Meeting): https://oa.org/find-a-meeting/?type=0

If, like me, you suffer from Fibromyalgia and ME / CFS, there are places that can offer support. In the first instance visit your General Practitioner for help and advice:

FIBROMYLAGIA RESEARCH GROUP (FACEBOOK): https://www.facebook.com/groups/753322534769373
CFS Support: https://www.cfshealth.com
ME ASSOCIATION https://meassociation.org.uk/
NHS BMI Calculator: https://www.nhs.uk/health-assessment-tools/calculate-your-body-mass-index/calculate-bmi-for-adults

GYMS & CLUBS

If you are not a fan of the gym, but force yourself to go, please don't lose that motivation to exercise because there are other options available:

PURE GYM: https://www.puregym.com
FITNESS FIRST: https://www.fitnessfirst.co.uk/
CLUBBERCISE: https://www.clubbercise.com/home
ZUMBA: https://www.zumba.com/en-US

If you would like to join a gym, contact your local authority for information on their memberships.

ABOUT THE AUTHOR

Marco Lewis lives in the Northwest of England with his long-term partner.

Working as a full-time writer since 2017, his creative mind has taken him in many directions, from writing Chewing the Fat, to crime fiction, horror and supernatural releases under his pseudonym, Marcus Brown.

For more information or just to touch base with Marco, you will find him at:

MORE FROM MARCO LEWIS

Find all my titles here:

MORE FROM MARCUS BROWN

Marcus Brown is the pen name of Marco Lewis.

From horror, to supernatural, and crime fiction, there is plenty to sink your teeth into.

Find me here:

Copyright © 2024 Marco Lewis / Marcus Brown
All rights reserved.

Printed in Great Britain
by Amazon

REAL ESTATE
UNFILTERED

HOW TO BECOME A
REAL ESTATE HIGH ROLLER

TATIANA LONDONO

Real Estate Unfiltered
How to Become a Real Estate High Roller
Author: Tatiana Londono
Published by: Tatiana Londono
All rights reserved. No part of this book may be reproduced or transmitted in any form or by any means, electronic or mechanical, including photocopying, recording or by any information storage and retrieval system, without written permission from the author, except for the inclusion of brief quotations in a review.
Copyright © 2017 by Tatiana Londono
First Edition, 2017
Published in Canada

I would like to dedicate this book to my parents. You are and forever will be my role models. To my father who is fearless and always encouraged me to take risks, thank you for inspiring me to think outside the box. To mother, your uncompromising work ethic and stoic nature have inspired me endlessly. I thank you both for your brave and selfless decision to move to Canada from Colombia. You gave me and Alex a future, and for that we are grateful.

To my beautiful children who were patient and understanding during the progression of my career. My love for you is fierce and unconditional. Know always that this is all for you.

To Oren, thank you for your loyalty and partnership - it has been invaluable.

To my brother Alex who believed in me when I didn't.

And to my wonderful David - your love, devotion and patience are appreciated more than you know.

Acknowledgements

I want to say thank you to:

Sunny Clarke and Allison Robins for all your hard work helping me with this book.

Philip Faith for the beautiful cover shots.

Phil Baker for his infinite patience and help.

Alex Londono for managing this project and making sure it reached completion.

Table of Contents

Introduction 13

    Tatiana, Unfiltered 18

    Dream Job! 21

    Real Estate Unfiltered 25

I. MASTER YOUR MINDSET 30

    Attitude Is Your Best Property 30

    Money Matters 32

    Awareness Inspires Your Development 33

    Rule #1 – Build Your Mental Frame 35

    Action steps: 36

    Rule #2 – Define Your Version of Success 39

    Action Steps: 42

    Rule #3 – Speak, Think, and Act Towards What You Want 44

    Rule #4 – Learn from Your Past Performance While Starting Every Day Fresh 49

    Rule #5 – Mindset Sets Your Image 51

    Action Steps: 53

    Key Points from Chapter One: 54

II. SEEING IS BELIEVING 56

Cruise Control Your Universe 56

Visualization 57

Set the Scene, Seize the Day 59

Meditate Into Your New Success 60

Attitude of Gratitude 61

Language 62

Overstating Your Case 64

Control Your Attention 66

Mental Dieting 66

Speak No Evil 67

Triple Play 69

Naming Names and Talking Numbers ... 72

Behavior Action Steps 72

III. BODY BASICS BOOTCAMP 74

Stress Will Test 75

Tat's Neuro Chemical Management Hacks: Succeed with Hits of Nature's Daily Dose 76

Your Image Management 81

Goals, Gear and Good Workouts 82

Tat's Top Six Get Fit Facts 83

Have a Ball with Budget Fitness 85
Sleep Deprivation and You 87
Body Basics Action Steps 89

IV. GOING FOR THE GOALS 91
Strategy Trumps Tactics 91
SMART Goals 91
W5 Goal Assessments 92
Strategy 94
Goal Worksheets 96
Goaltenders and Goalkeepers 99
Goal Setting 101
Goal Action Steps 103

V. REAL ESTATE 101 FOR HIGH ROLLERS 105
Real Estate Sales is a Full-Time Business ... 106
COMMITMENT is the reason why Realtors make big bucks! 108
Action Plan 116
Get in the Phone and Email Zone 117
ANSWER THE PHONE!! Double Ended Commission from a Sunday Call 119
Lunch is for Losers 121

VI. REAL ESTATE ABC'S 124
    Be in the Game 126
    Delegation is Your Duty 129
    Tat's Quick Tips 131
    Finance Facts.. 133
    Cash in on Coaching 136
    Capital 139
    List to Last 141
    Listing Agents Own the Market................... 141
    Making Dollars and Sense of Long Listings. 142
    The Price is Right 144
    Recap of Action Plan 146

VII. THE REAL ESTATE PROSPECTOR'S GUIDE TO GOLD DIGGING AND FIRST TIER MARKETING 149
    Digging for Gold 150
    Cold Callers Make Dollars 151
    Money Grows Like Trees............................ 154
    Prospecting Prep 154
    For Sale by Owner (FSBO) 158
    Network Your Way to Net Worth 160
    Schmoozapalooza 162

Network Notes 164

Professional Contacts 166

Reputation Redux 167

Ethics vs. Unemployment 167

Taking the Crazy with the Cream 169

Listen like a Pro 170

Tat's Tips for Active Listening 170

Networking Opportunities 173

Chambers of Commerce 174

National Real Estate Investor Association ... 175

Event Hosting Gives Value and Increases Authority 175

Education Nation 176

Networking Groups 177

Full of Facebook 178

VIII. HIGH ROLLER MARKETING 180

Marketing Choices 180

Introduction to Marketing by Alex Londono 181

How to Qualify Leads 183

The High Roller Marketing System 184

Unbranded Advertising 184

Celebrity Branded Advertising 186
Creating Content 187
Celebrity Video Marketing 189
    Types of Videos 190
Celebrity Branding with Photography 193

IX. REALTOR SOFTWARE FOR SUCCESS 196
Tracking Contacts with a Customer Relationship Management (CRM) Tool 196
Automation Software for Engaging and Following Up with Your Database 200

X. GETTING TO THE TOP AND HELPING OTHERS JOIN YOU 204
    Looking for Answers 205
    Integrating the Answers 207
    Developing Success Momentum 208
Shifting Priorities from Income to Impact 211
Achievement Levels Help Decide Your Charity Levels 213
Helping Others! 214
Your Turn to Create a Legacy 215
Recommended Reading 217
Bibliography 219

About the Author 222
Contact Information 225

REAL ESTATE UNFILTERED

How to Become a Real Estate High Roller
TATIANA LONDONO

Real estate is one of the few professions in which you go to school to earn a license, yet they don't actually teach you how to be a real estate agent. Like any top performer, to become a Real Estate High Roller, you need a coach.

Learn the methods that put me at the top of the real estate profession, with billions of dollars in sales, coaching thousands of realtors and even starring in my own hit television show, HGTV's The Property Shop. We live in an age when realtors can be rock stars – follow these steps and you can become a high-rolling real estate rock star, just like me!

Tatiana Londono
Billion Dollar Broker Sales Coach

Introduction

As a first-generation Canadian from a working-class, immigrant family, the experiences of my early years shaped my life and fueled my ambition. Each member of my small family worked long hours to make ends meet. We worked as housekeepers and kitchen staff, held yard sales for extra funds and managed micro-businesses, all to ensure the possibility of a bright future.

My ambition for what I knew I could become, and the work ethic I learned that allowed me to achieve my vision, were both heavily influenced by my always- devoted and tenacious parents.

My father came to Canada from Colombia with imaginative ideas and big dreams; however he did not have a clear plan of how to turn them into reality. He and my mother were married by proxy while he was in Canada and she was in Colombia.

Many months later, while my father was working as a dishwasher, my mother arrived in Canada, and they settled in the Greater Toronto Area of Scarborough.

My mother worked all throughout my upbringing, maintaining a steady paycheck while my father sought to build our fortunes through various business ventures. Like many immigrants, my parents were selfless in ensuring that my brother Alexander and I attended good schools in order to prepare us for what would be our upward journey on the ladder of success.

When I was 11 years old, my father dreamed of returning to his homeland, feeling hopeful that things would be different. So, we moved back to Colombia for the short time of two years, but upon the realization that some things do not change, we moved back to Canada and settled in Montreal, where I currently reside.

During that brief stay in Colombia, it was challenging for me to attend school in a country where I didn't speak the language, but I adapted. I knew only basic Spanish; however that didn't stop my parents from enrolling me in a native Spanish-language school. I had to sink or swim on my own. My tenacity towards conquering the language and facing cultural challenges helped me navigate that period of my life successfully.

By the age of 14, I had lived in three different cultures, speaking three separate languages, the last being French in Montreal. I learned to read body language out of necessity, as I struggled to learn foreign words. Most importantly, I learned to think on my feet and to react effectively in unexpected situations. The same ability is reflected now in how I negotiate on the fly in complex situations with all kinds of people – even when there are linguistic barriers.

My brother and I were always close with our parents; they taught us how we can control our life and overcome challenges. They encouraged us to stand on our own and to make decisions with long term goals in mind.

From my mother, I learned both gratitude and a focused, around-the-clock work ethic. My father fueled my ambition, encouraging me to become who I wanted to be despite how impossible it seemed. He taught me to stand up for myself, always defend my ideas, and follow my own path, a value system that I now imbue in my own children.

I am eternally grateful to my parents for nurturing the foundation of my eventual success and helping to solidify my firm sense of self. They have completely opposing personalities that, melded together, created the traits within me which determined my life choices and ultimately my business model.

My father is a dreamer. He always took enormous risks, because it's better to dream big and fail at times than to dream small due to fear of failure. While sometimes his grandiose dreams had negative effects on our family, he was a sincere and generous person, always eager to help those in less fortunate situations than his own. Sometimes, those people would prove they didn't deserve his help, but that never stopped him from trying to help the next person who came along.

My mother is more conservative and steadfast. She was always there to help support the family when my father's risks or generosity left him without a paycheck. Through their opposite approaches towards people and business, I developed my own thoughts around money and security. Namely, how hard it can be to make money, and how easy it is to lose it.

I have certainly taken risks in my life, just as my father has. I dream big, but the more skeptical filter I learned from my mother has made me look before I leap and understand that not everyone has pure intentions. Their two personality types have shaped my own, one tempering the other.

Much like my parents, I too worked hard to earn money in my youth. My brother and I were born entrepreneurs. We started small with lemonade and ice cream stands on the weekends, and by the time I was seven years old, I was running my own garage sales, successfully.

The only real problem with my sales activities was that not all of the items I sold belonged to me. Some of the items at my garage sales belonged to other members of the family, like my mother's wallet for example, which didn't go over well. I was just so anxious that I would sell whatever I found in my environment. It was such an intense force within me; I would even sell my own things for less than their value, at first, simply for the experience. I was educating myself on how to sell, sell, and sell! A strong entrepreneurial spirit is great when it comes to finding unique ways to make money. A downside is that the same drive can make it difficult to work for anyone else. My brother, Alex, and I were always determined to do things our own way. Opening our own business seemed inevitable.

Just as my upbringing had a tremendous influence on my business ability, so did the employment I pursued before becoming a real estate agent.

Tatiana, Unfiltered

When I was 19, I signed up for a stint in the military. That year had a lasting impact on me. The military taught me about discipline and ingrained within me the unwavering belief that you really can accomplish anything you set your mind to. It also taught me how to push my body to limits that I never thought possible.

While in the army, I got into the best shape of my life and ate ravenously the whole time. I was fit, young and felt ready to realize my potential. After boot camp, during my regiment's final drills, I actually picked up a guy much bigger than me and ran with him over my head in a simulated rescue operation! I didn't even feel his weight. Suddenly I realized how far I had progressed physically and mentally, following months of exhaustive physical training.

I remember running with this guy in my arms – as if I was saving a fallen soldier's life. It was a rescue drill in front of drill sergeants, making it a pressure-filled exercise. Afterwards, I wondered how I could have possibly accomplished that. Overcoming this physical challenge showed me that I could do anything if I just let go of doubt.

The value of being fearless in the face of obstacles suddenly became crystal clear.

Another thing I vividly recall from my time in the army was rising daily at 4 a.m. to ensure that our environment was up to par with military standards in order to avoid the wrath of their authority. Typically, my all-female barracks enjoyed watching our male counterparts faint from standing for hours while forced to listen to some seemingly endless, boring harangue. It was part of our training to be able to endure. Many of those silly soldiers would rise from slumber at the last possible minute, trading breakfast for shut-eye, only to then pay the price, face down doing push-ups hours later.

One particularly gruesome day, the Master Corporal decided to give our barracks the infamous "white glove test" despite the dusty, old building we were housed in. Our beds were impeccable and our gear was perfectly arranged. You could practically eat off the aged floor.

Not to be outdone by a troop of girls, the Master Corporal rubbed an ivory finger across the outside of the window pane which, naturally, left its mark like a dirty trick. To express his disdain with the results, our dear Master Corporal next plucked my already pitiful mattress from the top bunk and tossed it right out that very same window. The dilapidated mattress hung outside all day, an affront to our troop and a guilty reminder to the whole company.

The lesson stuck with me to this day. A real estate deal can go the same way as that lumpy, old mattress ripped from its uppermost perch – one smear and your deal can easily go sailing right out the window!

I learned some important concepts living under military rule including one we have all heard before: do not sweat the small offenses and do not take anyone else's behavior personally. Instead of focusing on the things you can't control, always focus on what you can.

To give you a perspective on my work ethic, I usually held two jobs, sometimes three. I typically worked seven days a week while going to McGill University full time.

A few days a week I worked part time at the McGill bookstore or the Center for Women Studies, performing administrative duties. When I was not attending university, I was working at a call center dialing for commissions from 8 a.m. to 5 p.m., and then I would shift to the customer service center for a steady hourly paycheck from 5 p.m. to 8 p.m. Weekends would see me either lifeguarding or at the university bookstore. I became a call center manager after six months, remaining in the industry for nearly four years.

Eventually, I opened my own call center where I earned a hefty paycheck. Eventually changes in the law made the business very difficult to operate. Suddenly, I had gone from making a top 1% income, to making nothing. My husband and I lost everything in a hurry. I was desperate to turn my life around after this financial and personal downfall.

Dream Job!

I have always been thirsty to grow and excel, to become better than before. My entrepreneurial father challenged me to take my sales success to a bigger playing field and join him in the real estate profession. I was eager for the next level. I took the formal licensing training and my father taught me the ropes of what eventually became a family trade.

Many mindset trainers, sales coaches, and business mentors have helped me to create a successful business career. Pieces of their wisdom are sprinkled throughout this book. The one I consider to have been of enormous educational and motivational influence for me and my way of doing business is Tony Robbins. I am a firm believer in his teachings and in Neuro-Linguistic Programming (NLP) systems because they dramatically improved my performance and my career.

    I remember being inspired by Tony Robbins to write out exactly what I wanted. Once I had my goal set and the image of whom I was to become, the rest was putting my intentions and my faith into action.

    Family, mentors, gurus, friends, teachers, employers and clients; these are the people who have helped me become the person I am today. They each framed, inspired or shaped my real estate career and for each I am grateful! Achieving can feel scary at times because with success comes huge responsibility, but carrying the fearlessness I learned from my father, along with the perseverance of my mother and the support and encouragement of my family eases the transition. That kind of strength helps you to ignore naysayers and pursue dreams all the way to fruition. In fact, it's the reason for this book, in which I will teach the elements that will help you create and sustain your own fearless work ethic.

It was my fearless mindset and personality – some might say ballsy attitude or chutzpah – that helped me find my way onto HGTV. *The Property Shop* opened many doors for me, and while it was a lot of work, the show doubled my already substantial success!

The steps toward *The Property Shop* took a winding road that required dedication. It was just a few, short years ago that I was walking through Toronto's Yorkdale Mall when I received a phone call from a television production company asking whether I would agree to appear on an episode of *Buy Me*.

It soon became apparent that the producers were asking just about every successful agent in town. While most said no, not wanting to waste time on something offering no cash payment, I sensed the value of both publicity and stepping stones, so I decided to buck the naysayers and agreed. Though others had advised me against it, I took my own counsel and followed my instincts.

The audience responded well and I was soon after asked to appear on a second episode. Before long, Cineflix called and offered me the lead role on *Property Virgins* in Toronto.

    I balked initially because of the distance from Montreal and how that increased the time commitment, but decided instead to leverage the offer from *Property Virgins* into another opportunity. Hans Rosenstein of Whally-Abbey Media responded with a commitment that, at his next opportunity, he would produce a show for HGTV with myself in the lead role. I stayed in Montreal, waiting, after passing on *Property Virgins*, expecting even bigger and better things.

    True to his word, as always, just two months later, Hans propelled my career to the next level, paying me handsomely in the process. (Thank you, Hans and WAM!) I offered up the name for my new television show because I had wanted to use it as my company name, but had been prevented by local language laws. That turned out to be something of a blessing in disguise, because *The Property Shop* was perfect for a new HGTV program.

    Filming *The Property Shop* was a truly wonderful experience. Even though the crew would follow me around all day and there was pressure coming from many sides simultaneously during tapings, I reveled in the challenge. The rewards are still flowing in from this intense period of my life.

Just as I did, you can learn to fearlessly achieve your goals by developing the right state of mind and applying a winning formula. You may not have a family history like mine or army training, but by reading this book you can learn how to use the strategies that worked for me and apply them to your own unique life situations. While everyone has a different starting point, we all wish for a similar sort of happy ending and there are steps and tools you can take to make it possible. And, of course, my whole team of experts, including my wonderful, long- term business partners, Oren Pinto and Alex Londono are always on the cutting edge of the industry and weighing in with their own expert advice.

Real Estate Unfiltered

Like most of us, I've learned a lot from my success, yet even more from my mistakes. I teach real estate agents the plainspoken, unvarnished truth about working smart to achieve their financial goals. I do so by highlighting what I have learned in my career that works, but also pointing out the pitfalls. Choose to learn the easy way in a day or two from an experienced billion-dollar broker, rather than from making mistakes the hard way.

Why waste time trying a bunch of strategies to see what sticks? The only shortcut that works if you want to be successful is to follow an expert's template. Any other shortcut works against your own best interests and wastes your most precious resource: time.

Everything you need to do to become a *Real Estate High Roller* is simple and step by step. It is not, however, easy. Achieving your most elevated dream of financial and business success is possible when you follow a proven path. You can do it. I am here to show you the way.

Absorb every scrap of information from this book that you can and put it to use immediately. Take the necessary steps laid out from beginning to end. With clear goals, a plan, diligence and the right mindset, anyone can accomplish what others may deem impossible.

From starting fresh faced and broke, recently divorced with two young children to support, I reached my original goal and more.

I am now the owner of a real estate agency called Londono Realty Group with a crew of top performing agents. I am also an active realtor, a real estate coach to thousands of up-and-coming realtors, and love living and breathing real estate every minute. It is far more than my job, it is my passion. Many of the people I coach in my *High Roller* and Master classes are real estate agents reaching for more in their careers. Much of the information in this book is tailored toward realtors, yet anyone in sales will benefit financially by employing the same or very similar elements to achieve *High Roller* rewards.

My proven system has already empowered over a thousand agents to become the best realtors they can be. With this book, you can be trained like one of my agents to join the top tier of business success.

I hire new agents, fresh out of local real estate school, as well as experienced agents. My company policy is to then mentor a real estate agent until they are ready to go out on their own. Londono Realty Group has become well-known for how we train and nurture our real estate agents. We are more like a family than a corporation.

Over time I've learned that I love sharing my knowledge and experience to help agents grow. Even after *The Property Shop* stopped airing, people still sought us out for our unique training. This book is a culmination of my experiences and the content of my training and webinars. Wherever you are, this template fits your local market. Selling real estate is the business of helping people with one of the most important transitions in life. I have the constant privilege of helping people find their dream homes. And now, I have the privilege of sharing how I have become a luminary in this glorious profession.

When you achieve a certain level of success and financial returns at my agency, usually over $120k in commissions, you achieve the status of a *High Roller*. Becoming a *High Roller* suggests that you have reached the top 10% of realtors. There are plenty of realtors earning over $1M in commissions per year and there is every reason to believe that you can join them as another member of the elite *High Roller* club.

Few professions offer the *High Roller* stakes and rewards that real estate does. Large sums of money are intrinsic to property trading for everyone involved in the transaction. Getting to that magical point when a transaction is about to be consummated, where all the details come into place and you are about to collect on your efforts, is show time for a realtor. This moment is the culmination of advanced training, following a proven formula, and taking the necessary action to put all the ideas into practice. Now you know how I got here and what you need to do to get to the top as well. Let's get rolling!

I. MASTER YOUR MINDSET

"Success is not the key to happiness. Happiness is the key to success. If you love what you are doing, you will be successful."
-Albert Schweitzer, Physician, Theologian, Nobel Laureate

Attitude Is Your Best Property

Location! Location! Location! is a familiar real estate declaration, yet contrary to popular belief, property sales result more from the agents who close the deals than they do from mere location. Sure, there are some markets that will sell almost no matter what, but those are few and far between. Deals are dashed with an undeniable regularity in every location in town whether good, bad, or ugly by unsuccessful realtors. Meanwhile, successful realtors are closing sales in all of the same neighborhoods, mostly by applying a different attitude.

"Your mind is powerful beyond imagining. In fact, your mindset is the cornerstone of all of your power."
-Tatiana Londono

Scaling new horizons begins with a finely-tuned mind and gathers momentum through diligent effort. Success results from a carefully cultivated attitude and systematically applied knowledge. Knowing your business and conveying that you are the master of real estate in your marketplace forms the foundation from which sales are made. Your first order of business is to learn your business, and then to develop your brand. To accomplish both of these tasks, you need the mindset of a *High Roller*.

A well-formulated mindset and unadulterated hard work pave the path to real estate riches. No matter where you are starting from in your journey, the resilience and strength of your own mind will narrate your future. Just like physical toning, exercising for a healthy mind creates energy and generates positive results. Your newly superior mind will be empowered to help you build your dream career in real estate.

A healthy intellect, unshakeable determination, consistent effort, and a truly positive attitude are my primary traits that helped me skyrocket ahead of other realtors.

In this first chapter, I cover the mindset shifts required for becoming a top realtor. Only after you have firmly planted these mental behaviors into your own psyche will you be in a position to apply the detailed strategies from the ensuing chapters.

Money Matters

"Money is portable power."
-Tony Robbins

Money can be part of building your attitude. Cash is king, with credit for its loyal queen. You can only fulfill a goal of financial security if you embrace wealth. As success guru Tony Robbins so succinctly puts it:

"80% of wealth is psychology and 20% is mechanics."

That has proven true for me. I'm here to teach you the mechanics of building sales and real estate wealth, but all these steps have to be executed with the right mindset to leverage your way to success.

By now, you might be grasping the invaluableness of why forming an empowering mindset sets the basis for achievement. We're going to cover the details of mindset building beginning from the state where most people start: without consciously deciding upon their mindset and going with whatever pops into their heads.

There is no theory or fluff in what follows because I have focused on the key elements that work. You can add more to these steps, but I recommend not eliminating any of them until you cement your new mental approach.

I presume you picked up this book because you want the most out of your real estate career. You want the most money you can possibly make, along with respect from your peers and your community as a leader in the field. You may also want to build your own high profit, high performance real estate agency. I completely relate to where you are because those were the thoughts that drove me to work more efficiently by developing techniques that moved me towards goals we almost certainly share.

This brief list of potential goals for your career all depends on one critical, and often ignored aspect of performance: make sure your mindset is serving you and not stifling you.

Awareness Inspires Your Development

By simply being aware of how important your state of mind is, you have already made a huge leap. Whether you are the top performer in your area or wondering if you're going to ever get another commission check, your mindset is producing the results. Like a master chef hidden in the kitchen, your mind is creating your life as a feast or as burnt leftovers. My goal is to get you into the routine of mindset development by first accepting how important attitude of the mind is. Reading about mindset starts you on the journey. From this moment onward, know that your first mission every day is pointing your mind in the right direction.

Congratulate yourself on learning the number one lesson that separates the top realtors or professionals in any field, from those that never reach their potential: our mind state defines our future.

Once you catch the mindset development bug, just like I have, your future performance is going to take a sharp turn towards superstardom. I know this to be true, because it is exactly what happened to me. I have also seen many of my coaching clients as well as employees turn their performance around when they address their mindset challenges.

Let's get you started on your new path with a mindset that knocks down walls, builds relationships, and fills your pockets with gold.

Rule #1 – Build Your Mental Frame

I started my real estate career with my back up against the proverbial wall financially. That on its own would have been a tough enough situation, but I had two children to feed as well.

Admittedly, I was depressed and scared before my father convinced me to try working in real estate. Being in a situation where you are not exactly sure what to do, but you know you need to do something, is incredibly stressful. You can probably relate to stress like this in some area of your life.

Once I agreed to take my father's suggestion and get my real estate license, I realized I did not just want to be successful. I had to be successful. There was no other option for me. I set the mission in my mind that no matter what kind of effort it took, what I had to learn, or what obstacles I had to overcome, I was on the success train. Nothing, and no one, was going to stop me.

This was the beginning of my "success is mine" state of mind. My mind state has always been the starting point of my success. Technology changes. Markets change. Your mindset, however, must always be pointed in the right direction as your secret weapon.

Your success is also based on developing the correct attitude with your own mindset. Simply acknowledging that your mindset is critical for your success puts you in charge.

Often, when I am coaching other realtors or mentoring one of my many agents, I find that students want tips, techniques and strategies for selling real estate. Learning advanced strategies and techniques for areas like digital marketing in real estate are unquestionably important. They are important though, after you get your mindset in the correct lane for success.

Here is how you can move from a state of not consciously guiding your mindset into a state of guaranteeing powerful energy.

Action steps:

1. Set aside time to develop your state of mind in the morning and in the evening. I include my mindset routine, which I will detail later, in my morning walk or run. When I return home at night, I take at least 10 minutes to show gratitude for my day, and rebuild my mindset from any blows I might have taken. I devote 10 minutes each morning and night to get into the mind state of achievement. Not a lot to ask for a process that will reshape your life.

2. Adopt the attitude of "Success is Mine."
During my brief time in the army, I never heard either an officer or an enlisted person say "I will try to…hit the target, try to carry the soldier on my shoulders, try to pass a test, or try to complete any other task assigned." Either you gave everything you had and achieved the results expected of you, or there were severe penalties if for some reason you fell short. Banish the word "try" from your vocabulary. You are now of the mindset that you will do whatever it takes legally and honestly to achieve your top performance. Success is now yours once you set your sights firmly on the crown. Adopting this mindset is more than mere words.

When you are confronted with challenges, you will now respond differently than the 80% of realtors who never reach their potential. If you do not have enough leads to prospect with, you take the responsibility of finding some immediately. If you lost a listing you thought you had sewn up, you forget about it and move on to get five better listings.

You become an unstoppable force. Keep the words "Success is Mine" or whatever close version resonates with you, imprinted on your mind at all times, especially in stressful situations.

When you are backed into a corner financially and cannot afford marketing, remember: success is yours. You will find some way to make success happen. Until you feel this attitude in your bones, you will not know how much potential you really have. Once you sell yourself on this key mindset, then your potential is completely unlimited.

3. Write everything down and create a routine of affirmations, gratitude, and visualizing your success. Small doses of mindset training are helpful, but they are not transformative. It would be wonderful if one dose of affirmations, or expressing gratitude or visualizing was all you needed to remake your mind forever. But that would be like brushing your teeth or bathing just once and expecting to done for good.

Consistency is your secret weapon. Be consistent in reciting your affirmations over weeks, months, and then years. Your affirmations will burrow deep into your conscious thought patterns. Then, these magic words of positivity will nestle into your subconscious. You will become your affirmations.

The start of consistency is writing down a formal mindset routine that you will engage in for 10 minutes in the morning and 10 minutes in the evening.

It seems almost comical that a 10-minute routine can launch your career in an upward trajectory. If I had not seen the results in my own life, with my coaching students, and with my own agents, I would agree with you.

The hard fact, I learned, is that the way in which you condition your mind every morning before you engage the marketplace will determine, in large part, how effective you will be that day. String together enough effective days, and you will have a stellar, high-earning year.

Rule #2 – Define Your Version of Success

My dream for my first year of real estate was to make $100,000. It was 2003 and $100,000 would have turned my life around completely.

Using the same techniques you are going to pick up from this book, I not only exceeded my $100,000 goal, but I did it in half the time I planned. In six months, I earned over $126k.

Even now as I recount this, I feel the thrill of having that money come in and financial stress from my life slip away with each commission check. Instead of being driven by survival, I shifted to a higher state of consciousness. That beautiful shift from stress to serenity was a luxury brought by financial success.

Transforming your own career works with a clear process that you may be familiar with but are not using. Essentially, you fixate your mind's eye on your life as though you have already achieved your goal.

You are mentally creating a set point of expectations for who you are, what you can achieve, and how you move through life.

Putting your mind into the ecstatic state of having achieved or surpassed your goal highlights the full power of this process. I would often close my eyes and rehearse what it would feel like when I had commission money coming in. I would almost shiver with excitement about being able to take care of my children the way I wanted to, pay off bills, and raise my family's lifestyle.

It was this kind of mental rehearsal that fueled me every morning. The same kind of mental rehearsal is going to fuel you. You may have already written down your goals, and I commend you for that.

The crucial next step is adopting the mindset that you have already achieved that goal and sensing how amazing your new level of success is. Feel it, as if it's already happened.

When you have that thrill vibrating in your body from thinking about already having achieved your new level of success, you are now drawing in the forces necessary to help you achieve your success in reality.

You may think this is all just a lot of fantasy thinking, so to speak. You are certainly entitled to think that. The proof that these steps work comes from the tangibility of my own achievements and those of the others whom I have trained to follow this routine.

Take this opportunity to enjoy the power that these techniques bring. All you have to do is open your mind just enough to engage in the exercising of your imagination. As soon as you feel the vibration and energy within you from imagining your new life, you have ramped up your state of mind. Your now energized mindset will motivate you to take all the business building actions in subsequent chapters.

Action Steps:

1. Write down your commission goal for the year on a note card or in a notebook that you will look at daily.

2. As part of your morning and evening routine, both recite your goal and feel as if you have already accomplished it. Feeling the excitement is as important as reciting. The feeling is what keeps you motivated through tough times.
Important note: I recommend not sharing your goal with others, unless they can help you achieve it. Keep all the steam in your mental engine for powering you towards your goal.

3. Assume you will achieve your goal. Here is an example of what this mysteriously powerful method looks like. Pick out the car you want to buy, or the home you want, or something else you plan to enjoy when you achieve your goal. With a car, I want you to go to the dealer and sit in it. Test drive it if you can. Smell the fine leather. Listen to the 16 speaker system (must be a Cadillac!) and savor every emotion of achievement you experience while in the car. Another example of this method for income goals is: Choose your income goal for the year; say for example, $200k. Remember, it has to be something believable for you. Choose a number higher than you think you can achieve. You are going to be getting help from the universe in ways you cannot imagine now, so think big. Post it where you can see it, and say it every morning and every night. "I am earning $200k this year." Use present tense as though it is happening now. Take a few seconds and feel in your body that you have already achieved your goal. When you are tingling with excitement and smiling, you are in the magnetic state you need to be in to manifest your goal. This feeling brings you into belief that you can and will achieve your goal. You have just created a magnetic force drawing you towards achieving your goal and getting your car, house, vacation, income, etc. Every time you sense doubt creeping in, or your motivation flagging, call up the experience of being in your dream ride or earning the income you set as your goal. Suddenly, making those extra calls and pushing yourself harder will come naturally.

Rule #3 – Speak, Think, and Act Towards What You Want

Unfortunately, most realtors or business people that are not achieving success have a lack of focus on their goals. They let too many distractions get between themselves and the destiny they wish to achieve. Instead of scheduling time for prospecting calls or hiring someone to do that, they are wasting time in a thousand different ways.

Sadly, those that cloud their vision with tasks, activities, and time wasters that do not get them closer to their goals become trapped in frustration. They are focused on things they ultimately do not want. Then the complaining begins about how unfair life is.

How often do we hear people talking about what they do not want in life? I admit that even I have engaged in negative thinking before I learned better. I talked about what I didn't want or what I was most dissatisfied with.

Every time I complained, or thought of problems instead of solutions, I summoned negativity and pointed my internal GPS mindset towards things that made me unhappy. I was directing my mindset towards my fears, away from a life of possibilities. Recognizing that you are being negative is pretty straightforward. Changing this behavior, however, requires being far more conscious of our words.

Our words are influenced by our emotions. Angry emotions trigger angry words, positive emotions trigger positive words, negative emotions trigger negative words. You get the picture.

Interestingly, we can also influence our emotions by our choice of words. Using negative speech reenergizes negative thoughts, building them into a bigger presence in our lives. When we speak positively about what we want and what we expect, we are energizing those pathways in our brains to attract these positive situations.

Wealthy people think about how to create wealth and build value all the time. People who are impoverished are continually thinking about why they are impoverished, asking themselves "why don't I have any money?" This is equivalent to giving your mind the order to come up with reasons why you will not have money. Your mind follows through and delivers reasons why you do not and will not have money!

The proper way to imprint this internal guidance system for realtors is as follows:

1. Challenge yourself not to utter negative thoughts or words. Go on a five day mental diet. Change: "I cannot afford...an assistant, a nicer car, and finer clothes." To "I am working harder and smarter to afford an assistant, a nicer car, and finer clothes." The same concept applies to any negative statements you tell yourself. You are pointing your mind towards improvement and achievement.

2. Recast your vocabulary to positive statements about your abilities and your expectations. If you ever listen to Donald Trump speak, he speaks positively about his abilities even though he has certainly taken his lumps. Oprah Winfrey also exudes confidence despite her well-publicized challenges. By staying focused on the positive, both of them were able to bounce back.
The same effect will occur with you. If you had a very unsuccessful year thus far, and you are struggling, then reframe your thinking, speaking,

and acting. Point your mind and speech exclusively towards positive outcomes and a positive approach to your own abilities. You will raise your performance dramatically.

Complaining and self-pity are luxuries that high performers never allow themselves. Examples of turning negative thoughts into positive ones:

Negative: "This market is too slow for me to make any money."
Positive: "Top realtors can make money in any market, and I am a top realtor!"

Negative: "Every prospecting call I make is either going to voicemail or when people answer the phone they doesn't want to talk to me. I'll never get any listings."
Positive: "I know there are prospects out there wanting to list their home and it will be fun finding them."

Even getting stuck in traffic is an opportunity for practicing reframing negative thoughts into positive ones. Exercising your positive thought forming muscles will turn you into an unstoppable force.

1. Create affirmations that support your goals and vision. You might even develop a mantra you rev yourself up with while you listen to music. Great athletes use affirmations and mantras all the time. It's your turn to be a superstar realtor and use the same mental tools as other superstars. "I am a prospecting machine." "I serve my clients brilliantly." "I am attracting listings." Any statement you resonate with will build your positive emotions.

2. Practice your mental dance routine to turn any negative voices that occasionally strike, into positive voices. As the Chinese saying goes, "we must constantly pluck the weeds of our mental garden to keep it beautiful, serene, and fertile."

3. Dress the best you can afford, drive the cleanest and most beautiful car you can, and carry yourself positively. Knowing you look good forms your mind towards an uplifting state. Acting positively, dressing like you feel great about yourself, and projecting success from every pore of your being attracts more of all the good things. More clients, more relationships, more deals, and more money.

Rule #4 – Learn from Your Past Performance While Starting Every Day Fresh

Past success does not guarantee future success. Every new day you must earn your position in life. You might think that the idea of starting every day fresh applies to people who have not been successful. The strategy applies equally to people who have been successful and to those who have not yet reached their full potential.

As an example, I still prospect every day I work. I also still put in long hours, even though I have a staff that can handle most of my operations.

When people become very successful, like a realtor selling several homes in a month, they are sometimes tempted to take their foot off the pedal. They stop prospecting as much or might stop putting in a continuous effort on their digital marketing program.

Just as night follows day, these successful realtors eventually see their performance drop. Whether you are a top performer or a struggling realtor in your agency, it's time to make every new day great no matter what you have done up to this point.

Following the steps I explain throughout this book, you are going to be a high achiever. As this new high achieving person, whatever your past performance was, it's now going to get significantly better.

Those of you who are already top performers may decide to launch a new agency, build a bigger team, or reach higher sales volumes through scaling the methods, which I will later explain.

Those of you who are struggling are now going to shut the door on your past performance. Move on. The new you with your improved mindset, dialed in motivation, and the techniques within this book are going to wash away any scars left over from your previous challenges.

I am not exaggerating the transformative impact of your new mindset routine. You have to point your mind, your language, and your actions toward your bright future. When you are fully committed to creating your bright future, you will not allow for any trips down memory lane. They are too expensive in terms of time and emotional baggage.

You are now positive and future facing. Whether you made $1000 in commissions last year or $1M in commissions, your mind focuses on what you will do in the future. Now is time to prove to yourself that you can build a better year with an improved, 100% positive, failure-proof mindset.

Rule #5 – Mindset Sets Your Image

Picture this: A woman gets out of a brand new Mercedes Benz convertible dressed in professional, high- end clothing. So far the picture sounds attractive.

Instead of seeing her stand up straight and smile, she surprises us. This otherwise attractive woman slouches her shoulders, her eyes point downward with a frown on her face, and her body seems like it has seen more couch time than gym time. All the effort she put into choosing clothing and arriving in style has just been thrown out the window. The world will see somebody projecting doubt, low energy, and negativity.

Our physiology works hand-in-hand with our mental attitude. Standing tall and looking up towards the sky and stars elevates our mood by elevating our sense of self. An elevated mood gives elevated energy. With high energy, we rightly feel entitled to success. We need to project entitlement for the business that we want.

One of the key methods to creating that sense of confidence is tuning your physiology. A common example of physiology reflecting a state of mind is depressed people tending to look downwards. Try looking upwards instead. You'll see what a difference it makes in your mood and your confidence, even if at first you have to force it.

When I present myself to a prospect, I have my shoulders back. I stand up straight with a big, sincere smile. I remind myself how much value I can bring to the transaction and how much I can help this person sell their home. My goal is to present an image of confidence, entitlement for the listing, competence, warmth, and positivity.

I carefully plan my image for my prospects. From how I dress, to my hair, my smile, and my physiology, I am tuning my mindset as much as presenting an image.

If I took the same outfit and showed up with a physiology that silently said I was depressed, full of doubt about my self-worth, and low-energy, my prospects would sense everything. How we stand and look people in the eye often impacts our closing ratios for listing presentations more than almost anything we say. Our physiology also impacts our mental state.

Action Steps:

1. Get on a physical fitness routine. More is not always better. Starting out by committing to a 10-minute walk every day is better than committing to an hour at the gym that you miss because it is too much time. Set a feasible goal for you to get in the ideal shape for your body type over a reasonable time period. Start today and keep at it, learning as you go. Waiting to find the perfect routine and the perfect diet will keep you stuck. Take action and learn as you go.

2. Practice standing up straight, smiling, and walking confidently in front of your full length mirror. You can even make a video of your presentation to see if there are any areas you want to improve on.

3. Monitor your breathing and keep it deep, slow, and regulated. When you are feeling stressed, all you need to do is control your breathing. There is a powerful breathing technique that helps calm nerves during stressful situations. It is called box breathing: Five seconds in, hold for five seconds, five seconds out, wait five seconds. Repeat. Use box breathing to remain calm, confident, and cool when you might otherwise feel anxious. Every client wants a cool-headed realtor during the stress of negotiating deals.

You are now well on your way towards being the realtor you have always dreamed of being. Success is yours when you take the right actions, as I will describe in the next chapter.

Key Points from Chapter One:

A. Acknowledging mindset as the basis for success, changes you immediately for the better.
B. Adopt the "Success is Mine" mantra to bust through any hurdles towards reaching your goal.
C. Create a morning and evening mindset building ritual along with your goals. This ritual should include your affirmations, gratitude practice, mental imagery, and energy building thoughts.
D. Speak, think and act towards what you want while steering clear of any negative thoughts.

E. Learn from your past and then focus 100% on creating your ideal future.
F. An energetic state of mind impacts your outward appearance and your outward appearance can energize your mindset.

II. SEEING IS BELIEVING

"Be the change you want to see in the world."
-Mahatma Gandhi

After reading chapter one, which covered the basics of developing a winning mindset, you are ready to learn how to visualize as an aid to achieve your goals. This process is called entelechy. As asserted by Aristotle, entelechy is the realization of potential. While some of this information might appear repetitious or similar, all of us, certainly me included, need frequent exposure to new ideas before making them our own.

Once you integrate the suggestions on visualizing, language selection, and other new behaviors, you will elevate your presence and performance.

Cruise Control Your Universe

To realize a higher level of reality, our perceptions and thought patterns must first change. New information changes our individual perception of reality. It can take time and practice to create a new way of thinking that informs and benefits our every move.

Crucial to the lessons of the old masters and the new physics of thoughts impacting reality is that change actually begins from within.

Are you:

- Happy?
- Tired?
- Impatient?
- Discouraged?
- Motivated?
- More proactive or reactive?

Do you act more commonly out of love or anger?

Many factors combine to form an individual consciousness. If you feel the need to make some changes in your life that are barriers to your success; it's in your hands and mind to do so.

Visualization

Freely and fully imagine yourself without fear. What does a fully satisfying life look like to you? What is the best outcome you can imagine with regards to your individual pursuits? Form a clear image in your mind; write it down on paper with statements in the present tense. Accept your desired outcome as your reality, and then take the necessary steps towards that outcome.

There is a massive difference between daydreaming and consciously using your imagination to shape reality. Day dreams do have value, like meditation, where outcome is not a concern, allowing the mind to refresh. Whenever you employ your mind to deliberately shape your reality, imagine only the very best possible outcome. Once your ideal is solidified in your mind, take action toward manifesting that outcome – the universe will catch up.

Begin by setting an intention in your mind and follow through with an action that supports your goal. For example, commit to getting 10 new listings this month (intention) then immediately schedule the time to get your first contact (action). You may already be doing this, either knowingly or unknowingly. To achieve a *High Roller* level of success, embrace the practice consciously and deliberately.

Set the Scene, Seize the Day

You don't need a sports psychologist like those employed by the US Olympic Team to know that visualization works. Even my television show, *The Property Shop*, on HGTV, began with me visualizing that I wanted my own TV show.

I star in an amazing TV show.

Ask for what you want. Mentally own it in the present to make it your present. Be specific. For example:

I am a well-paid star in a hit real estate TV show.

This will get you to your goal more closely than the first version. Should you share that same goal I once had, I look forward to being a guest on your new show!

Know your worth and own it for all time! It may take a few months for your bank account to catch up with the reality of your success-oriented mindset, but don't let that discourage you from knowing in your heart and mind that you are a winner who succeeds.

Choose to be successful right now in order to set the cornerstone building block of a wealth-building framework. You must create and maintain a positive mindset to achieve amazing things in your real estate career, and it all starts by accepting and knowing that success is yours whenever you are ready to claim it.

Being authentic is key to winning client loyalty and positioning yourself ahead of the pack. Pretending to believe in yourself is like falsifying information on a real estate contract... it won't stand up to scrutiny, so it will not stick.

Meditate Into Your New Success

Another method you may have heard of to help achieve goals by enhancing our beliefs is known in NLP as the Prometheus Induction, a combination of guided self-hypnosis and an NLP process. The technique is employed for relaxation, setting goals and to expand awareness. Seek out an NLP practitioner to guide you if you choose this option.

I believe in the power of NLP and call on practitioners when I need to tweak my own performance. You can use the Prometheus

Induction pattern or any meditation pattern you sync well with to get into a receptive state of mind for visualizing your new reality.

There are many methods that you might employ to reach a true mindset that enables success. Each individual should allow themselves to gravitate toward the types that work well for them because we each learn and grow in ways as unique as we are.

Whatever nurtures your positive mindset so that you can stick to the formula – get at it now! And whatever you need to feel fully focused and deserving of success, whether its yoga, meditation, NLP, affirmations, prayer, all of the above, or something completely different, devote yourself to it consistently.

Attitude of Gratitude

Another aspect of the success formula that you may be tempted to overlook is adopting an attitude of gratitude. Embrace gratitude, practicing it daily, to make all of your work count.

Often, highly successful people are grateful for all that they have, marking the difference between individuals who inherited assets and those who earned wealth. Express gratitude before you earn your fortune for the things that you do have in your life; and it is certain that we all have something to be thankful for – and continue expressing gratitude when you finally have your fortune, because this will help you keep it.

The best executives in any given field conclude company meetings with heartfelt expressions of gratitude for their team members and the contributions they make. As a result, they are able to assemble great teams because people love to work where they are appreciated. People thrive when they are made to feel worthy. Like attracts like and expressing gratitude has the effect of attracting the same.

Language

Most of us are not fully aware of the language we use on a day to day basis, both internally and externally. It's very important to pay attention to the words you choose. Adopt positive speaking habits. Learn to express yourself like a copywriter and reference what is positive rather than what isn't.

It may seem like a small task, but a habit of speaking positively will have a huge effect by reversing the negative impressions that you may not realize you have been making. After all, we attract what we give off to the world, so speaking with negativity will only attract more of it in your life. Try it my way. Catch and edit yourself from using negative language. It will become a habit if you let it.

Consider the nuances of:

"I'm late! I'm stuck in traffic."
Versus
"I'm on my way. I am almost there."

Which choice would you prefer to hear? Which is more likely to keep your appointment?

I learned from my own mentor that taking command of your language is a necessary tool to achieving goals.

Accept complete responsibility for your communication. If you are not getting the response you want, then adjust your communication. In sales, exuding knowledge and confidence with your words is absolutely crucial.

"If you don't believe you, who will?"

Always assert your value with your verbal presentation. Rather than saying, "If I don't believe in me, who will?" for instance, loudly, clearly, and repeatedly assert:

"I believe in my value, skills and expertise; so does everyone I meet."

Overstating Your Case

Knowing when to stop selling, stop talking, and when to simply listen is as important as the words you choose when you speak. To borrow a maxim from my children's father and business partner of many years, Oren Pinto,

"Never sell what's already sold."

When we do, we only sell ourselves short and deflate the momentum built with a client. Adopt appropriate silence as a part of your language. Practice substantial, fact-based communication complemented by a double-dose of listening.

To reiterate, we need not only pay attention to the type of language we use, but how and when we use it.

Physiology – Your physical experience of life, including the body language you display, can also influence outcomes. Pay attention to the energy your body is portraying. Engage it, along with your language choices, to command your mood by altering your physiology.

> *Walk like a fashion model.*
> *Keep your shoulders upright like a superstar.*
> *Smile like everyone is cheering for you.*

When you imagine your success in the present, your body will react accordingly, rewarding you with the chemistry of success. Imagine being a complete success in all that you do using the power of your own physiology to create and nurture your momentum.

On the other side of the coin, negative thoughts induce negative chemical reactions that undermine your success. Improve your mood by positively improving your physiology.

Momentarily stuck in a performance rut? Move. Change your perspective of the room and your surroundings. Often, just a small change can make a big difference – altering your posture, changing the light flow into the room, your seating, or simply good background music at a volume that enhances your work can all contribute to focusing your productivity.

Super stuck? Take a walk, or go for a run. Take up swimming or a fun fitness class, or both!

Physical activity is so useful in propelling us toward success that it warrants its own chapter. Any time you need a quick and sure-fire boost in the right direction, just choose an action from my suggestions on fitness for success.

Control Your Attention

All your hard work will not take you where you want to be without a razor sharp focus on your goals and both choosing and sticking to your methods.

Any time spent worrying about negative outcomes undermines your efforts in the present. Always stay focused on positive outcomes. Your brain will keep you stuck in negativity if you do not focus on replacing negative thinking with positive.

Mental Dieting

Positivism is a critically important part of your focus. You grow rich by thinking positively! You grow rich by taking ownership of positive outcomes. Whenever you begin a negative statement, whether in your mind or out loud, stop yourself and turn it around into a positive one.

Though it may feel difficult at first, adopting an optimistic mental diet will make you financially fit

"Real estate brokers and salespeople use Neuro Linguistics to enhance their communication skills and provide them with more choices when working in a difficult situation. . . it shows how we make sense of the world around us and communicate." - Roberts Dilts

Since the article appeared, a few converts became many and now NLP is a trusted tool for countless salespeople. With the help of my own life and business coach who is an NLP practitioner, I've learned to focus on the feelings of success and project myself into desired outcomes. NLP coaching has proven to be a key tool for me in becoming a *Real Estate High Roller*.

All the mental, physiological, and active steps that you take towards your success will work together, including focused, written and mental visualization in your mindset program that will lock in your highest states. These are effective systems that you can employ to achieve your personal form of success, exactly as I and so many others have.

Triple Play

Reinforce your positive mindset by focusing on your goals and creating an optimistic outlook on life. Most of us are so busy that we are used to doing double duty in many areas. Your road to success is probably no different. Affirmations are a fantastic way to solidify goals and create optimism. A busy lifestyle led me to communing with nature, regular exercise and the practice of affirmations.

The triple play of nature, exercise and affirmations truly fuels my fire on a regular basis. Rise to the top and stay there by combining your chosen affirmations with spending some time outdoors every day. Your outlook and productivity will benefit. Add your exercise routine to the mix and you'll have a winning formula.

Almost without exception, we each need to spend time outdoors. Fresh air and natural surroundings help relax the body and clear the mind while providing your brain with its main fuel: oxygen. It's as important to spend regular time in nature as it is to occasionally let go of whatever hurdles you may face. Allow your mind a chance to refresh, so it can do its work, helping to tackle whatever life challenges pop up.

Even if you only manage to step into the yard in your bathrobe some days, take those important personal moments to meditate and enjoy some time in nature. It's also a perfect opportunity for reciting your affirmations.

I begin affirmations as I cool down after jogging. I tell God and the universe, and anyone else who cares to listen in, that I am thankful and grateful for all that I have. I am a firm believer in developing and nurturing a spirit of gratitude, being thankful for everything I have in my life, including the goals I set.

When I say out loud, or even just think an affirmation, I speak and act as though I have already achieved my desired outcome. From first-hand experience, I know that a properly-focused mindset and the right script work together to attune your mind for success.

Commit to getting outdoors in nature a few times a week, then follow-up with affirmations as part of your cool-down. Take a walk. Someday sooner than you might imagine, that walk will become speed-walking, jogging, or some other physical pursuit altogether. For the winter time, you might choose yoga instead.

Naming Names and Talking Numbers

To begin, practice the spirit of gratitude by acknowledging what you do have and then include what you may not yet tangibly have, but want in place in your life. Assert a healthy mindset with the practice of declaring daily affirmations. Speak your truths out loud. Whatever aspirations you have, make them a reality with very specific wording. Name names and pay great attention to detail.

Start with affirmations of gratitude as discussed in the previous chapter for what currently exists and follow with the reality you are now building. Keep to the present tense and assert your statements with the full force of belief.

Behavior Action Steps

1. Determine that you are in charge of your life. Take full responsibility for your life and your success. You are in charge of your destiny.

2. Remove negative intentions from words and deeds.

3. Eliminate negative words and phrasing from your vocabulary. Think and speak in positive terms to alter your perception and realize your goals.

Avoid Negation, Embrace Celebration!

III. BODY BASICS BOOTCAMP

"Exercise is the magic pill... Exercise can literally cure diseases like some forms of heart disease. Exercise has been implicated in helping people prevent or recover from some forms of cancer. Exercise helps people with arthritis. Exercise helps people prevent and reverse depression."
-Michael R. Bracko, EdD, FACSM, Chairman of the American College of Sports Medicine's Consumer Information Committee.

So far, we've mainly looked at the essential component of success, which is creating and maintaining a healthy mindset. A solid mindset is a necessity that continues as a theme throughout this book but, before we get too far ahead of ourselves and overlook any basics, we also need to cover how living a healthy and active lifestyle supports a healthy mindset.

Real estate sales requires your interactive attention every day, and often right through the evening as well. That's why regular breaks are a necessity for any successful realtor. To keep pace, stick with a practical, daily fitness and nutrition plan so that you can perform, even in stressful circumstances.

Stress Will Test

Stress is inevitable in life and can be a positive thing when it moves you forward. That's why those special types known as adrenaline junkies enjoy stressing themselves to the limit as a way of both facing and overcoming challenges.

Stress can also be negative due to unwanted events. One thing is certain, though, stress is, by definition, a fundamental element of any effort, no matter how great or small. Be aware of the stress you feel as you master the world of real estate; allow it to both energize and inform you, but never let stress own you.

In the case of real estate, profit margins reward your hard work. The inherent stress of negotiating feels well worth it; allowing most realtors to quickly adapt to and even enjoy the special exhilaration that accompanies deal-making.

A good place to start is by developing and maintaining healthy lifestyle habits. You will achieve your goals through adhering to meticulous steps, which your body and mind will need to follow together.

Your mind and body alike require a great deal of care and maintenance, not unlike a valuable piece of real estate. Neglect it and the value crumbles along with the plaster and peeling paint. Its surface erodes like untended grounds, losing its curb appeal. Neighbors may even begin covering their noses and averting eyes as they pass by. This is not how you want to treat your most important property, your mind.

Tat's Neuro Chemical Management Hacks: Succeed with Hits of Nature's Daily Dose

As much as all of us would like to think we operate strategically, we more often than not are controlled by our primitive impulses. Getting a firm grip on the reins of our impulses means dealing with our hormonal triggers. In concrete terms, here is what operating on primitive impulses looks like:

- Spending work time on Facebook looking at images, surfing funny posts, and chatting with friends.

- Not prospecting when we know we should be because we have administrative tasks or cleaning up to take care of.
- Deciding to take a day off to "de-stress" when we are behind on our numbers for the quarter.

What's really happening is our hormonal system is aligned with the wrong activities. Our job, as top performers in real estate, is to make sure we understand how our hormones drive our behaviors.

Loretta G. Breuning's (Ph.D) wonderful book, *Meet Your Happy Chemicals*, explains our hormones (shown below in italics), with slight alterations to the definitions for the sake of clarity:

> *Dopamine: Gives you the great feeling that you will succeed at meeting your needs.*

Addictions are based on dopamine cycles that are misdirected. Instead of being addicted to social media, tune your dopamine production to something productive! When you make those prospecting calls, for example, you will feel a surge of dopamine from taking action that builds your career. Get over the internal resistance you feel, and glide with the dopamine rush that takes over once you start.

Low dopamine levels lower motivation. Along with your major goals, constantly set easily reached milestones and goals to keep your dopamine levels high. As dopamine releases with every accomplishment, no matter how small, celebrate having reached any milestone toward your goal.

From dinner at a favorite restaurant to a new bauble you've had your eye on – celebrate your accomplishments, big and small! You can easily manufacture dopamine on demand using this method.

> *Serotonin: This is your peaceful feeling that flows when you feel important.*

Most realtors feel unimportant when they think about prospecting, shutting down the feel-good chemicals.

Try my mental frame: making prospecting calls is going to make me successful, rich, and respected for both by achievements and contributions. I know I have instilled within myself that I am important before I pick up the phone or introduce myself at an event, because I am taking action. Action alone can deliver serotonin once you reframe the situation as I do.

Oxytocin: Promotes feelings of trust.

Our goal is to give our clients a burst of oxytocin when they meet us. We achieve this by being someone worthy of trust, developing a reputation for delivering on our word, and by setting the intention to help our client out to the best of our ability. Creating the environment of trust gives your business and life a foundation that nothing can destroy.

Endorphin: Gives you a sense of euphoria that makes either physical or mental pain.

Anytime we take risks and try something new, or push ourselves physically (e.g., marathon), mentally (e.g., learning a language), or psychologically (e.g., dealing with a high stress situation), we may enjoy a sense of pleasure during the struggle. We can use this to our advantage when confronting challenges that we feel are holding us back.

If you have a business project that has been on your to do list for a year, then push into it. Instead of sensing stress, imagine you are working to complete a business marathon that will raise your status and performance. All it takes is reframing the stress into an event, and your mind will dump endorphins into your system.

Now that you understand how hormones steer you, unless you choose to control their influence, you can make changes starting today. According to Dr. Breuning's book, expect your brain to trick you into wanting to return to your old ways for about 45 days. Once you have asserted your prefrontal cortex executive brain over your hormone production, your career will veer towards the stars!

Balance your body chemistry for success by eliminating any need for it to react to projected negativity. Instead, hack into Mother Nature's quartet of positive neurochemicals for a kick-start to your efforts. A good chemical balance is key to success, so get your DOSE – this is one chemical soup you'll want to have regularly to fuel up your fire!

Allowing yourself to reflect on past accomplishments isn't self-indulgence so much as it is self-care. Your brain doesn't know the difference between then and now in these cases, so it gifts you with serotonin anytime you allow yourself to feel highly significant.

Believing in your own healthy self-image also releases serotonin, dopamine, and enhances oxytocin. Self-esteem propels your efforts and helps you develop resilience. 20 minutes in the sunshine to absorb UV rays promoting vitamin D and additional serotonin production is your obligation to your body, even when the sun is masked by clouds.

Your Image Management

Are you someone most people would wisely trust a million-dollar home with? Do you look the part? If not, carefully examine and alter whatever barrier is present and then work towards elevating your presence to fit your target consumer.

For those of us living in fashion Mecca's and style-conscious cities, it's clear that all of the highly successful agents look great because they are well-groomed and conscious of their presence.

True beauty comes from within, but society likes you well-groomed.

The old saying, dress for success, was never so true as it is in real estate sales. Consider your physical presentation. In order to become a hot property yourself, you need to make the packaging as attractive as possible. You are a walking, physical reflection of your professionalism, almost like a billboard. Resolve to be consistently well-groomed in every way, and that includes your scent as people have complex relationships with aromas that can work for you or against you. Want to make a million dollars? Look like a million dollars. This is especially true for sales professionals as before you can sell a product you have to sell yourself.

Look like you respect yourself and so will others. It's better to wear the same well-tailored suit every day, so long as it's clean and pressed, than to opt for a casual presentation with clients or prospects. Buyers and sellers are expecting you to look the part and you should.

Goals, Gear and Good Workouts

Getting into better physical condition is a gradual process and your determination may waver from time to time. What's important is that you stick with it.

Tat's Top Six Get Fit Facts

1. Set goals. Goal setting should be at the top of the list for any new objective. A strong and focused effort to meet specific and realistic goals is the most effective method of changing behaviors and outcomes. Start simple and pace yourself. Taking a brisk walk for twenty minutes three times each week is a healthy start if fitness has not been part of your weekly routine. Swimming is another highly accessible and effective way to exercise and have fun. Add more ways to work out each week until you reach the level of activity that both exercises and energizes you. Personally, I treat my jogging and spinning classes as a mental and physical fitness effort. I start my day by listening to music and saying my affirmations. By the time I finish my workout; I am mentally pumped as well as physically invigorated.

2. Have a fitness test. Your physician or local fitness center can provide access to simple testing that underlines the areas you most need to improve upon, like cardiovascular, muscle strength or problem areas.

3. Choose for you. Don't follow fads. Stick with tried and true exercise routines and research. Consider your personality and pick the path you are most likely to follow. For instance, are you more inclined to do yoga at home, alone, with a recording to guide you, or in a class with a live instructor? Being true to yourself will make it easier to stick with. .

4. Join a fitness class, gym, sports team or event. For many people, team sports can provide motivation. Gyms offer fun group fitness classes that incorporate dance and music, which can kick-start your own efforts; group physical activity such as charity runs, rowing, softball and bowling offer networking opportunities as well.

5. Keep a daily exercise log. Keep it simple by using your calendar. Record your walks and other exercise. In a few words, jot down the level of challenge, the specific type and amount of exercise and how you felt before, during and after.

6. Dress for fitness success. There's no need to drop large chunks of change on fitness gear, but having proper safety equipment, like a cycling helmet or decent running shoes, along with a couple of stylish and durable workout ensembles will add to your incentive and keep you comfortable.

Have a Ball with Budget Fitness

Walking and running are only the tip of the iceberg when it comes to free fitness. Jumping rope is another quick, accessible home remedy to physical inertia, and its fun, too! Strengthen your cardiovascular system, burn calories, tone thighs, calves, abdominals, back, chest, and shoulders. A jump rope is affordable and light enough to carry.

The exercise ball has grown into a huge, inflatable boon to home fitness. You can find a sturdy, plastic exercise ball at a discount store for fewer than twenty dollars. Most people prefer a 24 – 28 inch ball.

The internet is brimming with video tutorials on how to turn this simple piece of equipment into an entire fitness regime. It's also a favorite for anyone with back pain. At my house, the whole family likes to roll around on them whenever we watch a movie. When it's over, our backs feel better instead of cramped!

Libraries also stock fitness books and DVDs that you can borrow free of charge. YouTube offers every form of exercise video you can think of. All you need to do is dedicate a few minutes every day to getting in shape with whatever works for you. Devote the energy to fitness and fitness will deliver energy back to you in spades.

Success also requires energy. You may have already come across the idea that a healthy lifestyle encompasses a trinity of good health consisting of adequate exercise, rest and nutrition on a regular basis. A healthy mind supports a strong body, and vice versa, because they exist in a symbiotic relationship. Neglecting one often comes at the cost of harming the other.

Looking for some kind of fountain of youth to rejuvenate your skin and add a healthy glow? You may even encounter some on your walks: Water!

Toss aside the expensive creams and pricey concoctions. Simple water is that "magic potion" we all need in order to look and feel our best. The Holy Grail, if you will, of good health is simply adequate H2o. We are born 75% water, yet few people manage to maintain that high a level of moisture in their systems – the average is closer to 65% for adults.

So simple, yet so often overlooked, be sure to drink six to eight glasses of water every day. A pitcher of water with lemon is like a magic potion for your personal 'body of water'.

Sleep Deprivation and You

Like water, a minimum daily intake of sleep is necessary to the high-performance life of a *Real Estate High Roller*.

Highly successful people in every industry typically wake up between 5:00 A.M. and 6:00 A.M. and are often the first ones to get to business, be it inside or outside of the office. If you get to bed at 10 p.m., then waking up early will not be a problem, in fact it will likely happen naturally. People who want to party half the night are not destined to become *Real Estate High Rollers*.

Imagine how good and confident you'll feel when you arrive at work refreshed by a good night's sleep, fresh air and exercise in the morning, a healthy breakfast and a luxurious shower. This relaxed pace flows because you got up early enough not to have to rush your way into each day; starting the day right increases the chances of it continuing right.

For some, the commitment to becoming an early riser is a big one. So is the commitment to becoming a *Real Estate High Roller*. No one wants to look back on their life only to see missed opportunities they didn't get out of bed for. We all owe it to ourselves to show up for our lives, our jobs and our families; the earlier, the better!

Many of us have difficulty sleeping. You cannot become highly successful at half-mast. If you suffer from even mild insomnia, then the time to take action is now.

The quality of your sleep is even more important than the quantity. Consult your healthcare professional if you have sleep issues because good quality rest essentially dictates the quality of your waking hours.

There are many highly effective methods for establishing good sleep patterns, from implementing regular bedtime hours to herbal teas and hydrotherapy. Try what appeals to you the most. If your own remedies do not work for you quickly, then it's time to see a sleep specialist because you owe it to your quality of life to get a good night's rest.

So, get your beauty sleep for the sake of body, mind and your bottom line.

Body Basics Action Steps

How can you improve your diet and exercise?

- Do you need to eat out less?
- Do you need to cut back on fast food or double lattes?
- Do you need to get up at 5 a.m. so you can go for a run before you take your kids to school?
- Do you need to get a family membership at the local pool and combine two things closest to your heart – your loved ones and your arteries?

I know that I love to jog and I love my spin classes. While some people have to force themselves to exercise, I love the exercises I have chosen, so taking care of my body becomes a joy rather than a burden.

Focus first on what you will enjoy doing, rather than how to lose weight or tone up quickly. Exercising is a lifestyle and not a three month event. You will be doing this activity every week for the rest of your life, so why not love it? Pick walking, jogging, rock climbing, bicycling, rollerblading, weightlifting, Barre, or aerobics. Just make sure you are having fun.

IV. GOING FOR THE GOALS

Strategy Trumps Tactics

When you embark on a real estate career, it's not unusual to feel a little overwhelmed. David only beat Goliath because he had good strategy. Strategy tends to defeat even a superior tactical position. Goals are the targets that define which strategy to apply, making it critical for you to set your goals wisely.

SMART Goals

The system I recommend when setting goals is the SMART one. You may already be familiar with Specific, Measurable, Achievable, Relevant and Time-Bound goal- setting strategies. When your objectives meet the SMART Goal mold, you will be more likely to achieve your aims and fulfill those goals.

Management Review Magazine published the concept of SMART Goals in 1981, outlined in an original article by consultant and former Director of Corporate Planning for Washington Water Power

Company, Mr. George T. Doran of Spokane, Washington.

Doran's "There's a S.M.A.R.T. Way to Write Management's Goals and Objectives" is now indelibly woven into the annals of North American business culture.

As George Doran suggested, not every single goal you set may meet all five criteria, since not every goal is as easily measured. Simply aim for the highest possible agreement with the five SMART specifics. This formula will guide you to make excellent choices and informed decisions.

W5 Goal Assessments

Measure each goal you craft with the time-honored W5 tools at hand: who, what, where, when and, perhaps most importantly, why?

A key aspect of SMART Goals is that it prompts you to specifically define your goals, which will increase your chances of being successful. You must define and outline your objectives clearly before setting out to work on them.

Carefully considered and organized goal-setting truly helps achieve better outcomes. Work smart and think SMART to turn your goals into your reality.

High Roller success is an all-or-nothing proposition.

You are in it to win it, right? Give your mind the goods it needs: a firmly positive mindset and goals to aim for.

Now, write down your reasons for wanting a particular goal. Be specific. Once you write down what and why, write down a specific strategy to achieve that goal. Then, devise a backup plan (Plan B) to achieve that goal. Truly and fully examine your feelings about each goal.

Do it now!

Successful application of these defined principles requires constant dedication and paying strict attention to the specifics. Writing your goals down and speaking them out loud are essential in creating the reality of abundant prosperity enjoyed by *Real Estate High Rollers*. Below is an exercise that will help you get started.

Now (yes, right now!) write down two important professional milestones you most want to reach in the next two years.

Strategy

By now, you have your goal and you've written it down. You've also written down your reasons for wanting to meet these goals. The next step is to come up with a specific strategy that outlines how you are going to go about achieving them.

It is similarly important to write down more than one strategy, as in life, as we all know; sometimes things don't always go as planned. In the event that things veer off path, you need a plan B.

With any goal, your number one priority is to devise the first step that you can take immediately to help you meet that goal. A typical realtor's example is the strategy of prospecting at least six hours each week in order to make $150,000 this year.

Another step may be to make sure that you attend one event every week in order to network and keep yourself current and relevant. You may also add other steps, such as educating yourself about real estate every other night. All of these strategies need to be as specific as possible so that you can complete them. Your milestones matter and they keep you moving on.

Action steps are also a great way to test your strategy and make sure that it's realistic. Your steps have to be feasible or there's a good chance that you'll become frustrated or experience feelings of defeat. This might make you quit trying to meet your goals. It's ok to dream big, but don't expect to get there all at once.

Believe in the power of baby steps and collecting small achievements. Working with this model will bring whatever your mind can fathom - you simply need a realistic plan to accompany your drive to get there.

Practice this simple and highly effective method diligently. Taken to the next level, a freshman agent might have the realistic goal of hitting the $100,000 mark in commissions. The goal is achieved by first, writing it down.

Goal Worksheets

GOAL:

I receive $100,000 in real estate commissions this year.

STRATEGY:

1. Engage a successful real estate coach that I want to emulate. Define my brand and consistently display and support it.

2. Devise an effective marketing plan that appeals to homeowners. Network with buyers, sellers and other agents.

3. Hold regular open houses and attend all office home tours.

4. Study my local real estate market until I know it like the back of my hand.

5. Enroll in continuing education classes and workshops.

BACK-UP PLAN:

1. Add original marketing concepts to plan, ie:
    - Sponsor local team and/or neighborhood contest.
    - Create or outsource relevant real estate content.
    - Volunteer at a senior recreation center.
    - Host a charitable event, or a homeowner property staging workshop.

2. Work with a partner or as a member of a real estate team.

3. Ask my real estate coach for more suggestions.

Be Positive

You now have your goals, your strategies and the words written down in front of you. Now that you have everything in place, you need to project the idea that you have already achieved that goal.

Close your eyes and use your imagination with as much vivid detail as possible to picture what it will feel like to achieve your goal. Imagine that you made it.

It's the end of the year and you've earned $160,000 in commissions. How do you feel right now? Be specific. What emotions are you experiencing? How does your body feel now that you accomplished that goal? Take that feeling, make it come to life by visualizing it to the point that it becomes almost visceral, and use it to help you achieve the goal.

That is how you create a positive mindset. You have to assume the sale. You know that you're going to meet that goal because you've already done it. Trust me, it works.

Being a product of your attitude means that you can feel successful anytime. Consider how lucky it is that confidence can be instantly manufactured by a focused mindset. Use the tools at your disposal from Chapters One and Two.

Goaltenders and Goalkeepers

If setting goals is old news for realtors, then why are so many failing after five years? While setting goals is straightforward, actually achieving them is the challenging part.

There's an interesting study conducted by Dominican University's Gail Matthews, which revealed the best kept secret for turning written goals in to achieved goals, demonstrating the powerful effect of setting our intentions in writing.

In Dr. Mathews' study, those who wrote down their goals and made them accountable to another person on a regular basis achieved close to twice the success rate of those who didn't write down their goals. They had a much higher success rate than those with no third-party accountability.

Having a goalkeeper makes you the goaltender that is required to report your own progress. Think of your coach or mentor as an ally to your success. The best teacher is able to act as a mirror, reflecting the intricacies of your sales career back to you with added clarity and experience. According to the study, goalkeepers significantly bolster success rates.

Any reliable ally is a boon to your success. *High Roller* sales success today requires an effective coach, as shown by the Dominican Study. The 77.5% improvement in accomplishing their goals realized by the test group that documented and shared them with a trusted advisor, versus those with unwritten goals, underlines just how powerful a tool you have at hand.

The act of writing your goal on paper also helps your body support your mind concerning the action, as writing something down is much like a contract in the form of an agreement that you make with yourself.

Success can be anything you want it to be. We each have our own definition and ambitions. We can achieve whatever our minds can achieve. The common thread is to be specific about your goals and always be diligent about writing goals on paper!

Skipping steps just because they are simple is a natural tendency for most of us, but *High Rollers* follow even the most simple of steps, overlooking nothing. Penning your goals is too accessible and effective a tool to be dismissed.

I got involved with coaching because I realized by practical experience the same principle the

Dominican Study verified: we all need mentors and coaches to keep us moving forward towards our goals.

My own coaching program, *Real Estate High Rollers*, keeps realtors focused on their goals with astounding results. From new realtors to those with a decade of experience, when I teach new techniques, get my coaching clients to define their goals, and keep them accountable for performing them, something amazing happens. Everything comes together and they have their best year ever!

The program fills up quickly, but you can learn more about the specifics of my *Real Estate High Rollers* mentorship program at www.realestatehighrollers.com

Goal Setting

Since most of my readers are realtors, here's an example that realtors often use as a definition of success. You cannot simply say, "I want to be a successful real estate agent" and think that that's going to cut it. You need a specific goal, such as "I want to be a successful real estate agent making $160,000 in commissions this year."

Alternately, you might phrase a goal this way, "I earned $1,232,000 in commissions this year." Always use the present tense and remember that the more specific you are with your goals, the more success you will have.

When I completed real estate school, I wrote down three specific goals:

1. I am the top real estate agent in the city.

2. I am as successful as _____[top agent in area].

3. I will bring in $100,000 in commissions this year.

With no money coming in and two young children to support, failure simply was not an option. Success was my birthright. I succeeded at achieving my goals and even knocked number three out of the park. I continue to set new goals for myself as my life and career evolve. Writing down a specific goal is one part of creating a successful mindset. You also need to decide why each goal is important to you and a good reason in order to truly believe in your goal and make it work.

Wanting to make $250,000 this year because you enjoy the perks of wealth or, worse, to show others of little faith just how well you are doing are not good reasons. A good reason inspires and gives you the drive needed to meet that goal. If you have a good reason, it will furnish crucial inspiration to see it through and not give up along the way.

Goal Action Steps

1. Write down a specific goal. Note one particular goal you want to accomplish. Make sure you include a time frame, whether it is the next three months, six months, or one year.

2. Write down why you want to achieve that goal. Be as specific as possible. This is personal, so make the reasons personal and do not be afraid of what others might think of them.

3. Write down steps you are going to take. How are you going to make your target number in commissions this year? Write down every idea you can think of that you can use to reach that goal.

4. Include one action you can do today. What can you do today, right this minute that will put you on the path to meet your goal?

Do it now!

V. REAL ESTATE 101 FOR HIGH ROLLERS

The world of salespeople is mainly comprised of those who do and those who do not have a winning success formula. Once you possess the right formula, you can add yourself to the success equation. A big part of that equation is setting and monitoring goals.

If you've picked up this book before becoming licensed to sell real estate for instance, then your first goal would be: Become a licensed real estate agent.

Attaining your goals is anything but a passive process. You have to always be working for it, and when you have it, you have to work to keep it. The myth of "overnight success" is just that - a myth. Success is born from years of practice, patience and dedication, which combined create the opportunity to become a sensation.

Being attracted to the real estate profession probably means you have already figured out not to rely on chance to create your success in business, or in life. The reality of being a *Real Estate High Roller* is the achievement of hard work applied to a proven successful formula.

Real Estate Sales is a Full-Time Business

Want to reap *High Roller* rewards in the real estate profession? Set your mind to work mode. You definitely have to climb your way to this pinnacle. Like ascending any hill, even Everest, it is really just a matter of constantly moving forward, one step after another, leading to great reward.

Your commitment to becoming a *Real Estate High Roller* must be strong and unwavering. Being a million dollar dealmaker means acting like one, so:

Start now!

To claim your place as a *High Roller*, you need to be at the top of your game. 'Real estate sales' is not a job for the faint of heart, or the weak of will. It's the perfect profession for people who are curious, love solving problems and enjoy dealing with other people. That describes a lot of individuals. Yet, the only ones who thrive and endure in high-yield sales careers are the ones who have a formula for success.

You cannot become a *Real Estate High Roller* from a part-time commitment. Like any other business, to succeed where many others fail, you will need to make real estate sales your full-time career. You must devote yourself entirely. This means working in excess of 50 hours a week. Even 80 hours a week is not unusual for an up-and-coming agent.

Real estate is not a get rich quick business. In order to build a successful business and become a master in your trade you have to dedicate yourself to it full-time. Typically, as a *Real Estate High Roller*, I will have listing presentations on the weekend. Then, on week nights, since most people work until 5:00 P.M. or 6:00 P.M., they will want to meet afterhours, at 6:30 P.M. or 7:00 P.M. That can be difficult on a family, so I make it a point to balance my schedule very carefully.

If you are a mother, like me, and you want to cook dinner for your family, yet are also offered an appointment for a listing presentation, what are the options? Either you're going to have to give up making dinner for your kids, or you are not going to go to the listing presentation, which is their bread-and-butter, too.

COMMITMENT is the reason why Realtors make big bucks!

You are in launch mode and it's not a joyride. All of you lucky parents with family members to help raise your children – keep the appreciation flowing for that necessary support. Plan your life around work so that your personal life gets regular maintenance, opting for quality. Weekday breakfast time, for instance, can be a daily family ritual that's much easier to accomplish than dinner – that's worth getting up a half hour earlier for, don't you think? The dividends will be huge and long lasting.

We are blessed enough by technology that we can count on cell phones to keep us in direct touch with our loved ones, wherever we go. If you have older children, consider getting in the habit of using Skype or face time with them for quick and easy eye-to-eye time when life gets hectic. Finding balance in your life will be a challenge at first, but don't let that throw you off.

If you are a parent, consider your timing carefully and be sure to choose the right moment for you and your family to embark on a real estate career. Think about what and how much you are willing to sacrifice and how much outside help you have for your children.

One of the major things I would have done differently when I was starting out is to have delegated all administrative work from my first sale onward, so I could spend more time with my children. I wish someone had tipped me off to that concept at the very beginning. I could have sacrificed a lot less time with my kids.

Thankfully, I had a supportive spouse but, I wish I had been there more when they were small children. At the time, I felt that I had to put everything into my new business in order to pay the bills, and I just didn't know any other way to succeed.

Almost everyone who has to earn a living sacrifices time with their children in order to support them. Do not despair people, because there is a big, bright light at the end of this particular tunnel. Once you become successful, you will be able to delegate and to pay other people. Fortunately, that time is in your very foreseeable future.

Whenever I am working with my mastermind students if they are ready to commit and have children I tell them, "You had better get a good babysitter because once you use our systems; you are going to be running a million-dollar business. You will need support at home." It's just logical that you can't be all things to all people at all times. Balance your priorities from the outset or hard lessons will be had.

Within your first year alone, you should hire one or two staff members. Within three years, you'll be able to delegate a lot to those you have been working with, whom you have groomed to suit your exact needs. Then, you get to spend more time with your family. I was successful right away but I didn't take that next important step for a little too long.

Parents launching real estate careers definitely need a reliable personal support system, along with a business plan and coping mechanisms. The extreme conditions of any business launch are temporary. If you focus and follow the formula, it can be a relatively short phase before you will be able to hire a support staff to help you so that you can have more work/life balance.

A good friend and colleague, who is a million-dollar realtor, demonstrated the wiser choice when he hired an administrative assistant within three months. I made the mistake of waiting because I felt that I had too much on the line.

My husband and I had just closed our previous business and had no income, so I wasn't willing to risk paying someone and then not having enough money for my family. However, that was my biggest mistake as a new agent.

When you launch, aim to delegate almost immediately; administrative work makes you no money and steals time away from prospecting and selling homes. If I had hired a secretary within three months, like my friend, I would not have had to be out on the streets working day and night. It's not necessary to go through unhealthy extremes when you know the tricks of the trade discussed in this book.

Should you somehow see "paperwork" somewhere on that list – call my editor, because that would be a big mistake! Paperwork matters of course, especially the legal documents, but obtaining listings, selling a home, and customer service trumps all.

The 80-20 Rule, also known as the Pareto Principle, is well-demonstrated in real estate, where only about 20% of new agents make it to the top. Those 20% of all agents typically control 80% of real estate transactions.

Just over a century ago, in 1906, Italian economist Vilfredo Pareto realized that just 20% of the Italian population owned 80% of all land in Italy. Pareto then observed a similar 80-20 pattern in both nature and European economies. As odd as it seems, he even discovered that 20% of the pea pods in his garden yielded 80% of the peas.

Though largely anecdotal, evidence mounted, continuing to support the 80-20 Rule. During World War II, a business consultant named Joseph Juran unearthed Pareto's work and began applying the 80-20 Rule to business practices. Since then, the 80-20 principle has ruled the day for sales managers and become integral to successful business strategies.

How do you join the top 20%? Every successful top 20 agent in my firm got there by following this structure:

- Get the achievement mindset / Self-Discipline
- Set SMART Goals
- Focus on Prospecting

1. Self-Discipline. Successful self-employment requires discipline. Top 20 Agents are able to set income goals and make action plans that will lead them to their goals. They have the discipline to stick to their plan: they set their alarm clock, get up early and achieve what needs to be done each day. Becoming a "Top 20%" real estate agent and earning commissions of over $100,000 per year takes persistence and dedication. Follow the formula and, very soon, you'll be earning those same commissions.

2. Paper Lions. Top 20 Agents are on intimate terms with the legalities and paperwork of their profession. Hence, they are able to delegate much of that work and simply oversee paperwork. Real estate law is complex and dynamic in every location. Continually educate yourself and your staff.

3. Niche Marketing. Today, everyone wants to work with an expert. Through concentrated study and data collection, top 20 agents position themselves as experts in their field. It's always a good idea to gain a specialty by farming particular neighborhoods, housing types, or niche markets, like first-time buyers or seniors for example. It's worth the extra time and efforts to learn everything you can about your chosen niche and capitalize on that in your marketing efforts as much as possible. The bottom line is that experts earn more than amateurs; a lot more.

4. Contractual Ties. Top agents know that time is money. Working with buyers without a Buyer's Agency Contract is risky business, often wasting your time. Agents who make over $100,000 per year typically don't commit to buyers who won't commit to them. It's also important to have a written agreement with one's broker to avoid any misunderstandings.

5. Lust to List. They work with both buyers and sellers, but focus, foremost, on obtaining new listings. Listing equals control. You own the contract and people have to come to you. Your ROI is much quicker and bigger; double end by representing both buyer and seller in order to make the full commission.

6. Sales Cycle Savvy. To a Top 20 Agent, an individual sales cycle begins when a potential buyer or seller begins looking online, often before a decision to buy or sell has even been made.

7. Careful Qualifiers. The top 20% of prospects result in 80% of a top 20 agent commissions. Top 20 agents are well- aware that some prospects are simply too much stress and/or maintenance, so they pass on them and send them over to new agents. A system that screens and hones in on the "low-hanging fruit" yields prospects most likely to result in a commission. This is fundamental to the success of cold calling and prospecting in general.

8. Delegate. Delegate. Delegate. I truly cannot impress upon you enough that every minute spent doing administrative tasks sets you an equal amount of time further away from your goals. Focus on listings and training your assistant to be like your right hand – the hand that does the paperwork!

9. Invest in Digital Marketing. Create content. Repeat! Today, 90% of people begin looking for real estate online. Increasingly, agents earning over $100,000 annually are dedicated to creating new content consistently. Write about your marketplace and your specialty. Write about everything local to your clientele. Schools, new businesses, restaurants and events are all rich sources of material. This is all about providing potential buyers and sellers whatever information they might be searching for. Most top 20 Agents are too busy to write anything but sales contracts, so hire freelance ghostwriters to pen engaging posts.

Action Plan

1. Figure out Your Expenses: Write everything down including rent/mortgage, utilities, food, gas, car payment – everything you need to keep a roof over your head, food in your belly and to get you around to your listings every day.

2. Figure out Your Business Costs: We went over some of them in this chapter but only you know what you need to run your business. Add it all up.

3. Multiply it by Six: Add your living and business expenses up and multiply them by six to determine how much money you need to set aside before you should begin a career in real estate.

4. Take a Look at Your Home Situation: Make it a good, hard look. Remember, you will be putting in 60-80 hours a week for the first three months. Do you have someone to help you at home? Do you have a jealous boyfriend or girlfriend who won't want you out all the time? Make sure you have a strong support system at home that will help your loved ones make it through until you can afford office staff.

5. Decide Right Now to do it Full-Time or Not at All: Your mindset has to be full-time or go home. Don't waste your time or your money with a half-baked attempt at jumping into the real estate business.

Get in the Phone and Email Zone

Like most professions that offer great rewards, real estate is not the kind of career that ever lets you simply coast in the first few years. This profession is not flexible when you start; that's earned. You have to show up early, stay late and always be around to get ahead as an agent. You even have to answer the phone.

Answering your phone is one of the most important things you do for your business. Unless you're speaking with a client or a potential client, someone else could be doing whatever else you're doing for you. Your mobile device and a wireless ear piece should be your constant companions.

Your focus is always sales. Connecting with people and fulfilling their needs is the lifeblood of sales. You can only do that by calling prospects and by listening and being available. And, if you're not, you can bet there are other agents ready and willing to do that for them.

Cell phones allow us to keep our clients close in those spare minutes while we're waiting for an appointment or driving. Hands-free technology truly is an agent's best friend. In sales, if you want to be successful, you make calls and answer your phone. If you see your phone as a dreaded leash, a tether, rope or chain …you are in the wrong profession.

I have experimented to see what kind of an edge always answering the phone actually does give me. One day, for instance, I called six realtors in two major cities with a varied amount of listings on their rosters, ranging from five to 60. Only the one at the top of that heap answered the phone, and the other five went to voicemail. A live assistant would have been a marked step up from that.

What do potential clients do when they're calling realtors who don't answer? They call the next number on the list, of course! There's never a shortage of real estate agents, but there's usually a dearth of agents overlooking the simple client connector that their marketing efforts bring them by making their phones ring. Ring! Ring! is the exact sound of money being made in a real estate office.

ANSWER THE PHONE!! Double Ended Commission from a Sunday Call

A true story shows how valuable answering even one phone call can be. I was driving along on a Sunday evening when my phone rang. Most realtors don't answer on Sunday but naturally, I picked it up, even though I did not recognize the number. Keep a human touch and answer. Do not use voicemail when you are available. I am driving along, already a successful realtor, and I take the call.

"Hello, I have a house I want to sell. You are the only agent out of three that I called who answered!"

I told him, "That probably means I will be the only one that sells your house." He had a beautiful home, and I sold it and represented the buyer. I made $33k. Then he bought a $1.5M house and I made another 2.5%. I made $65k in commissions by picking up the phone on a Sunday!!!

I am as busy as any other agent in the city, but I make sure to pick up my phone whenever humanly possible. This is so simple, I wonder why other realtors do not follow the same principle, but I'm not complaining, for had they picked up I might not have made that sale!

Smart phones, laptops and tablets are like a gift to realtors. The various software we use on our portable devices allows us continual access to both our clients and to up-to-the-minute information. Momentum has always played a valuable role in closing sales and today's technology can fuel it faster and further. Embrace it.

As necessary as it is to know your way around your devices, surround yourself with technically adept support staff or you'll spend too much time trying to keep up with the ever-changing IT world at the expense of making sales.

Staff will help you take your business to the next level in every respect. A big mistake I made early on in my real estate career was to try and do everything myself. Neglecting to delegate non-client-facing tasks within the first three months of my career came at the cost of my personal life; a good misstep to avoid.

If I was allotted a do-over, I would have hired an assistant almost immediately, having learned the hard way that it isn't necessary to do everything on your own, even at the beginning. Get an assistant, even two days a week, at first, if it's all you can afford, because administration doesn't make sales – salespeople do.

Lunch is for Losers

One thing that may come as a surprise to newer agents is that, in real estate, lunch is for losers! Successful realtors do not have time for lunch. Sure, we eat lunch, usually at our desks while reading trade information.

What *Real Estate High Rollers* often do, though, is enjoy fine dining at A-List restaurants. We happily indulge our highly deserving palates after work, not during the work day. Fancy fare at five-star restaurants is a favorite indulgence of society's most successful people. How else would so many thousands of fine establishments stay in business year after year?

In real estate, when you are on, you have to be fully tuned in and energized. Not wondering about the lunch special at your favorite time-wasting café. When you are off, that is when you are free to relax. Enjoy your downtime and you'll see that your work time will prove to be more rewarding. When you have a whole day off with your loved ones, always turn off your phone, and set your email to an automatic vacation responder:

"This is Tatiana. I'm out of the office today, but I sure do want to speak with you! Leave your name, the time and date, and it'll be my pleasure to call you back tomorrow. If this is an emergency, please contact my colleague, Joe Schmoozie, at xxx-xxx-xxxx. Thank you for calling and have a beautiful day!"

Rare as that message from a *Real Estate High Roller* is, when it's time to play, be in the game. The rest of the time... answer that phone!

Once you have your mindset in shape, your positive visualization and verbalization practice, your physical health routine, and your goals, there is only one thing left:

Do It!

VI. REAL ESTATE ABC'S

"Nothing will work unless you do."
-Maya Angelou

I've witnessed amazing professional transformations with these techniques. Not only have I been able to achieve success, but I've been able to help other realtors who work at my agency and in my coaching business to do the same. The agents I work with achieve their goals because they have a successful mindset, regardless of who they were before or what they did prior to coming to my agency. They followed my formula, worked hard and they became *Real Estate High Rollers*, too.

You must be willing to do the following:

- Put the hours into prospecting, finding listings, and making sales, every day.
- Make 'follow up' a priority in your business.
- Find ways to attract and connect with more buyers and sellers.
- Implement processes and systems in your business.

- Delegate administrative work.

I still do all of those things today, despite being successful, because in order to keep success you need to work as hard as you did on day one and keep that feeling of hunger and motivation close. If I wanted to I could technically retire today and receive a passive income, but that's not who I am and that is certainly not how I define success. I get out there, I work hard, and I make deals. I keep my brand alive and thriving. Keep reading to gather the tools for your own success.

There are no get-rich-and-be-lazy schemes. You cannot make a million dollars in commissions without putting in a million dollars worth of effort, hoping that listings will miraculously find you. You've got to get up in the morning and you have to be willing to stay up late as well, when needed. Welcome to the fast lane. The brass ring doesn't fall into your lap – you have to want to:
1

Work It!

High Rollers work very hard and dedicate enormous amounts of time into achieving the type of income that you picked up this book hoping to obtain. True success is earned. You gain it by first understanding what every billion-dollar broker knows: It takes a lot of work and is not by any means a passive process.

Be in the Game

Only when you put 100% of your efforts into real estate sales and marketing will you reap and sustain *High Roller* rewards. If you try to do it part-time, you'll more than likely fail at the profession. In fact, one of the most frequent mistakes made by people who want to become successful real estate agents is trying to do so part-time.

In what other profession do people attempt to run a business without full-time commitment? Whether you're opening a medical clinic, a hair salon or a restaurant, no professional launches their business thinking, "I'm doing this part-time and expect it to be successful." Yet somehow, in a time-consuming, paperwork-laden profession like real estate, people have the notion that they can succeed without 100% devotion. This is mind-boggling!

Many seem to confuse the reality of flexible hours with working relatively few hours, just by virtue of controlling their own schedules. Not having to report to a superior has no bearing on your workload. Besides, in reality, your clients have as much influence over your schedule and your accountability as you do at this stage.

Like any other new business, not only do you have to support it full-time, you have to do it all the time. You have to live and breathe it. When you're opening your business, there's no 9-to-5. Rather, you should expect and be prepared for 8-to-8, six days a week, if you're well-organized, and good at delegating; otherwise, it could even reach closer to 80 hours a week and beyond. You need to decide if you are willing to give 100% of your time, no matter how much time that might mean.

In real estate, anything less than a full-time commitment is just an elaborate exercise in wasting time and energy, if your intention is to make a living in the profession.

Why work so hard? Because you want to build enough wealth to achieve financial freedom and true independence for a lifetime. You want to be a *Real Estate High Roller* and that's how you get there. Some people with other sources of income attempt real estate sales on a part-time basis. Sure, they can close a deal here or there, but you can't make a living from that and you won't ever become a truly successful realtor. Be prepared, because it's very challenging in the beginning. Be ready and willing to put in the hours. Yes, it's hard work. And, yes, it's worth it!

Becoming a master at anything requires full-time focus. Many of my biggest deals came through working when other "part-time" realtors had already set their phones down for the evening. I was still prospecting, taking calls, and flowing with enthusiasm to make the most of every opportunity. I was all in.

Treat real estate as though you are in a race. Like any race, you have competitors next to you attempting to cross the line first and take your clients, your commission, and ultimately, your future. Are you going to let that happen?

Early on I committed to pushing myself as hard as I could to get into the real estate race with a strong start. As I progressed and won clients and deals, I started implementing business processes that my competitors were not. Instead of running at a full sprint every day, I could depend on the business organization I built to help carry me along to victory. You can follow the same path.

When you are not there watching and making sure that your business processes are being attended to, it is very possible that the business will fail. That may account for why so few agents make it to the top and why so many fail in the profession.

Your mindset determines how focused you are on achieving your full potential as an agent. If you devote 50% of the time and effort compared to someone else running against you, your earnings most likely won't even reach 50% of their earnings. You would be lucky to earn 20%. Devoting yourself completely to achieving your wildest income goals gives you power far beyond the hours you work because clients can tell a true professional from someone dabbling in real estate.

Go all in like I did. The rewards you will enjoy more than compensate for the initial lifestyle adjustment you will need to make. Eventually, after you have developed an organization around yourself, you will be able to work less while reaping an income that 'part-time realtors' cannot even hope to approach.

Delegation is Your Duty

"There are people who have money and people who are rich." -Coco Chanel

You need to learn how to delegate your non-client-facing and administrative tasks quickly. Otherwise, you will spend a lot of your time chasing your own tail instead of securing the listings that pay all the bills.

It is a lesson I may have learned a little late in life, but I've learned it. You have to let go and divide some of your work up amongst bright, loyal people so that you have time to be with your family or just enjoy life and recharge your batteries. You need to maintain the proper balance in life so that you can not only be successful, but have the time to enjoy the success.

When you delegate, both your quality of life and income go up. You can't become a *Real Estate High Roller* in a vacuum. Creating a winning real estate practice all by yourself means you'll make fewer deals while your quality of life diminishes.

Too many people merely appear successful, whether on paper or on the red carpet, when, in fact, they are miserable. Their spouses are unhappy and their kids are upset because they seldom have the simple luxury of relaxing around their parents.

What benefit is there to wealth if you can't enjoy it with your family and the people you care about? Delegate administrative tasks from the outset and be conscious of maintaining a healthy work-life balance. Your children will thank you because, not only will they get more quality time with you, they'll learn from your example.

Building that wealth in a real estate sales career is achieved by sticking to a winning formula, like the strategies in this book. Stay the course with these key elements to sales success:

Tat's Quick Tips

The Five-Fact Formula for High-Stakes Sales Success

1. Work Hard: It's not easy to become an expert and succeed in a high-ticket, competitive profession. You have to meet the challenge of working smart and working hard, while staying strong. Commit your time and body to your success. If hard work isn't on your agenda, choose a different profession.

2. Be in Business: Treat real estate like what it is: your business; hire experts. Implement a system and follow it. Show up, get to work, prospect, answer the phone, follow through, and earn commissions.

3. The Client is Correct: Follow the old adage that "the client is always right". Your most valuable sales tool is your reputation. Right or wrong, your clients need to feel validated by you.

4. Create Your Brand: Consistently presenting your value with branded ads online, engaging with emails, postcards, or offline channels will help keep you as the top of mind realtor.

5. Delegate: Doing it all yourself only guarantees that you'll make fewer deals while your quality of life diminishes.

6. Reward Yourself: With every commission check, treat yourself to what you need most: time off. Real estate sales may consume your time when you're working, but don't let anything consume your whole life all the time. Rejuvenate, reconnect and fuel your fire. You earned it.

Finance Facts

"If you're looking to save money, you're in the wrong business. If you're looking to make money, real estate is the top business to be in."
-Tatiana Londono

Like any other professional career or business, you need some seed money. Business and personal expenses have to be covered or you'll be under so much stress that you are likely to get stuck in a no-agent's-land of near-deals and missed commissions.

"The lack of money is the root of all evil."
-Mark Twain

My right hand, Dale, for instance, borrowed $20,000 to launch when he started out. He was in his twenties and had never had a real job before. His mother lent him the money because she believed in him. He never looked back, and six months into working with me, he was able to pay his mother back in full.

Every business and every realtor has expenses. You'll need to pay for your licenses, memberships and broker fees; you'll need to cover general expenses like food, medical and transportation. You will need to put gas in your car and keep up with insurance and maintenance. Being a full-time agent requires an investment of time and money.

Stick to the formula. The money you invest in yourself during your first year will be offset by the income you make in your second year.

Since you're a full-time salesperson, you will need savings, a loan or another source of family income during your first year in business. Depending on your lifestyle, you may need to trim the way you spend on a daily basis, or, if you are unwilling to cut your budget, you can maintain your ways by taking a loan from the bank.

So many of the tools you need to start out cost money, from basics like business cards and your mobile device, to marketing and beyond. Advertising for both your business and any listings that you acquire will be your responsibility. You'll have to pay for whatever it is you need to fully and properly service each listing: signs, ads, flyers, postcards, photography, graphic design and more. From business cards to being able to buy your clients a coffee, there will be ongoing costs, as everyone knows, because (and this news is ancient):

> *"You must spend money to make money."*
> -Titus Maccius Plautus 255-185 BC

You must have presentable clothes and a decent car. You can't show up in a dilapidated minivan to a listing appointment and expect the meeting to go your way. To become highly successful, you must behave and present yourself as a picture of success. When you're just starting out, you've got zero, yet you must show the world that you're a million-dollar broker.

I've seen new agents exercise creative solutions to obtain use of a presentable vehicle by doing things like trading off with a relative during the workday and even renting a car when a lease is not obtainable. Later, when you can afford a little more, they'll often be happy to sell you a car from their fleet, and may even finance such purchases in-house. The car you get does not have to be fancy, just clean, presentable and reliable.

There are good reasons why statistics show that most agents will quit within the first five years. In fact according to the North American

Realtors Association, *87% of realtors leave the profession after five years.* It's because new agents are not prepared with sufficient savings, a plan, and the commitment to put their plan into action. It is therefore important to prepare for the initial investment and obtain some form of financing for your first year before you get started.

If, within six months of real estate work, you have not obtained a sale, there's a serious flaw in your system. One year is the most it should take anyone to become self-supporting in residential real estate and you can only get there on a path that is funded.

Cash in on Coaching

Your initial investment should include a real estate coach. You have to use the tools that are out there in order to not waste time and effort struggling to learn on your own what others can help you with.

The formula I recommend is to list and add up your monthly, quarterly and annual expenses, then add to that the cost of doing business in your chosen real estate market, and then multiply the sum total by six months.

Keep your records in a file on your personal computer or laptop and save regularly to an external memory. Backed-up files are the only files you can count on as an agent.

Keep in mind that in six months, though you may make several sales, there is a waiting period between the time an offer is accepted and its closing. Then, there's another short wait until your commission is in hand.

Six months of full financial support is the minimum you will need to get underway and, with my formula, you should be able to start making sales within your first four months. My first sale was within my first six weeks, but you only need to be able to make a sale within your first three or four months in order to launch a lucrative career as a real estate agent.

You may quite likely need a fair bit more than my VP of Sales. The boy wonder who had borrowed $20,000 to get started was able to live frugally on that amount because he had few obligations and his rent was under $600. He never worried about paying a high rent while he was in launch mode and you shouldn't, either. Once you're past the launch stage, you'll acquire the income to pay the mortgage, and then some.

Full-time initially means you eat, sleep and breathe real estate. When you first start out, accept the fact that it will be difficult, like any other new business, because you work hard and put in long hours. If it were a cakewalk, everyone would be doing it. You're going to be working day and night. It is a challenge, but the rewards are well worth it!

Whether you are planning for a career in real estate or are already a realtor, you will need to have a start-up fund to reach your next level of success. You have two choices: reduce your expenses to save money, or increase your income. By far the more enjoyable of the two is increasing your income, however, a combination of cutting expenses and earning more will fill your coffers the fastest.

If you are already working in real estate, then your focus must be on getting as many commission checks in a hurry as possible. I am primarily speaking to those getting ready to launch their careers when I say, plan for several dry months by having a six-month savings cushion. Still work like you will not be eating if you don't manage to get a few prospects every day, but have the resources to keep you sane and financially sound while you begin winning deals and earning income.

Income tax, like hourly wages and commission splits, must be paid. Always set aside the portion of your commission checks that will be due for taxes – not doing so is a common, frequently tragic mistake that new agents and newly self-employed people too often make. Do not set yourself up for undue stress as that costs you, too.

Taxes are a painful part of business and personal life. I am sure you agree, it is not enjoyable having a huge portion of our incomes taken from us after all the effort required to earn it. Until something changes and we get relief from the burden, all of us have to plan early by setting aside money for our future tax payments from each check. The consequences of not preparing early for tax bills can wreck your business. You have a brilliant future to create, and you cannot let the tax man get in the way!

Capital

Of course, as previously touched on, no one can start a business without capital, so it's inevitable that you'll need some financial resources to start a real estate career. Aim to make your first sale within your first three months and allow for closing time so that you have an income at the six-month mark.

You have to act as if you're a million dollar broker in order to become one. This is not a fake-it-til-you-make-it proposition; when your mindset truly reflects (in the present tense) the outcome you desire, fulfillment is enabled.

Use the right tools for the job; a quick web search on Google will deliver a vast array of free budgeting templates you can use to project expenses. Be sure to include all of your essential tools of the trade and list the expenses associated with each.

Once you have your survival fund ready, you can begin taking the steps to avoid using it. Every day, your main job is prospecting. You don't want just any prospect though; you want those that are most likely to put the greatest amount of money in your pocket in the shortest time possible with the highest probability of a deal.

List to Last

"Agents who list, last; those who don't, won't."
-Tatiana Londono

It's self-evident that the more listings you have, the more people will see your name. The more people see your name, the more people will think of you when buying and selling. The more listings you get, the more revenue you earn. I'm sure you're getting the picture. So, what do you do? You get those listings, of course!

Listing Agents Own the Market

The dominate realtor in any market is the one with the most listings. By focusing on acquiring listings in your market you will earn far more money. In order to become a *Real Estate High Roller* you need to list.

The advantages of listing properties:

- Representing sellers guarantees you a percentage of the commission when a property sells whether you sell it or any other realtor does.

- Advertising your listings attracts more sellers. They see you are actively selling homes.
- Advertising your listings attracts buyers. They want to see your inventory.
- When you find the buyer for a property that you have listed you earn a full commission with no split, also referred to as double ending.

Focusing on getting listings does not mean you ever neglect a buyer. In fact buyers are frequently a source of listings. Almost half of buyers have homes that they will need to sell too. Offer them a great service by helping them find their next home and they will reciprocate by listing their current home with you, another opportunity for two commissions like double ending.

Making Dollars and Sense of Long Listings

The longer the mandate to sell a specific property the more likely you are to sell that property, it's that simple! I've sold many properties on the last day of a listing.

There may also be offers that don't go through that take up a lot of time before failing to materialize to your seller's satisfaction.

If you assume the sale and behave as if the terms you seek are within the norm, your chances of obtaining those longer terms rise exponentially. Remember, you are the real estate professional therefore you have the obligation to offer logical reasoning as to why you need a longer mandate. This includes sufficient time to market their property, sufficient time to show their property, sufficient time to conduct showings with buyers and lastly, sufficient time to go through the sales process.

Ultimately, you should not be signing mandates for less than six months. The longer the mandate and the longer you have to do your job, the better the chance you have of selling the property. Being factual is your best resource in situations where sellers balk at lengthy listing commitments.

The Price is Right

The number one reason a home does not sell is because it's priced too high. Home sellers love to assume that "there's a buyer for every home", but they forget to add "…. at the buyer's price". The truth is that buyers, not sellers, ultimately determine the price of a home.

The top dollar that a willing buyer will pay is the right price. Nothing else qualifies a price point more properly than the purchase price. By paying attention to listed and sold prices, it doesn't take long to learn realistic pricing. The bottom line is that well-priced homes sell the fastest.

When you ask for an unrealistic price, chances are it will burn the listing. Convince your sellers to price their home properly – that's your job.

Having a complete and well-rounded knowledge of the price points of your marketplace with respect to sales along with sold and expired listings makes all the difference in negotiating asking prices with your sellers. In many cases, they give only a cursory glance at written comparisons, which you provide. So, having local market figures on the tip of your tongue is what's most convincing.

Your client has to know that you know price. You are guiding them through a complex process, so be equipped to lead the way, confident in your base of knowledge.

When you have a client that is very difficult to convince that their price is too high, try agreeing to their price for an initial trial period then lowering the price if it hasn't sold. This is the last resort; they are trying out an inflated price on your dollar, so seek the most realistic listing price possible.

Remind them that listings sell fastest when they are priced right. Sitting on the market and later lowering your price often costs more, rather than making more. Remind them of how much you'll market their property as soon as the listing goes into effect.

I once had a listing for a beautiful condo in Old Montreal, which had not sold with a previous agent. I told them their price of $389,000 was too high. However, the potential clients believed that since they had a garage while most units in their complex did not, their property was worth more. They were adamant. After much (aggravating) back-and-forth, I quickly regrouped and took another path, saying: "If you're not happy, I'm not doing my job right. Let's work together and sell this place!"

That small redirect allowed us to then find a common ground. The solution I offered was based on their specific sticking point: the garage. The creative solution was to list the property and garage individually. Since in most condo projects the garage is sold separately, what I did was remove the garage from the price of the property. In Old Montreal, where the prices of garages are high, I was able to remove $40,000 from the asking price. By doing this, the seller was able to agree to a reasonable asking price of

$349,000, which the market would respond to. Within two weeks, I got an offer on the now reasonably priced condo and the buyer offered to buy their garage for $35,000. In the end the seller made more than he would have when it was overpriced (if he would have gotten anything at all). Don't fool yourself. Buyers are very price sensitive.

Recap of Action Plan

1. Get a Makeover. It does not require a lot of money to be well-groomed, but you need regular haircuts, manicured nails and a clean, neat, professional appearance. Be sure to include a power suit in your wardrobe. You may only be able to afford one well cut suit, but make sure it's a nice one and make sure it's always tidy. When you can, get another one. By all means, get a professional make-over if you can afford the service. It's a legitimate expense when you are a client-facing professional as presentation is one of your most valuable sales tools.

2. Maintain a Comfortable Office and Car.
Ensure that your client is comfortable in your office, whoever they may be. A vehicle's presentation is equally important. Your wheels don't have to be expensive, but your ride has to be presentable and reliable. And like you, it should smell good!

3. Delegate. Assign all administrative and support tasks as soon as possible so that you can both spend your time securing listings and maintaining a healthy lifestyle, enabling you to build long-term wealth and security for your family. Be prepared. Get into the habit of knowing all about the neighborhoods you work in. Subscribe to local publications and newsletters. Know the information about the school district, important and insider details about the area and of course, any property you work with. Research and be sure to have your act together before you show up to a listing presentation. Appearing scattered will without a doubt work to your detriment, especially since bad first impressions are difficult to reverse.

4. Behave ethically. Avoid short cuts; never mess around with your clients or their interests in any way. A mistake is a mistake; a repeated one is a choice: make that commitment now and keep it if you want to last in the real estate profession.

VII. THE REAL ESTATE PROSPECTOR'S GUIDE TO GOLD DIGGING AND FIRST TIER MARKETING

"Do the one thing you think you cannot do. Fail at it. Try again. Do better the second time. The only people who never tumble are those who never mount the high wire. This is your moment. Own it."
-Oprah Winfrey

The agents who make it and last are listing agents. The power of a listing is amazing, while representing only buyers doesn't afford the same benefits. Signs, advertisements, open houses and MLS are all working for you when you have a listing.

To get listings, like in any sales job, it's about prospecting. Listing success comes down to simple numbers: the more calls you make, the more listing appointments you will book and the more listings you will get as a result. No prospecting means no listings, so treat the process like digging for gold, not like mining for coal.

Early in my career, every time I picked up a phone to call a potential client, I'd remind myself of two important facts:

1. The opportunity to make thousands of dollars comes with every homeowner who answers the phone.

2. That opportunity just takes making a simple phone call!

Of course, I was eager to fully accept those opportunities as they arose, with my calendar in hand, ready to schedule a listing presentation that included a viable marketing plan.

Digging for Gold

Listings truly are the goldmines of real estate. Once you have accepted that prospecting is like digging for gold, you will have leapt over the mental hurdle which impedes 85% of realtors from reaching success. Here is the not-so-secret formula to being a successful listing agent:

Cold Callers Make Dollars

Your marketing efforts bring you prospects that need your type of expertise and assistance. Accept that you are not the problem; instead, you are the solution. Embrace your helpful self and dial that phone, because ultimately that is your path to wealth!

One of the most common ways that sales agents undermine themselves is by avoiding the lifeblood of their income: prospecting. Your first and main job is keeping your calendar full of listing appointments by making regular prospecting a part of your routine.

Separate your ego from the deal you're trying to make. You are not the commodity or house, so don't take anything about the transaction personally, especially at the prospecting level. It's not you being rejected rather consider it a prospect that does not understand your value. Move on to greener pastures. Look through the windshield ahead, not in the rear view mirror.

You are not the first sales agent to struggle with rejection and you won't be the last. In order to grow rich in real estate, you must prospect regularly and successfully without being affected by the process. It's crucial that you deal with your feelings in this area from the start, rather than wasting time learning the hard way.

If I had to credit one reason for my success, the ability to pick up the phone and make gold-digging calls daily would be it. That's how important it is.

> "High Rollers succeed in business because they don't take anything personally – especially while prospecting." -Tatiana Londono

While prospecting, you have to put on a tough shell to deflect any rejection. You need to know your value whether or not the person on the other end recognizes it.

> "Nothing others do is because of you. What others say and do is a projection of their own reality, their own dream.
> When you are immune to the opinions and actions of others, you won't be the victim of needless suffering."
> -Miguel Ruiz

You may have to adjust your attitude thoroughly and reset your thinking about calling potential clients. A diligent practice of affirmations can get you there quickly, if you stick to it.

Try these affirmations:
- I love calling potential prospects.
- I am great at prospecting.
- I know that I will help my prospects.
- I can realize my dreams when I consistently prospect with joy, with passion, and with focus.

Practicing these affirmations repeatedly before prospecting will allow you to take full control of your perspective and your reality, helping to create a destiny of success.

Prospecting is ultimately what paves your path to riches. There are a lot of rocky bits to get through in order to discover the few gems. The prospects you win shine all the more when you unearth them through your own diligence. Cold calling will expose you to a variety of people, some of whom will become clients, others of whom will refer clients, and some of whom will hang up on you mid-sentence. Don't dwell on the ones who don't show interest, remember, the next homeowner you call just might.

Money Grows Like Trees

Think of the business cards you hand out as tiny seeds that can grow into mighty green. By green, of course, I mean money. Every card you hand out has the potential to connect you to a homeowner.

Keep your cards handy at all times, whether at the gym, jogging, social gatherings, picking up your kids or out on the town. Bring them with you everywhere.

I keep cards in all of my purses and workout clothes. Whenever I meet someone, I let them know right away who I am, and what I do. Being a realtor is more than a profession. Being a realtor is our identity!

Make a commitment to yourself right now to always be prospecting. The office doors may close but opportunity lies beyond the walls. You can be as successful as you choose to be once you realize that.

Prospecting Prep

The first rule of prospecting is to set yourself up in such a way that you are comfortable on the phone; schedule private, regular phone time four to six days per week to prospect. It's very important to note that your surroundings matter. Make sure you have privacy, a proper pen, crisp paper, a clear phone and a comfortable chair to sit in or room in which you can pace. Don't call prospects before eight o'clock in the morning or after eight o'clock in the evening.

> Prime-time for cold calling is between Monday to Friday, 8:30 A.M. – 10:30 A.M. and 3:30 P.M. – 7:30 P.M.

1. Set Goals. Milestones allow you to reach goals, motivating more of the same positive behavior. Setting daily prospecting goals of about 50 - 100 calls keeps you focused and gives you some of that hormone dose of dopamine mentioned in previous chapters.

2. Comfort Counts. Are you most comfortable at home in a familiar chair, settled in front of your computer at the office, or do you think best on your feet? You will sound more energetic if you speak while standing up. Set yourself up for success by controlling your atmosphere and surroundings. Ensure that you are in a comfortable and quiet environment so you can focus on the call, not the distractions around you. Noise, and even a disagreeable chair, have the power to distract you just enough to lose focus when speaking with a potential client. Whatever enhances your focus, employ it now, because the better you feel, the better you'll communicate with others. Turn your consciousness towards your breathing. It sounds simple, yet many people have a tendency to hold their breath when they feel challenged. In doing so, we deprive our brain of fuel by limiting its oxygen. If you tend to feel nervous while prospecting, practice breathing techniques to help you keep your breath and voice under control when you're on the phone or networking with others.

3. Practice. Build confidence when you start out by talking to everyone. This is how you will eventually become comfortable with the task, and this is also where you will pick up on your strengths and weaknesses. Practice with a friend or coworker to make your pitch perfect. Being relaxed and natural is key. Practice before every cold calling session until you lose those nerves. Remember to get ready, smile and breathe. People can hear you smiling. Use a mirror and the recorder on your phone to review your calls. Watching and listening to ourselves recorded informs us on what aspects of our delivery need to be tweaked, and how we can elevate our communications.

4. Script It! Familiarity breeds comfort, especially at first. Once you attempt the scripts with live prospects, you'll soon find yourself making changes and edits to better suit your local market, creating something uniquely your own.

5. Speak Once, Listen Twice. The reality of prospecting is that you should not need to say all that much. Urging prospects to talk, particularly about their motivations, is really what contact is all about. To become a *High Roller*, you need to listen at least twice as much as you speak. Our eyes and ears seem to function at their peak when our mouths are perfectly still.

Expired listings often show the homeowner's name and even their phone number. The amount of research required is, therefore, quite minimal. Call expired listings first – you know they almost always want a sale! Choose natural lead-ins:

"I'm calling about your house on Street. I see your sign is no longer up". "Are you still selling?"

"I'm a realtor. If I were to bring you a client, are you still willing to pay a commission?"

"I really don't want to waste your time, so could I come by and have a look at your property to make sure it's what my buyers are interested in?"

The only other question you may want to pose is: "What do you think went wrong with your listing the first time around?"

When you reach out to potential clients, be sure to have done your research on their address, ensuring that the property has not already been re-listed.

For Sale by Owner (FSBO)

I've saved the best for last. Simply put, properties that are currently For Sale By Owner (FSBO) are the prime, low hanging fruit ripe for the picking in the real estate industry.

FSBO owners have already decided they want to sell. What they lack in most markets is access to the multiple listing service (MLS), which is the top tool for selling properties. Get online to visit local FSBO databases via their public websites and be sure to check that the database isn't owned by a real estate broker. Only call the ones that are not, that is, when you aren't calling the numbers from FSBO signs that you've seen while out in the neighborhood.

The number one reason that sellers try to sell on their own is because the owner does not want to pay a commission. My company was built by tackling that main hurdle in the script we use for FSBOs.

"Hi, I'm calling about the property you have for sale. Is it still on the market?"

Speak naturally, conversationally, and take charge of the inquiry by asking two questions,

"I was wondering... what kind of view do you have and do you have covered parking with your condo? ...are the kitchen and bathroom in your house renovated? And, is the basement finished? "I'm a real estate agent..."

They may hang up on you then, but save their number to reach out again a couple of months later. In the meantime, move on.

"I don't want to pay a commission".

"Why is that?" Whatever the answer, a version of this is usually persuasive:

"I have a unique system from the other realtors out there. Depending on how much money you want in your pocket, I work the MLS to make my commission on the side of that."

What if they are adamant that they don't want to sign a contract?

"I'll just handle the MLS side of it, if you don't want to be locked into a contract. That way, you can cancel at any time and, if you do sell it yourself, I'll be the first to congratulate you and shake your hand. Statistically, the MLS makes more money than any other property sales method."

If you want specific strategies and solutions on how to handle client objections, visit RealEstateHighRollers.com for more scenarios.

Network Your Way to Net Worth

Networking is an invaluable method of prospecting. Once you become systematic about it, you will quickly learn that networking is both powerful and empowering.

Real estate is a people business that emphasizes who you know. Each one of us has valuable life experiences and a lifetime of connections. Our networking foundation is already existent to some degree and may even already be strong from years of cumulative personal and professional interactions. Every person you know forms your network and is a potential source of referrals that can help grow your business.

Who cuts your hair? Do they know that you're a realtor who specializes in their area? Do they have your business card? Who mows your lawn, teaches your children, and leads your yoga class? Talk to everyone, including the below:

- Shopkeepers
- Insurance agents
- Nail technicians
- Postal carriers
- Librarians
- Crossing guards
- Ministers
- Bookkeepers
- Coaches
- Restaurant staff
- Everyone

Practice networking to create new opportunities as well as revenue streams. Make every effort to understand the needs of individual sellers and to form personal bonds with them. Unearth each potential client's own desires as you make them aware of how you can help them.

Schmoozapalooza

Unless you're a natural extrovert, sign up for classes that might help you come out of your shell, like amateur improve comedy, singing or even an acting class. The arts offer many methods of dealing with jitters while providing a supportive and inspiring forum to enhance your natural communication abilities in the real world. If the thought of presenting yourself in public seems intimidating, it's a sure sign that you need to learn to face the challenge of an audience. Why not do it in an environment tailored to encouragement and camaraderie while having fun with trial and error?

Those of us who are already well-acquainted with our gift for gab could skip this recommendation, although it might still be valuable in enhancing your comfort and confidence.

In life, as in business, there are daily networking opportunities where you can engage with others and gain an understanding of their specific needs. Buying and selling each begin with desire. Unveiling and understanding individual needs and desires are crucial to developing an effective database.

Focus your networking efforts on two basic relationship types:

- Potential home sellers and buyers.
- Industry professionals to work with and/or those who can also refer clients.

While establishing both kinds of connections, you'll find that the second group of industry professionals will be enormously helpful in expanding your contact list and client roster. They may even do so, in some instances, without costing you a penny! I still give out gift certificates, if not finder's fees to people that refer clients. It's the right thing to do, and it keeps the good karma flowing.

Whether seeking buyers, sellers, agency referrals, lenders, or even an introduction to the new president of the neighborhood association, warm introductions are the heart of our interactions.

If you do not have a large social circle, increase your social and professional presence by nurturing existing relationships and actively forming new ones. Every single relationship potential can lead to multiple real estate transactions. This is called the "network effect".

Even if your direct connections are not the ones buying or selling properties, they can refer others to you, and referrals are one of the cornerstones of a stellar sales career.

Network Notes

As we've said, nurturing relationships is the basis of all networking. One connection may mean little, but each is valuable in that it is filled with possibility. You will become a marketing maven and networking master by taking one step at a time, each of which begins with some kind of gesture directed towards one individual.

Begin by establishing trust between yourself and any new contact through connection.

Exude:

Camaraderie – openness, attention, friendliness, curiosity, integrity.
Caring – an offer of information, introduction or service for another's apparent or stated need.
Commonality – find common ground like a club, organization, school, mutual contact, hobby, or neighborhood.

Think about what value-added service you might provide to your network. You might connect sellers to trustworthy home repair or cleaning services, or offer something as simple as emailing them another party's contact information. You might find a link that matches their interests especially well. People are more likely to accept a call to action from a source they already feel connected to in some way.

Start networking today with every single person you meet. Relationship-building is a daily occupation for sales professionals and soon becomes second nature through constant practice.

Following up with connections grows your network, whereas dropping the ball on a new contact may end the relationship as quickly as it began. Be consistent, make notes of any actions you need to take on behalf of others and always, without doubt, follow up and follow through. It will not go unnoticed.

Professional Contacts

Every person you will encounter has intrinsic value and a unique skill, yourself included; adding value to someone else's skill set is the most direct and accessible way to further bond and solidifies a relationship.

Connect with effective and successful individuals who not only may have skills that could at some point benefit your enterprise, but connect with those individuals whose recommendations tend to influence others.

Other influencers, such as realtors, investors and contractors are prospects that you should include in your database. Every single real estate broker you'll ever meet is an entrepreneur – that's why they became realtors!

Entrepreneurs work together to build even greater wealth. In North America, only licensed real estate brokers and their employees - also known as agents and their salespeople - may legally represent or collect property fees from a sale when there is no personal interest of ownership.

Reputation Redux

When you're comfortable in your own skin and believe in your actions, people are more drawn to you. Other people find it easier to trust you when you trust yourself and show your true human nature. Building on that dynamic has a charismatic effect. Networking can be powerful and fruitful when handled with integrity and consistency, so try things like volunteering in your community. As your reputation grows on this foundation, so will your referrals.

Ethics vs. Unemployment

The second part of protecting your reputation is ensuring that you're doing everything ethically. You need to ensure that the people with whom you are associated are doing the same. Make sure you are following the rules, that you abide by a business plan and that you are organized.

Create for yourself a solid and admired reputation by behaving morally. This will help with racking up referrals. When I do my prospecting, people already know who I am and what I am about. Establishing a respected reputation by doing things the right way (not the easy way) from the onset of your career will save you more time and earn you more money than you can imagine. It takes years to build a reputation, and just a second to destroy it. Nothing is worth it.

I'm not saying that you're not going to get into trouble. Once in a while you are going to deal with difficult clients. It happens. Handle any situation that arises with as much respect and diplomacy as possible because your reputation is everything, so take care of it. There's a lot of temptation in real estate because there's the potential of making a lot of money, but I promise, cutting corners doesn't work. Money that is not rightfully earned will never last, so don't waste your time.

Women, be aware that there are a lot of men in the real estate industry. Be mindful of your interactions with them, and be sure not to exchange yourself in any way, shape or form for a listing. This is not to say that you will encounter a problem, but it's a good thing to keep at the back of your mind. Most importantly, do not date your clients. This will damage your reputation beyond the point of repair.

In so many words, the underlying suggestion here is to always be aware and always think ahead. Ask yourself, "If I do this, will there be repercussions? If I make this decision now will I get into trouble later on?" Whenever there is an ambiguous situation, stop to think before moving ahead.

Taking the Crazy with the Cream

Obviously, no one will impress 100% of people all the time. Even those with the best reputations are sure to encounter people who are simply impossible to work with. I have dealt with some "crazy" people in my career. If you have ever watched *The Property Shop*, you've seen me deal with some of them in front of an audience on reality television!

While it may be risky to work with such people, eventually they develop their own reputation as a problematic client who is impossible to please. So, your reputation will remain unblemished, pending that you maintained your respect and dignity throughout the entirety of the transaction (to the best of your ability given a specific situation).

Listen like a Pro

Sales stars know how to listen empathetically to read the intention with which words are spoken by interpreting visual cues and other emotional information. Listening for clues is one of the most finely-tuned skills of the highly successful sales pro. Understanding body language and really listening will lead to the development of emotional intelligence.

Genuine listening requires an open mind. Using the time when your conversational counterpart is talking to contemplate your own next set of words is the opposite of active listening. By the same logic, also resist any urge to offer solutions before a consensus on a certain issue is reached. Investigate first; listen actively and observe, then think and offer qualified solutions.

Tat's Tips for Active Listening

1. Focus on the speaker.
Be present. Though difficult in our busy lives, active listening means you stop doing all else and simply listen. This requires eye contact and your undivided attention. Set aside all distractions, including electronic ones. Clear your attention of

anything you can that removes focus from the person you're conversing with.

2. Listen to their story, not yours.
Too often, listeners pretend to listen while instead they're formulating their own next remark. Listening means not interrupting and not developing opinions until the person speaking has finished. Each person thinks and speaks at their individual pace. Quick thinkers with agile tongues have the responsibility of slowing down enough for thoughtful discourse and genuine communication. Some of your clients will simply require patience. Allow them their voice and their time.

3. Walk and talk the body lingua.
Breathe. Relax. Lean in, nod appropriately now and then and maintain eye contact. Notice the speaker's stance, cues and tone of voice. Facial expressions, gestures and their eye contact all communicate more clues. You'll gain insight through experience as you practice active listening, a valuable skill when negotiating a contract.

4. Ask relevant questions.
Asking clarifying questions, no matter how simple they are, lets the listener know you're paying attention and it demonstrates your own engagement in the discussion.

5. Re-word, Repeat.
No matter how well you may think you understand the speaker, restate their message in your own words. When the person you're engaged in conversation with finishes speaking, paraphrase their words and repeat them back to ensure that you heard their intent above all.

Networking is truly simple, yet it takes energy, dedication and sincerity to network at a level that will significantly boost your business. Whether you're shopping, taking your kids to the park, or attending local events – be prepared to meet people and let them know you're here in their neighborhood, and are ready and able to sell their house when they need it sold.

Your milestone task is to personally hand out more than 20 business cards each week. Always keep a supply of business cards in your car for restocking. Count at least 25 of them into your wallet or purse every week and see what's left each time you do. None is something to celebrate.

Networking is as much about the 'where' as it is about the 'how' because in real estate, we often sell where we live, whether or not you live in your exact marketplace. Does everyone on your block know you're a realtor? If not, you have your first networking assignment.

Devise a creative approach to meet your neighbors and make sure they know what you do. Who better to sell your street than you? No one – so make sure your neighbors know that, too! Everywhere you go, every group you walk into, is an opportunity to schmooze your way into people's memories.

Networking Opportunities

Because there are so many networking opportunities available, careful planning and time management are necessary. Take advantage of every chance you get to connect with others and become pro-active about seeking out new avenues of social interaction. However, still be selective about where you spend your time and efforts.

To quickly expand your network, attend local events and join organizations that hold regular meetings. Attend as many real estate or investment events as possible, even if you suspect that there may be nothing new for you to learn there. Your real purpose is to learn the name and contact details of the new connections you make!

Chambers of Commerce

Search on Google for your city or regional Chamber of Commerce to find the business association nearest you. Visit your local Chamber to sign up; you'll find that most of the major players with a business license in your community already have.

The Chamber of Commerce can act as a lobby group in the interests of the local business community and hold or sponsor local events that afford realtors countless valuable networking opportunities. Become a sponsor, whenever possible, to place yourself in an even more advantageous position with your fellow Chamber Members.

National Real Estate Investor Association

(National REIA) Every major city has one or more clubs and associations of real estate investors who network in your area. Attend gatherings frequently to both build a rapport with others in the industry and to remain knowledgeable regarding your marketplace by networking with colleagues. Offering meeting space to pockets of local investors is a common winning strategy in this scenario.

Network with any organization's leadership; find the most active of buyers, sellers, landlords and various real estate professionals in your area. Give your business card out as much as possible and ask for the cards of others as well.

National Association of Independent Landlords: Landlords, of course, are real estate buyers and sellers who may be in the market for new holdings. It never hurts to network with real estate investors.

Event Hosting Gives Value and Increases Authority

Want to be the real estate expert in your area? Teaching others is a networking tool with profound effects. Distinguishing yourself as a leader and educator makes you a local expert in your field. Giving a helpful presentation is a unique opportunity to inspire trust and to interact with potential buyers and sellers from a position of friendly authority while showcasing your expertise.

Meet and follow up with each participant to cultivate your network. Be sure to hire a capable photographer to shoot those all-important social media sharing photos without being obtrusive. Encourage attendees to join in group photos, bringing them further into your sphere.

A flattering picture of you in your element posted on social media sites is the golden ticket of networking. Take advantage of any worthy photo op.

Education Nation

Education and self-help is one of the fastest-growing market niches in America. Hosting classes, workshops or seminars present a myriad of opportunities to expand your network. Look to local civic organizations for the niche in need of your skills. Home Selling 101 or Home Staging for Sellers might bring just the right clients your way.

Discover a need and fill it with your informed and skillful presence.

Depending on your geography, topics and experience, a regular workshop or an online webinar might be your logical next step to regularly furnish you with new contacts. Don't forget to have handouts for attendees and a plan for an informal coffee hour afterwards, encouraging interaction.

Networking Groups

In most areas there are groups of professionals meeting regularly to network with others in their own and complementary industries.

A Google search will easily locate clubs and groups in your area, like those found using Facebook and MeetUp, through which you can network with potential buyers, sellers, financiers and entrepreneurs.

A useful hint is to use Google to search out social media-based groups by using terms such as "real estate investment group" or "real estate investment club" and adding your city, state or region – the more local the better. Try it for various social media sites; Google may prove quicker to filter to your needs.

With Facebook in particular, there may be a temptation to over-socialize and under-network. The trick to doing business through social media is to maintain "clean hands" with regards to professional decorum, resisting any urge to display social controversy or inappropriate imagery on your page or in your personal comments.

Full of Facebook

Facebook and social media marketing will be fully covered in the next chapter. These tips are for online networking, not for creating an automated marketing system.

It's best to separate your personal profile and your professional profile when seeking to attract clients through Facebook. Don't mix business with pleasure, as they say. Think of your professional Facebook profile as a booth at a trade show.

LinkedIn is an especially useful social media platform as it is strictly devoted to business networking. It has become a major hub of real estate and investment information, much like Facebook.

Join LinkedIn Groups that reflect your real estate market, then access their membership lists to connect with individuals who are likewise interested in real estate. Within the membership list, simply search for "real estate" to target the contacts you seek.

Send a personal message in context to the Group and mention that you have buyers or sellers (or both) in their market area. Save your message on a Word document, making it your template to copy and paste to members of various groups you want to connect with.

Obtaining contacts is the first step. Creating and maintaining an ever-expanding database of clients and potential clients is how we turn those contacts into gold. Working your database is fundamental to your success and should be thought of, along with prospecting, as the backbone of your sales work.

VIII. HIGH ROLLER MARKETING

Marketing Choices

In the beginning of my real estate career, like most agents, I handled everything myself. My marketing knowledge was limited, so my focus was on picking up the phone and make prospecting and follow up calls. To this day, making these calls is my best return on investment for my time spent.

While the latest marketing strategies and technology will bring you more leads than ever before, unless you have the phone and follow up skills as I developed early in my career, and the commitment and organization to respond to all prospects in a timely manner, you will not reap the benefits of marketing.

Not that long ago, when I started in real estate, the choices were limited to direct mail, radio, or print ads. Today, the number of channels through which we can market ourselves and our businesses is endless and overwhelming. Choosing the right marketing channels that will actually produce leads is the primary goal.

According to data from Realtor.org, 90% of home buyers search online during their home buying process. Developing the right online marketing strategy has never been more critical for realtors than it is today. The right strategy is the one that positions you as the expert 'go-to' realtor in your marketplace; a strategy that places you in the minds of prospects first, the moment they even consider buying or selling a home.

So how can you accomplish this without having to spend most of your time at the computer?

The solution is simple. Don't try to do this yourself! Hire an expert. You need at least one technical person on your team to help you.

The head of my marketing team is my brother, Alexander Londono. Alex has years of digital marketing experience under his belt. He has a passion for staying on the cutting edge of the latest real estate marketing technology. He has contributed the next two chapters to share his expertise with you. Alex gives you an inside look at how he runs the marketing systems for me.

Introduction to Marketing by Alex Londono

Thank you, Tatiana. Helping your readers is my pleasure. As Tatiana mentioned, there has never been more choices for marketing which can be challenging for realtors. In order to build a successful marketing system, you need a multi-channel approach that uses what I call:

The Four M's" of Modern Day Marketing

>**M**essage: The right message
>**M**arket: To the right market
>**M**oment: At the right moment
>**M**edia: Using the right media

As we discuss more and as you get involved in marketing, you will see and understand the value of "The Four M's" approach. You need to know how to choose the right channels and form the optimum strategies. Then you must collect and interpret marketing data and track results to know how to make the right decisions on where to invest your hard earned dollars. You must hold all campaigns or ads accountable to produce positive ROI's (Return On Investment.) If you cannot track it you shouldn't do it. If a campaign or ad fails to produce than you must stop it. I have seen too many realtors continue to throw away money on marketing that is not getting results.

Marketing is about generating leads. Most realtors generally have one of two issues (or both) with leads; either they are not generating enough leads or they are not converting enough leads to appointments. When realtors are not generating enough leads they find themselves chasing any prospect that comes their way. This results in wasting time with unqualified prospects, not making enough money, and becoming very frustrated. Converting these unqualified prospects will be close to impossible.

How to Qualify Leads

It's important to know that not all leads are equal. The quality of a lead is based on the prospects' timing and motivation to make a move. Why are they moving? How soon do they want to move? The answers to these questions will help you qualify if a lead is worthy of your time now or should be categorized and followed up at a later date.

Until you have a constant flow of leads, you will always be at the mercy of whoever comes your way. So now I will share how you can generate an overflow of qualified leads to have the luxury of choosing who you want to work with and who you don't.

The High Roller Marketing System

After extensive research and spending several million dollars in advertising I developed '*The High Roller Marketing System.*'

This system consists of only two specific types of advertising; unbranded advertising and celebrity branded advertising. Each group has a unique objective.

Unbranded Advertising

The objective of unbranded advertising is to produce leads for low cost. These types of ads do not include your name, company, and/or face. Due to the bombardment of marketing messages and constant requests for personal consumer information, people have developed high buyer defense mechanisms. The purpose of unbranded advertising is to generate new leads without raising buyer defenses, to gain trust, and develop a connection with your eventual prospects.

This type of advertising provides free informational materials as a service for your prospects.

The information can include:
- Lists of homes for sale
- Average days it takes for a home to sell in the area
- Local home prices
- Recent sales
    - School district ratings
    - Market trends
    - Financial data on mortgages

Giving away this type of content starts a conversation, engages prospects and builds relationships. This informational material needs to be concise, relevant, and valuable to your target audience. The objective of providing free information is to cause buyers and sellers to make contact with you in the early stages of thinking about buying or selling a home. By delivering valuable information for free you create good will and enact the law of reciprocity. When the time comes for them to buy or sell a home, you will more likely be the first realtor that comes to mind. This is when you introduce prospects to your celebrity brand.

See some samples of our unbranded advertising at:
www.RealEstateUnfilteredBook.com/bonues

Celebrity Branded Advertising

The purpose of Celebrity Branded Advertising is to convert leads generated by the unbranded ads to appointments and stay top of mind as the 'go to expert' with your contact list. This type of ad tells your prospects about who you are and establishes you as a knowledgeable trusted authority and celebrity in your marketplace. These ads include your face, name, message, and logo. Your celebrity brand must have a clear simple message of what's in it for them and why they should choose you over every other realtor. In the marketing world this is called your "Unique Selling Proposition" or USP.

Leads from unbranded advertising come in tenfold for every one lead you get directly from your celebrity branded advertising. However, the leads from your celebrity channels will close at a far higher ratio than those from your unbranded advertising. This is because they are closer to making a move and are ready to speak with a realtor. That being said, both segments are equally important as unbranded advertising generates leads and your celebrity brand converts ready now leads (within 6 months of making a move) and nurtures those not ready yet (beyond 6 months.)

Ultimately, you need both types of advertising to thrive.

After coaching and training hundreds of realtors and other business professionals, I have learned that the biggest challenge with creating a celebrity aura and brand is the mindset shift. You must see yourself as a superstar first. Once you perceive yourself as a celebrity realtor, then all the steps that follow will come easier.

If you have cold feet about creating content and putting your name and face out there you are not alone. For example, some people are hesitant to put themselves in videos or speak in public because they are shy, intimidated, or do not like the way they appear. However in the real estate business, you must publicize yourself. Don't take yourself too seriously, and I promise, the more you do this the more comfortable and confident you will become.

Creating Content

Content can be articles, blog posts, videos, podcasts, flyers, and letters. You want people to find value in your content and cause prospects that are looking to make a move to identify themselves. Do this by following a formula of presenting valuable content that describes a problem, proposes solutions, and presents the benefits of working with you. All content must include an offer such as:

- A free home valuation
- List of recently sold homes in the area
- Current homes for sale in the area

And in every content piece you need to tell your visitors what to do next; this is called a CTA (call to action).

For example:
- Call now
- Text this code
- Click this link
- Sign up
- Access now

The primary purpose of all content is to generate leads that eventually convert and turn into money.

Celebrity Video Marketing

Creating videos is almost like cloning yourself for prospecting and making a great impression in your market. Making videos is easy, quick, can be fun, and you need nothing more than a Smartphone. The most important points to note in creating effective videos are the following:

- Make them engaging
- Ensure that they are easy to watch and hear
- They must be relevant to your prospects
- They must be branded with your logo and contact information
- They must have an offer and call to action

You can create familiarity, connect with your market, and add clout to your brand by filming at a popular location, event, business, or at a recognizable landmark in your area. These videos also present the opportunity to build relationships with local business owners. By including their establishments in your videos you will be promoting them. Remember, selling real estate is all about relationships.

Keep your videos short (three minutes or less) and sweet, and at a high-energy level to maintain the viewer's attention.

The key is to get started and be consistent.

Types of Videos

Testimonial Videos

These are by far my favorite type of videos to shoot. Capturing your client's appreciation for the services you have rendered, is great for lead generation and can make you money for years to come. As consumers, one of the factors we give heavy weight to is past customers' reviews. This is one of the most powerful forms of advertising. Testimonial videos can be created quickly and can be as short as a few statements.

Videos of clients 'attesting' to their experience working with you can answer questions that your current prospects have. Hearing from someone that has been in the same place in the moving cycle where your prospect is now, and how you helped them, can be very reassuring.

Timing is important when approaching clients for testimonials. While you can go back to your past clients for testimonials, one of the best times to get your clients accolades is at the point when all contract conditions have been met or when the contract is 'clear to close'. At this time they are usually the most excited and are not yet busy with their relocation.

Listing Videos

Listings videos are the most engaging. People love touring beautiful and interesting homes. If you have not had a professional virtual tour created for your listing, you can just hold your phone and do a walk through. However I found that a better way is to use the same professional pictures you already took for the MLS. Choose the 5 or 6 pictures that best showcase the home and with video editing software create panning and zooming effects with the pictures to produce a walk through feeling.

The Realtor Advertising Myth

One of the biggest realtor myths is that promoting listings is the way to sell homes. Ads do not sell homes. Very few people ever buy a home because they saw it advertised. In fact you might never sell that property because you created a video or did any other type of listing specific advertising for it. Then why spend the time and money advertising your listings?

Advertising your listings promotes you, your services, and gets you more buyer and seller leads.

Every ad has your brand, logo, name, and contact information. Every video shows you are active, professional, and offer a unique specialized service. Your ads tell potential sellers that you will do more to sell their home.

Do's and Don'ts VIDEOS

These videos outline the 'do's and don'ts' when buying or selling a home. These are some of my favorite because they are easy to make and position you as an expert in your market. Offering tips for selling homes faster and for more money and how to save money when buying a home is valuable information to your prospects.

Examples:

The Top 7 Mistakes Home Buyers Make

6 Costly Mistakes to Avoid Before Selling Your Home

Discover How to Save Thousands When You Sell Your Home

The 5 Most Common Home Buyer Traps

These videos are easy to make, simple and short. You can get the ideas from similar articles on the web. Include who you are, your contact information, and an offer or call to action. Then focus entirely on presenting high value information.

Celebrity Branding with Photography

Professional photography is an important part of your celebrity branding process. Schedule an appointment with a professional photographer at least once a year to get head shots or other images for marketing. These photographs are imperative for your brand and will be used for all of your celebrity branded print and digital marketing: We use professional photography of Tatiana on:

Billboards: Tatiana uses billboards frequently and strategically, resulting in an increase in phone calls. Negotiate hard and pick the top spots to get the biggest branding impact.

Business Cards: Strongly consider whether or not

you want your picture on your business card. If you choose to include your picture, make sure that you portray yourself in the most professional light possible.

Flyers: Use full color flyers to broadcast your presence in a neighborhood. They are an excellent way of letting other homeowners know that you are active in a neighborhood and have been successfully selling homes.

Postcards: We mail celebrity branded postcards once a month to the areas we are farming.

Social Media Covers: Facebook, Instagram, Linkedin, Twitter, Youtube, and you name it. All of these channels should have your best photography, name, and logo. You want to make a great impression.

Email Newsletters: We send newsletters once a month to our list with a celebrity branded email header.

Pictures such as 'Selfies' or shots of you and your friends or associates at an event have their place. They are a great way to help your social media audience stay up to date and feel connected with you.

The *High Roller* Marketing System is based on strategy that requires some specific knowledge of technology. Once you properly implement *High Roller* marketing you will be generating a steady stream of new leads and opportunities. In order to manage all of the data you will need certain technology in place. In the next chapter I will reveal some of the software we currently use.

IX. REALTOR SOFTWARE FOR SUCCESS

There is a plethora of software programs available for the realtor and more being produced all the time. There is software or an app to manage or do anything you could possibly imagine. Trying to stay up to date with the latest and greatest programs and choose the right one is time consuming and difficult for realtors. If I had to recommend just one type of software that is a must, it is CRM (Customer Relationship Management). CRM will help you effectively manage your business communications.

Tracking Contacts with a Customer Relationship Management (CRM) Tool

Most established brokerages will have a CRM package for you to use. If that is not the case in your organization, or if you are starting your own realty business, you should choose one right away. This will be where you centralize and manage all of your contacts, interactions, and data. You will be able to track everything that is happening with your contacts and initiate follow up sequences. A CRM system isn't just a list of names and contact information. With most CRMs today you can write emails, send text messages, and make and record your phone calls.

The Benefits of CRM:

- You can use the dashboard, calendar, and schedule to see who to follow up with every day, have records of each communication, and use a tracking system that reports where people are in your sales pipeline.
- You can automate email campaigns.
- A CRM tracks your follow ups; you see the who, when, and why of contacting each person.
- A CRM makes training an assistant and building a team much easier.
- You will be more productive and make more money. And as you grow, all this information can be entered by, shared with, and viewed by you and your team.
- You can tag new leads, track their sources, identify level of responsiveness, and score each lead.

- The score for prospects can be based on the parameters you establish such as a buyer or seller, prospect potential, how soon they plan on making a move, and whatever you can think of.
- You can follow and track deals and clients as they move through the buying or selling process.
- You can manage all communications with prospects and clients from one location.

In time, by examining your data you will be able to see where you get the most leads from and their quality. You will also be able to determine what personality types you work best with and ultimately optimize your operation. You will have peace of mind knowing you can see what is happening in real time with your business.

When you are starting with a CRM, you can tag people in your database. Here are four basic classifications that I recommend:

<A> Your biggest Raving Fans - Clients, friends and family, or prospects who have referred you, or done business with you in the past.

<B> Clients or Prospects that have stated they would do business with you in the future and/or refer potential prospects to you.

<C> Prospects/Clients who have not referred leads to you and may or may not do so in the future. These are new leads or prospects you are following up with and have not yet spoken to regarding future referrals.

<D> Prospects/Clients who you really don't want to work with.

As new leads are generated I recommend further classifying these leads as follows:

<Ready Now> People ready to buy or sell now.

<Future Business> People not ready yet but have expressed interest and will require follow up.

<No Business> People that are unreachable, or not interested.

Using a CRM takes a decision and commitment. Then you will need to develop the habit of using this powerful tool on a daily basis. Like most changes you will probably resist setting up and learning how to use a CRM. But believe me, it will be worth every minute of your time. We contribute a great deal of our success to using a CRM.

Automation Software for Engaging and Following Up with Your Database

Prospecting is a contact sport. Automation technology will enable you to reach out to the contacts in your database without the heavy lifting realtors once had to do. For example, without email marketing software, you would have had to write and send individual emails one at a time. With automation you can broadcast a message to thousands of recipients with the click of a mouse.

Automation saves you time, gives you a competitive edge, allows you to reach many more people much faster, and tracks prospect data that gives you valuable insights. For example, you can track your prospect actions such as who opened your letter, who clicked on a link in your email, who viewed your video and more.

As the technology officer at Londono Group, part of my job is to research and evaluate new automation technology. Here are my current top five technologies we are using:

1) Email Marketing Software: This software helps you send out email broadcasts to segments of your database all at once. There are two types of emails:

1. Auto-responders: Where visitors take a specific action such as entering their email address on a web form and receiving an automated response from you.
2. Newsletters: These are time based broadcasts scheduled to go out on a specific date.

2) 1-800 Info Lines: These are toll free phone lines where people can call in and receive a prerecorded message from you that provides reports, services you offer, or even information on your current listings. At the end of the message you give them another call to action such as "for immediate assistance or to speak to me now enter 0" or "if you would like more information and pictures sent to your Smartphone now press 1". This provides people information that are engaging with your advertising that might not be ready, all without being forced to interact with a sales agent. This gives you the opportunity to capture the people that are ready now and those that are not quite ready yet. You are also initiating reciprocity as you are providing free information which will inspire them to contact you when they are ready to make a move.

3) SMS: SMS marketing software is the technology that allows you to reach people on their mobile devices via text messaging. SMS is the new preferred method of mobile communication. SMS has a high (99.9%) read rate.

4) Voice Broadcasting: Voice broadcasting software enables you to call a list of numbers and leave a message. Broadcasting voice messages to your list saves tons of time. Rather than calling people individually one at a time you can call an entire list at once. Some voice broadcasting software allows you to skip ringing the person and go straight to voice mail.

5) Live Streaming Video: This is a new way for people to join you in a live environment on social media. The experience is currently novel and inspires a feeling of inclusiveness on an intimate level and encourages people to interact with you.

This is a brief review of some of the realtor software available. Technology is a powerful tool for lead gen, management, and compelling people to take action, but will never replace direct contact with you, the realtor. You will still need to meet with prospects and sell. However technology will bring you more and better qualified leads and free up your time to focus on the high income producing activities in your business.

Additional resources:
www.RealEstateUnfilteredBook.com/bonues

X. GETTING TO THE TOP AND HELPING OTHERS JOIN YOU

"Non nobis solum nati sumus."
Not for ourselves are we born.
-Marcus Tullius Cicero

The journey we have been on together through the previous nine chapters will lead anyone who applies the information to the top in their market. Applying the information means working consistently and with focus while using the tips and technology that I have proven creates a successful realtor. My own history is proof enough, but the hundreds of realtors that I have trained at Londono Realty Group, as well as those in my *Real Estate High Rollers* program, have confirmed that this system truly works and produces top realtors.

Before concluding our journey together, I am going to summarize and explain the transition that hopefully you have gone through from the beginning of the book to your new beginning as a star realtor.

You can expect to pass through three general stages while raising your performance to new levels.

Stage 1: Looking for answers for how to make it to the top

Stage 2: Integrating the answers and forming new habits

Stage 3: Developing success momentum to carry you to the top and keep you there

Knowing what to expect as you transition through these stages will help you make swift progress with a low level of stress.

Looking for Answers

Depending on whether you are an experienced realtor or somebody who is new to the business, you probably have more questions than proven answers. So long as you are open to taking input from somebody who has achieved success in your chosen field, you will leap ahead of all those realtors not reading this book or being coached.

Even though you have already read this book, it is only the beginning. You must integrate the beliefs, activities, and structure which I have explained. Reread the book to get deeper insights and cement the new beliefs. Study it like you would a map taking you to a treasure chest filled with gold and wealth beyond your wildest dreams.

The critical activity at this stage is taking the advice and techniques within this book as proven formulas for earning a top 10% income as a realtor. Engage your mind as though everything is possible, and you are capable of working this program. With these two internal beliefs working for you, as opposed to engaging with a critical internal voice that will hold you back, you will be able to get in the flow of new habits, new ways of thinking, and new levels of success.

Your first mission is adopting the learning mindset for implementing and adapting the lessons within this book. I suggest that you keep the book on your desk and go through it as you are conducting your day. Not only will it remind you of your journey towards the top, but it will keep you on the narrow path of success where you avoid distractions.

Becoming successful in any endeavor is equal parts performing the correct activities as it is avoiding the incorrect activities. Stage one is your chance to open your mind, accept the lessons, avoid all distractions that could hinder you from performing each of the tasks explained, prospect like a professional, and turn your dreams into reality.

Integrating the Answers

You have the playbook to success in your hands. Like a recipe that requires certain ingredients processed in a specific way, you are now the master chef of cooking up deals. A lot of the tips and techniques are not going to feel natural to you at first because you have not been doing things this way. Accept a level of discomfort during this integration stage.

Discomfort when learning and adapting new methods means that you are growing. You are growing towards your full potential as a realtor and as a person. Expect challenges along the way while you are prospecting and developing your new marketing system, or as you transition your mindset to feeling that you deserve an exceptional life. Welcome to stage two, the integration period of expanding your capabilities.

Now that you understand that these new methods will not automatically feel right for you, you can look beyond the initial discomfort to the point where your new sales muscles have become stronger and more capable.

Developing Success Momentum

Stage three is where strategies begin delivering increased activity and the indicators of success. The first time you use my prospecting script and get directly to a listing presentation, you are building success momentum. Just sitting down to prospect for two hours, which might be a new sort of discipline for you, helps you build success momentum.

These strategies work directly as a function of how hard you work. I have had brand-new realtors closing deals within their first month of working with my agency. These are deals that pay commissions of $10,000 and more, providing a new realtor sufficient income to hire an assistant and begin building a team almost immediately. Success momentum enables that kind of rapid growth.

Unfortunately, if your efforts are sporadic and hit or miss, you are not going to develop momentum. This is a key concept that requires devotion and consistency, day after day, week after week, and month after month.

Fully engage your mind on the singular path of achieving your real estate dreams with consistent effort, and you will float to the top based on always prospecting for new leads and closing deals.

Rather than having a good month and then a bad month, you can expect to have good months, better months, and great months. Your results will initially depend on telephone prospecting. After several months, and when you have a steady income, you can build a premium online marketing campaign that will double and triple your results following the blueprint from the marketing chapter.

All the basics for becoming a top 10% or higher realtor are within this book. As you progress from Chapter One all the way through to Chapter Nine you are moving through levels of new capability as well as new income levels. With more income you have the ability to hire team members and specialists to develop business processes.

As you expand your team and the sophistication of your business processes you may decide to become a broker or open an agency. I chose this path and it has led to more opportunity, more income, and more growth than I could have imagined. Making the most of your higher income, successful career and ability to give back is the next step.

Whether you decide to open your own agency or to build a team that makes your life more enjoyable and more profitable as a realtor, the ultimate destination of success momentum is freedom to express your dreams. Many of you have dreams outside of real estate and view being a realtor as a means of achieving those non-business related aspirations. The idea of being able to support causes that I am passionate about, help charitable organizations, take care of those in need, support religious beliefs, or provide for loved ones has been one of my strongest reasons to succeed.

Once you are making a certain amount of money, the extra income does not bring you more joy or less stress. After meeting your basic needs, have funds set aside for emergencies, for retirement and for investing; it is time to look outside yourself for reasons to increase your income.

Shifting Priorities from Income to Impact

Anticipate that your priorities are going to shift as you close more deals and make more money. You become comfortable with your prospecting schedule as well as your marketing program and building a successful team. Instead of being worried about paying bills and whether or not you will be successful, you envision you will be successful and have plenty of money.

At some point in the near future, you will arrive. You will have satisfied your desire for a certain income and to become successful in your field. You are no longer constantly wondering whether or not you have to do something differently or improve certain aspects of your business. You are officially successful in your own eyes and throughout your community.

What do you do then to keep your motivational fire burning to reach more people and create more impact in the world?

I faced this crisis of shifting motivation after about six months into my career. The financial challenges I encountered when I started in this business were no longer a problem. I was able to take care of my family and myself while saving money towards a brighter future; if my only motivation had been to make money than I would have stagnated at that point. For a substantial percentage of realtors, stagnation hits the minute they become successful at a certain level.

I looked around and decided that the next step up for me was to become an agency owner, requiring me to get my broker's license. This was my new goal that formed the growth pattern in my evolution towards the highest performing person I could be; having big goals leads to big motivation and big action.

Getting my license and building an agency took years. A lot of this activity made it onto TV during my time with HGTV on *The Property Shop*. Eventually, I reached the point where I considered myself a successful agency owner. I had processes in place to continue the success momentum with my team handling most day-to-day activities.

You can certainly expect to achieve the same kind of life transformation I did, as long as you are willing to work as hard as I did. And, once you achieve this level, your priorities might shift dramatically towards helping others achieve their own level of success.

Expect and embrace the transition wherein you become a mentor. My own experience has shown me that helping others achieve success is as satisfying as achieving success for yourself.

The rest of this chapter focuses on what I consider to be some important causes that I chose to help in my community, and how I have approached the art of giving back.

Your new priority is making the most of your position as a successful realtor and enabling others to become successful, raising the standard of your entire community.

Achievement Levels Help Decide Your Charity Levels

If you become a successful realtor with a small team, then you are in the position to donate a certain amount of money to causes that you consider worthy. Once you become a broker with other agents working for you, you can probably afford more money for charitable gifts and to devote company resources towards helping the community.

For me, the goal of being able to give millions of dollars to causes that I believe in feeds my passion for building my achievement level to the point where I can make massive contributions. Your desire to give back can be one of the greatest motivational thought engines, rushing you towards your highest expression of self, financially and charitably.

Helping Others!

Some of my greatest sources of joy are my family, business partners, team members, and those I have touched through scholarships, charity, mentoring, coaching programs, and inspiring.

I will share with you my own experience about choosing to give back and impact my community. Since education has played a critical role in forming my personality and ability to learn what I needed to learn in order to become successful, I provide scholarships to several learning institutions in my area.

Some of my scholarships provide tuition for girls from single-family homes to attend top schools that will prepare them to enter top universities. These scholarships allow deserving girls a chance at an educational path they would otherwise not be able to afford.

I also fund programs for children to experience the outdoors while attending a sleep away camp. My inspiration for this comes from knowing the character traits that being on your own and exploring nature can build early on in a child's life.

I am similarly passionate about working with Athena house, a shelter for battered women. I have joined the board of directors to help ensure that women have a place to go where they can feel safe and get back on their feet.

While there are many charitable causes that I contribute and devote my time to, the single biggest area of satisfaction for me is mentoring, training, and coaching. Every time I help a realtor become successful through my training program, I feel the greatest reward.

Your Turn to Create a Legacy

Success in itself, whether financial or by community recognition, brings temporary joy. Helping others from all walks of life move towards a higher plane of existence by sharing your wealth, time, and expertise sews satisfaction into your spirit for eternity, not just your bank account.

My fondest wish for those reading this book is for you to quickly achieve your goals regarding income, recognition, and contribution with the strategies I covered. Then, share your new wealth and energy with the world by elevating the lives of others with your example, your resources, and your spirit.

To the best you can be..

If you want to become a *Real Estate High Roller* go to:

www.RealEstateHighRollers.com
and
www.RealEstateUnfilteredBook.com

Recommended Reading

Release the Giant Within: How to Take Immediate Control of Your Mental, Emotional, Physical and Financial Destiny! by Tony Robbins; Simon & Schuster, 1992.

Little Red Book of Selling: 12.5 Principles of Sales Greatness by Jeffrey Gitomer; Bard Press, 2004.

The Power of Now: A Guide To Spiritual Enlightenment by Eckhart Tolle; Hodder and Stoughton Ltd, 2005.

The Four Agreements: A Practical Guide to Personal Wisdom (A Toltec Wisdom Book) by Don Miguel Ruiz; Amber-Allen Publishing, 1997.

The Four Agreements Companion Book: Using The Four Agreements to Master the Dream of Your Life (A Toltec Wisdom Book) Amber-Allen Publishing, 2000.

Law of Attraction: The Science of Attracting More of What You Want and Less of What You Don't by Michael Losier; Grand Central Publishing, 2003.

The Moral Molecule: The Source of Love and Prosperity by Paul J. Zak, PhD: Dutton, 2012.

The Secret by Rhonda Byrne; Atria Books, 2006.

~ Tat's Tip: be sure to see the film version of this one!

Bibliography

Sir James Jean, English Physicist, Astronomer and Mathematician, *The Mysterious Universe:* Cambridge University Press, 1930.

"Compassionate Intention As a Therapeutic Intervention by Partners of Cancer Patients: Effects of Distant Intention on the Patients' Autonomic Nervous System" by Dean Radin, PhD, et al: Explore The Journal of Science and Healing, Volume 4, Issue 4, July 2008.

"Quantum Physics – His Holiness the Dalai Lama Participates in the 26th Mind & Life Meeting at Drepung"

"Let NLP Work for You" by Robert Dilts: Real Estate Today: Volume 15, Number 2, February, 1982.

"There's a S.M.A.R.T. Way to Write Management's Goals and Objectives" by George Doran: Management Review magazine: Volume 70, Issue 11, November 1981.

What They Don't Teach You at Harvard Business School: Notes From A Street-Smart Executive by Mark McCormack: Bantam, 1984.

"Goals Research Summary" of Goal Study by Gail Mathews, PhD: Dominican University of California, 2007.

The Moral Molecule: The Source of Love and Prosperity by Paul J. Zak, PhD: Dutton, 2012.

DISCLAIMER: Data presented herein are deemed accurate without guarantee. Figures are for illustrative purposes only and reflect the true life experience of Tatiana Londono as a licensed real estate broker. The information provided is not intended to substitute for any legal, real estate, tax, or other professional service. Individuals are duly urged to consult with a professional in the respective legal, tax, accounting, real estate, or other professional area before making any decisions or entering into any contracts pertaining to real property. Please check with your physician before starting any exercise programs described in this book.

About the Author

Tatiana Londono is the Founder & CEO of Londono Realty Group Inc, one of the largest residential brokerage firms in Montreal, with more than 100 agents and 3 offices located in Montreal, the West Island and through a joint alliance in Miami, Florida. Londono Realty Group primarily focuses on residential purchases and sales but also offers a vast number of real estate services, including commercial transactions and retail leasing.

With over 15 years of experience in the real estate industry, Tatiana started her successful career as a broker for Re/Max Du Cartier, followed by a period at Sutton Group. Her determination to succeed on her own then led to the founding of Londono Realty Group in June, 2007.

Tatiana's background (which includes time in the Canadian Military and a degree from McGill University) and strong negotiation skills have given her a unique outlook and drive to constantly find new ways to grow her business and improve the efficiency of her sales team. Her vision brings something fresh and energized to an old and tired business. In a few short years, Londono Realty

Group has become one of the most successful independent offices in the country.

In 2008, her bright smile and blond curls caught the eye of a television production company who offered her an opportunity to be the star of her own show *"The Property Shop"* on the popular HGTV network. The show was an instant hit which led to three complete seasons and continues to air today while also being syndicated around the world. As a result of her TV popularity, Tatiana has been able to attract a vast international clientele. Specializing in residential properties, Tatiana and her dynamic team offer a professional buying and selling experience throughout the greater Montreal area.

In 2014 Tatiana launched *Real Estate High Rollers* – a coaching business for other real estate brokers. Whether just getting started in the industry or an experienced professional trying to take their business to the next level, Tatiana and her team have developed a detailed, step-by-step intensive program to help brokers achieve their goals.

Outside of her success in the professional world, Tatiana has taken a leadership role in numerous philanthropic causes and non-profit organizations. She established the Tatiana Londono Gratitude Bursary giving opportunities to young women from single family homes to attend Marianopolis College and is also on the board of Bouclier d'Athena – a shelter for abused woman and mothers. She has also taken great pride in helping send underprivileged children to sleep away camp in the summer months, as well as being active in other community organizations.

Tatiana is a mother, an entrepreneur and a born leader. With her drive, down-to-earth business sense, impressive sales skills and natural street smarts, she is a true role model to others. Tatiana dreams big and along with her loyal colleagues, she has built Londono Realty Group into a billion dollar real estate brokerage firm.

Contact Information

Author: Tatiana Londono Address: 4150 Sherbrooke O. Suite 100 Westmount, Quebec, H3Z 1C2, Canada

Get Your Free bonuses, downloads, and additional resources:
www.RealEstateUnfilteredBook.com/bonues